What Every Woman Needs to Know About Menopause

What Every Woman Needs to Know About

Menopause

THE YEARS BEFORE, DURING, AND AFTER

Mary Jane Minkin, M.D.   Carol V. Wright

Foreword by Frederick Naftolin, M.D., D.Phil.

Yale University Press   New Haven and London

Published with assistance from the foundation established in memory of Calvin Chapin of the Class of 1788, Yale College.

Designed by Nancy Ovedovitz and set in Monotype Joanna by The Marathon Group. Printed in the United States of America by R. R. Donnelley and Sons, Harrisonburg, Virginia.

Library of Congress Cataloging-in-Publication Data
Minkin, Mary Jane.
What every woman needs to know about menopause : the years before, during, and after / Mary Jane Minkin, Carol V. Wright.
p.   cm.
Includes bibliographical references and index.
ISBN 0-300-06573-6 (cloth : alk. paper)
      0-300-07261-9 (pbk. : alk. paper)
1. Menopause—Popular works.   2. Middle aged women—Health and hygiene.   I. Wright, Carol V. II. Title.
RG186.M57   1996
618.1'75—dc20   95-52665
                    CIP

A catalogue record for this book is available from the British Library

The paper in this book meets the guidelines for permanence and durability of the Committee on Production Guidelines for Book Longevity of the Council on Library Resources.

10 9 8 7 6 5 4

The information and suggestions contained in this book are not intended to replace the services of your physician or caregiver. Because each person and each medical situation is unique, you should consult your own physician to get answers to your personal questions, to evaluate any symptoms you may have, or to receive suggestions on appropriate medications.

The authors have attempted to make this book as accurate and current as possible, but it may nevertheless contain errors, omissions, or material that is out of date at the time you read it. Neither the authors nor the publisher have any legal responsibility or liability for errors, omissions, outdated material, or the reader's application of the medical information or advice contained in this book.

Although the case histories have been drawn from Dr. Minkin's medical experience, the names of the patients have been altered to protect their privacy.

Contents

Illustrations

Figures

Tables

Boxes

Foreword

The subject of menopause receives much attention both from the medical community and from the press. The vast amount of information available—in books and articles, on radio and television—can be overwhelming, medically unfounded, even frightening.

Dr. Mary Jane Minkin, who is my colleague and friend, and her coauthor Carol V. Wright have written an authoritative, comprehensive book about menopause that reassures and informs women. In a single book, *What Every Woman Needs to Know About Menopause* explores the known medical and alternative approaches to menopause. Issues range from who is a good candidate for estrogen replacement therapy to when is hysterectomy the right choice. Also discussed are remedies for menopausal anxiety, depression, and mood swings; effects of caffeine, alcohol, and diet; concerns about intellectual performance; changes in sexuality; links between estrogen (or hormone) replacement therapy and cancer and heart disease; the possibility of bone loss; such midlife annoyances as fibroids and the onset of incontinence; and the challenges and satisfactions of menopause. The contents cover the period from when a woman first becomes concerned about menopause to the time when she is comfortably into her postmenopausal years and has "just one more question."

This book not only educates women about the many choices available for noting the signs and treating the symptoms of menopause but also encourages them to participate in their own health care. Dr. Minkin urges women to review their options with their gynecologists or other health care providers.

What Every Woman Needs to Know About Menopause reflects the wisdom of Mary Jane Minkin's long practice in obstetrics and gynecology. Over the past twenty years she has built up a treasury of important facts and misconceptions about menopause, and here she shares them with the reader. Carol Wright, a patient of Dr. Minkin's and a professional writer, is the logical coauthor: their collaboration began as conversations between doctor and patient. The authors have combined their strengths to produce an intelligent book that is easy to read. The style is a classical Socratic approach to teaching: questions (frequently those of patients) are asked and answered. To make the reading still more to the point, Dr. Minkin has included short anecdotes about her patients. She sets out to teach women about themselves and she succeeds.

Mary Jane Minkin was an honor student at the Yale School of Medicine and a star resident in obstetrics and gynecology during her training, and she has never lost her zest for knowledge and for teaching. She lectures about menopause to Yale medical students of obstetrics and gynecology and internal medicine. She gives talks to various medical and nonmedical groups, among them Planned Parenthood, the Red Hot Mamas, and the Connecticut chapter of Operating Room Nurses. And she speaks frequently at bookstores and on public radio shows.

What Every Woman Needs to Know About Menopause covers nearly half a woman's life; it can serve as a personal guide through good and not-so-good times. Written in a lively style, it will remain current as you return to it again and again.

Frederick Naftolin, M.D., D.Phil.
Chief, Department of Obstetrics and Gynecology, Yale-New Haven Hospital; professor and chairman, Department of Obstetrics and Gynecology, and director, Center for Research in Reproductive Biology, Yale University

Preface

As a culture we have become sexually liberated in many ways, but menopause remains one of the last taboos. Perhaps that is because we revere youth so much, or because women who are approaching midlife fear the superstitions that surround what used to be euphemistically called the change of life. Hot flashes (or "flushes," as they are called in Britain) are still an embarrassment to many women—although visible pregnancy, once cause for dismissal from a job, is today a source of pride. While the modern woman may be comfortable talking about her experiences with childbirth, surgery, or even cancer, she may find herself unwilling to discuss menopause with friends or family, or even to articulate her feelings about it.

Because of this wall of silence and the influence of a culture that has often valued women primarily for their sexuality and their fertility, virulent myths have sprung up. They imply that menopause means the end of youth and sexuality, and that it lays waste to women's minds, their memory, and their emotional stability. Furthermore, this view suggests that menopause brings instant wrinkles, extra weight, and overall dowdiness, which consign anyone over 50 to the scrap heap—or at the very least to the sidelines.

In the past few years, however, the barrier of silence has begun to crumble.

After decades, even centuries, of an obscurity that makes benign neglect look like intense public scrutiny, menopause as a topic of interest has leaped into the headlines and onto the talk shows. The woman who is today approaching menopause may not even have been aware that her mother was going through "the change," but she can certainly flick on her television set and listen to her contemporaries talking about their hot flashes.

The fact that the women of the "baby boomer" generation are currently perimenopausal certainly has something to do with this new openness. The oldest of these women, a large, well-educated group born in the years following World War II, are now approaching their fifty-first year, the average age of menopause; an estimated 40 million American women will experience their last menstrual periods in the next twenty years and will have to deal with the increased health risks and change in social rank (real or perceived) that menopause brings.

The best-seller status of recent books on the psychological and sociological implications of menopause shows the wide interest in the subject. Women's magazines, occasionally even business magazines, feature articles on menopause. In addition, menopause support groups that offer information and psychosocial support are mushrooming. One such group, the Red Hot Mamas, founded three years ago in Connecticut, already has more than seven hundred active members in the Danbury chapter alone.

At the turn of the century the average life span of American women was forty-eight years. Put crudely, this statistic means that in 1900 the average woman died only a few years after the end of her childbearing years. Today that same average American woman is the beneficiary of antibiotics, better nutrition, better public health measures, and better medical care. She can look ahead to thirty or even forty comfortable postmenopausal years—years that, despite the cultural bias against older women, may be among the most productive and enjoyable of her life. There is even an acronym, PMZ (postmenopausal zest), that highlights the renewed energy and liberation that many women feel at this stage of life. It is crucial, however, that women know how to maintain their health if they are to optimize these years.

Women also need resources to guide them through menopause, a time of profound change socially and psychologically as well as physically. Gynecologists who take care of women in their premenopausal years recognize this concern; they report that the question they are most frequently asked by patients in their forties is, "What is menopause going to be like, and what can I expect will be happening to me in the next few years?" While it is difficult to predict the course of menopause for each individual woman, there is a range of possible symptoms or signs of which all women should be aware.

Since some of the signs of menopause at first glance seem to have little to do with the female reproductive system, women should know which are normal and which should be cause for concern. Few women, for example, associate insomnia with their ovaries, yet the two can be closely linked. A woman is unlikely to report spontaneously to her gynecologist that she is not sleeping well, and her internist may have no idea that her insomnia is related to menopause. In this case, as in others, informed women can participate more fully and intelligently in their own medical care.

Today there is an increasing body of scientific knowledge about menopause and the maintenance of health throughout life. Certain information is incontrovertible. Exercise basically is good for everyone. Stopping smoking and limiting drinking are good for everyone. Some calcium intake is good for almost everyone.

In other areas no clear choice is immediately obvious. Estrogen replacement therapy may benefit many women but is not necessarily right for all. The subject of estrogen replacement therapy has become complex, for reasons that are political as well as scientific. Consumer advocates and feminists alike have rightly emphasized the long neglect of women's health care issues. Research on diseases that affect only women has historically received inadequate financing; not until 1990 was a women's health research bureau formed at the National Institutes of Health, a government-supported organization whose funding often reflects national priorities. Although major studies on the long-term effects of estrogen replacement therapy at last are under way, their results are not yet known.

Furthermore, feminist and consumer activists have pointed out the huge profits accruing to a pharmaceutical industry that presses on women drugs and treatments that may not be necessary and may even be harmful. The controversy and subsequent litigation over the health risks of intrauterine devices and the charges and countercharges surrounding silicone breast implants have undermined faith in both the medical profession and the pharmaceutical industry. From the 1940s to the 1970s physicians routinely prescribed DES (diethylstilbestrol), a synthetic estrogen, which they mistakenly believed prevented miscarriage; in 1971 researchers discovered that the daughters of women who had taken DES were at increased risk of cervical and vaginal cancer and other conditions. Today women want to know whether a given treatment (estrogen replacement therapy in particular) will be safe in the long run or will turn out to be another DES.

The relations between women patients and their physicians have come under scrutiny as never before. Increasingly, women feel uncomfortable in a role where their physician, male or female, sits behind a desk dispensing prescriptions and dogma. Nor can many women accept the formerly widespread custom, symbolic of the politics of the relationship, whereby physicians addressed their patients by first name and patients responded respectfully with title and surname. In short, women nowadays hope for a physician-patient relationship that reflects respect for the individual. While the adversarial relationship with their physicians that women have often experienced is being alleviated as more women enter the medical profession and as the profession in general becomes more responsive, women still need to be armed with information about their own bodies in order to seek out the best possible medical care.

Furthermore, even with the best doctor-patient relationship, the traditional annual office visit of fifteen minutes hardly allows time for education about menopause and discussion of personal menopausal issues. Pregnant women visit their caregivers at least monthly and attend special classes to prepare them for a comparable major life change. As changes in the health care system pressure doctors to see more and more patients in less and less time, the situation will get worse. Not surprisingly, the American woman who receives estrogen replacement therapy but is not educated about it stays with it for an average of only nine months.

Despite legitimate complaints against the health care industry, modern medicine does offer today's women significant benefits unavailable to their mothers and grandmothers. To take advantage of these possibilities, women must be able to find a middle road, a course with which they are comfortable. For many this path lies between the do-it-yourself feminism of the 1970s, which treated the health care industry and the medical profession as one vast conspiracy, and the traditional unquestioning acceptance of what someone else prescribes. Women must be vigilant about their own well-being; they must have accurate, up-to-date, understandable information that will help them know what questions to ask in order to make intelligent decisions on their own behalf.

If you are approaching midlife and menopause, or perhaps are already there, the chapters that follow have been written for you. One of us (M.J.M.) has been a practicing gynecologist for almost twenty years, talking with and listening to thousands of women as they go through menopause. This book is based on what these women have wanted to know—on their concerns, questions, and experiences at midlife. We have written in question-and-answer format, trying to anticipate what you might ask your own physician, given the luxury of time. Although there are two authors, the "I" who answers and discusses the questions is M.J.M., the physician.

We hope this volume will help you understand the physical and emotional changes that you are probably feeling as you approach menopause. It will tell you why you feel as you do, if medical science has the answer. It will inform you about what we know scientifically, and it will tell you what we do not know. Obviously there are important questions you will have to answer for yourself, but we hope that this book will give you the information you need to make wisely the decisions that will ultimately affect the rest of your life.

Many people assisted us in the preparation of this book. We thank Dr. Kristen Zarfos for helping with the section on breast cancer and Sue Weiser, Registered Dietitian, for reading the sections on nutrition. Dr. Donna Criscenzo and Dr. Mary Scheimann suggested the guidelines on general medical care. Dr. Fred Naftolin, who read the manuscript pencil in hand, made thoughtful suggestions on the sections devoted to the physiology of menopause. We are also grateful to Miriam Wilkerson for typing the manuscript and to Andrea Champlin for her work on the illustrations. Without our agent and friend, Mildred Marmur, this project would never have gotten off the ground. Jean Thomson Black of Yale University Press provided judicious editorial advice, as well as enthusiasm and encouragement.

Closer to home, we would like to acknowledge the important, sometimes extrascientific contributions of our families, Allie, Max, and Steve Pincus, and Fred and Catherine Wright.

M.J.M.
C.V.W.

◼ The Physiology of Menopause:
How It Happens

Menopause represents the end of about forty years of monthly menstrual cycles. After producing, nurturing, and sending out an egg cell every month—except during pregnancies—your ovaries finally wear out and cease functioning. Unlike labor, a process that has three well-defined stages, menopause has only one well-defined end point, your final menstrual period. The changes leading up to this event, however, may make themselves evident to you for as long as ten years.

In order to understand what happens during menopause, you need to understand something about the years that preceded it.

Basically, the ovaries have two functions: to make eggs and to make sex hormones—mainly estrogen and progesterone, but also a few others.

The Ovaries and Their Functions

The ovaries make estrogen in several forms, of which the most important is estradiol. Other forms are estriol and estrone, but all three are usually grouped under the single name "estrogen." This hormone is important in changing a girl into a woman, in contributing to the growth spurt of adolescence, in the matu-

A.

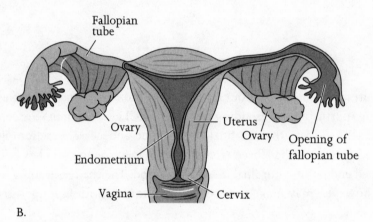

B.

Figure 1. *The female reproductive organs.* *A. Lateral view.* *B. Frontal view.*

ration of the uterus and other reproductive organs, and in the development of female sex characteristics. It also plays a major part in regulating the menstrual cycle, and it influences other organs that are seemingly unrelated to the process of reproduction. The second important ovarian hormone is progesterone, which along with estrogen regulates the menstrual cycle.

In addition to these hormones, generally known as the female sex hormones, the ovaries produce very small amounts of male sex hormones called androgens, including testosterone. In women, testosterone seems to have a role in the female sex drive and in assertiveness, and it may account for certain "masculine" traits (such as facial hair) in postmenopausal women.

The other important function of the ovaries is to produce eggs. The ovaries are formed during fetal life, as are the egg cells within them. Early in fetal life the future baby girl carries within her immature ovaries about a million eggs, her full complement for a lifetime; at birth this number has dwindled to perhaps four hundred thousand. Only a small fraction of these, perhaps four hundred, are destined to reach maturity; the others degenerate at some point in their development, and at menopause only a very few remain.

This state of events means that a woman's egg cells are the same age she is, a fact that is important to older women who are seeking to bear children. Consequently, the eggs that are available to be fertilized when a woman is aged 45 are twenty-five years older than the eggs that were available for fertilization when she was 20. Statistics have confirmed that certain birth defects, in particular Down syndrome, result from chromosomal changes that take place in the eggs as they age.

The Physiology of the Menstrual Cycle

By the time a girl reaches puberty, more than half of the million eggs that were formed prenatally have been lost. The remainder are at rest, encapsulated in structures that will form the ovarian follicles. In their simplest or primordial state, the follicles consist of the egg cell surrounded by a single layer of cells called granulosa cells. When the ovaries become more active at puberty, the eggs begin to develop. Every month some of the follicles start growing. In each growing follicle the granulosa cells divide and reproduce many times so that soon instead of a single layer, layers and layers of them surround the egg cell; these granulosa cells make the majority of the estrogen in the body. At this stage of development, the follicle is called preantral.

The cells in the ovary around the outside of the follicle make a contribution too, causing the outer layer of the follicle to grow and its cells, in turn, to differentiate. Then when the follicle reaches a certain size, it develops a fluid-filled pocket, the antrum (from the Latin word meaning "cave"). As the cycle continues, the antrum gets bigger and bigger.

About a week into the menstrual cycle, a selection process takes place. The biggest follicle of the group that is growing and differentiating is chosen to be "follicle of the month"—in scientific terminology, the dominant follicle. It con-

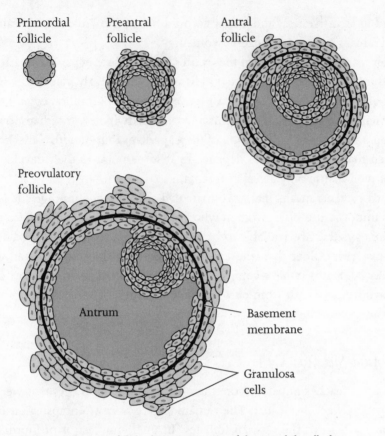

Primordial follicle

Preantral follicle

Antral follicle

Preovulatory follicle

Antrum

Basement membrane

Granulosa cells

Figure 2. A developing follicle, showing maturation of the egg and the cells that surround and nourish it during the first half of the menstrual cycle.

tinues to increase in size while the other follicles degenerate and die off. (Once in a while the signals get crossed and more than one follicle continues to develop, creating the possibility of fraternal twins.)

When the dominant follicle reaches a certain size, it ruptures. The egg cell and some of the surrounding granulosa cells burst through the wall of the ovary, an event that is known as ovulation. This happens on about day 14 of the twenty-eight-day menstrual cycle. If all goes well, the egg cell is swept into the fallopian tube. The ends of the tube have specialized cells whose hairlike projections sweep back and forth, beating in waves and propelling the egg cell toward the interior of the tube. Once in the tube, the egg may or may not be fertilized. This part of the cycle, which deals with the development of the follicles, is called the follicular phase.

Meanwhile, back in the ovary, what is left of the follicle starts to become active again. It changes into a glandlike structure called the corpus luteum, Latin for "yellow body," which indeed is the color of the follicle remnant. If the egg cell in the fallopian tube does not meet any sperm and get fertilized, the corpus luteum reaches its maximum growth in about ten days (day 24 of the cycle) and in its turn begins to degenerate. But during its short life span (in a nonpregnant woman), the corpus luteum is very active and secretes large amounts of both progesterone and estrogen.

All of this action taking place in the ovaries brings about changes in the uterine lining, or endometrium. As the follicles within the ovaries enlarge and develop, the lining of the uterus begins to thicken and proliferate in response to the estrogen produced in the ovaries. After ovulation takes place, roughly on day 14, the estrogen level again rises. The additional progesterone produced by the corpus luteum acts on the endometrial tissue to stabilize it and turn it into a hospitable environment, ready to receive an egg, should fertilization occur.

If fertilization does not occur and the once-active corpus luteum degenerates (on about day 25 of the cycle), there is a sudden shutdown in the production of both progesterone and estrogen and the endometrium is deprived of its support system. The uterine blood vessels constrict, so that the lining has a diminished supply of oxygen and of nutrients. The muscular tissue of the uterus begins to contract rhythmically. Soon the uterine lining disintegrates and is sloughed off as menstrual blood, except for a thin deep layer that will start regenerating the endometrium for the next cycle. This part of the menstrual cycle, from ovulation on day 14 to the onset of menstruation on day 28, is called the luteal phase.

This routine is complex, at least as carefully organized as an intricately plotted murder mystery. The organizers or controllers — the agents that start and stop the different actions of the cycle — are hormones, and in fact the very name comes from a Greek verb meaning "to urge on," or "rouse." Although the ovaries are the chief producers of the female sex hormones estrogen and progesterone, they do not do their job in isolation but are part of a chain of command that begins (to the best of our knowledge) in the brain.

The remotest roots of the sequence seem to be in the cerebral cortex, the mass of gray matter that is known to play a role in memory, language acquisition, and motor control. The exact action of the cerebral cortex in the hormonal regulation of the menstrual cycle is not yet known, but such changes as the loss of periods during times of stress seem to be influenced by the cortex.

The next player in the sequence is the hypothalamus, a small region of the

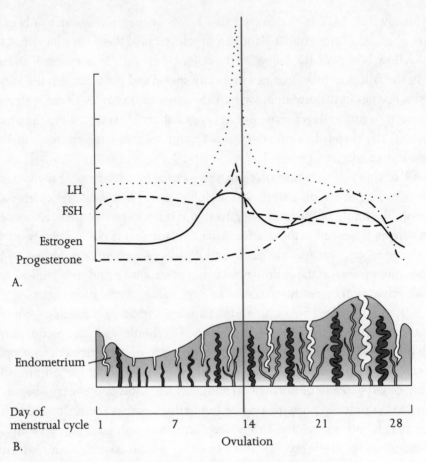

LH
FSH
Estrogen
Progesterone
A.

Endometrium

Day of menstrual cycle
1   7   14   21   28
B.   Ovulation

Figure 3. *Hormonal and uterine changes during the normal menstrual cycle.*
A. Bloodstream levels of pituitary and ovarian hormones.
B. Maturation and thickening of the lining of the uterus and its blood supply.

brain that lies above the pituitary gland (and below an area called the thalamus, as the name suggests). Though tiny, the hypothalamus has a role in regulating the internal environment of the body, for example influencing the water balance within the cells and tissues, eating behavior, and the daily sleep and waking cycle. The hypothalamus also releases the hormones that will trigger menstruation.

Starting around the time of puberty, the hypothalamus begins the ovarian cycle every month by secreting a hormone called GnRH, gonadotropin-releasing hormone. The gonadotropins, which are luteinizing hormone (LH) and follicle-stimulating hormone (FSH), control the ovaries, the female gonads.

(The word "gonad" simply means an organ that produces reproductive cells—eggs or sperm.)

The chemical messenger GnRH alerts the appropriate region of the pituitary gland, geographically a close neighbor of the hypothalamus, to secrete its hormones, LH and FSH. The hormones from the pituitary will in turn stimulate the ovaries. The FSH does just what its name suggests: it stimulates the follicles to develop. The LH, whose presence in the blood surges at midcycle, causes the dominant follicle to release the egg cell, culminating in ovulation.

All of this regulation is governed by a control system called negative or reciprocal feedback, which works more or less like a thermostat. After you set the thermostat in a room at the desired level, the device senses the temperature and turns the furnace off or on to keep the level where you want it. Within your body the regulating factors are chemical, rather than thermal, but the principle is the same. There is a constant reciprocal feedback loop between the brain and the ovaries, and the brain continuously responds to the levels of estrogen that it senses being produced. For example, a lack of estrogen in the blood causes the LH and FSH to rise, during the menstrual cycle and also after the menopause.

What Happens at Menopause

Your ovaries, like many of your other organs, peak at some time in your late twenties or early thirties. Thereafter their production of estrogen and progesterone begins to decline gradually and finally stops altogether. Researchers surmise that this has to do with the depletion and finally the absence of follicles. It is estimated that you have five thousand to ten thousand follicles left when you are 40 years old; the number declines precipitously after that. Researchers also know that with aging either the follicles become less responsive to the gonadotropins that formerly urged them to action or the smaller number of follicles started at each cycle results in lower estrogen and increased LH and FSH.

At some point, most likely when you are in your early forties, your menstrual periods will probably become irregular in response to these declining estrogen and progesterone levels. You will begin having occasional anovulatory periods, that is, periods in which no egg is released from a follicle. (Your ovaries are producing enough estrogen to build up the endometrium, but not enough to fully mature a follicle.) Because ovulation does not occur, there is no corpus luteum to make progesterone. And because there is no progesterone, there is no way to stabilize the uterine lining; nor is there a signal (the withdrawal of pro-

Figure 4. The hypothalamic-pituitary-ovarian feedback loop. The hypothalamus manufactures GnRH, which stimulates the pituitary to make FSH and LH. These in turn stimulate the ovaries to make estrogen. The presence of estrogen inhibits further production of GnRH. When estrogen levels fall, the hypothalamus makes more GnRH.

gesterone) for the shedding to take place in an orderly, controlled manner. Instead, the uterine lining keeps on building and building, eventually breaking down only because it outgrows its blood supply.

Another scenario for the menopause is that your ovaries may be producing some estrogen and progesterone, but not enough to keep the cycle going at its usual rate; the process may take longer than usual, and while you may still have ovulatory cycles, your periods may be more widely spaced. Sooner or later you will have your last menstrual period. A year afterward, you can safely say that you are menopausal.

2 Signs and Symptoms

The first questions most women ask about menopause are, "What is it?" and "How do I know if I'm having it?" In the medical literature menopause has a clear definition: the cessation of ovarian function, which results in the permanent cessation of menstrual periods. In this sense, menopause is analogous to menarche (the onset of menstruation), which marks the beginning of a woman's reproductive life; menopause, and with it the end of menstruation, marks the conclusion.

In life things are seldom as straightforward as they are in literature, and so this definition is not entirely helpful. In the first place, it is useful only after the fact. Because most women skip a few menstrual periods before they cease altogether, you can't be sure that you are truly menopausal, that your periods have stopped and will never return, until you have gone a year without one. In other words, you don't even know that you are menopausal until a year after the "event" has happened.

In the second place, the medical definition suggests (as do some of the afternoon TV talk shows) that menopause is a single event, something that happens once and is over. Actually, the process that ends in menopause, the decrease of ovarian function to the point that menstruation ceases, happens over a period of years beginning in one's midthirties and continuing for the remainder of life. (Incidentally, this extended period is called the climacteric.) What concerns most women is not that final menstrual period or the time thereafter, but the changes in long-established physical and psychological patterns that come about in the five to ten years on either side of menopause—the period known medically as the perimenopause. Also important to women and to their caregivers are the long-term issues, when the menopausal symptoms have passed.

At what age can I expect to go through menopause?

The average age of natural menopause in this country is about 51, a statistic that has remained remarkably constant over the years. The normal range of age at menopause is about 45 to 55, but among my patients I see a range from about age 35 to 58. Any individual woman can begin experiencing the symptoms of perimenopause as early as her midthirties or as late as her early fifties.

The relative stability of the average age of menopause has a couple of interesting implications. First, it stands in contrast to the average age of menarche, which decreased slightly between the turn of the century and the 1950s, probably because of improved nutrition; in Western industrialized countries we seem to have reached a plateau in the age of menarche, which has remained stable for the past four decades or so. Menstruation doesn't usually begin until a girl weighs somewhere between 95 and 100 pounds. Since children in financially comfortable families nowadays are likely to be optimally nourished, girls probably reach their adult weight sooner than their mothers did. Body-fat percentage also plays a role in triggering the onset of menstruation, so lean, athletic girls may begin menstruating later than rounder, plumper girls.

Second, while the age of menopause has remained the same, the life expectancy of American women has gone up to about age 81 for white women and to about age 76 for women of color. Thus the average American woman, who begins menstruating at age 12 and goes through menopause at 51, spends more than one-third of her life as a postmenopausal woman. The significance of this fact to her health is tremendous and will reflect the care she takes of herself during the perimenopausal years. Fred Naftolin, chairman of the department of obstetrics and gynecology at the Yale University School of Medicine, points out that "the perimenopause casts a long shadow."

Each year hundreds of thousands of women, many of them not near the age of natural menopause, experience surgical menopause—that is, removal of the ovaries—at the time of hysterectomy. Surgical menopause, if not followed by estrogen replacement, often leads to more profound menopausal symptoms than does natural menopause.

How can I predict when I might experience menopause?

The best way to predict the age of your own menopause is to check your family history. If your mother was menopausal at age 42, then it is likely that you will have a relatively early menopause (though not necessarily at age 42). If she had a late menopause, you can probably count on having yours later than the average.

The onset of perimenopausal symptoms, hot flashes for example, does not necessarily predict the actual coming of menopause. If you begin noticing peri-menopausal symptoms at the age of 42, there is a chance that you might not be fully menopausal until you are 50, especially if your mother and older sister did not experience menopause until that age.

The classic dogma used to be that if you began menstruating late, say between the ages of 14 and 16, you would reach menopause early. Conversely, if you began your periods early, before the age of 12, you would reach menopause relatively late. The notion behind this theory, presumably, was that if your ovaries weren't the most robust to begin with (accounting for late onset of menstruation), they would give up and stop functioning early. While some gynecologists still find some relevance in this theory, my own clinical practice does not support it.

Studies have shown that smokers have an earlier menopause than non-smokers. To put it bluntly, smoking destroys your ovaries. That is the bad news; the good news is that if you stop smoking you may buy yourself a few extra years of ovarian function. So if you are concerned about preserving your fertility, perhaps wanting to delay childbearing until you get your career on track, you should quit smoking immediately.

Can a sudden, stressful event bring on menopause all at once?

I have talked to many women who said that menopause came on them suddenly without any warning symptoms.

Natalie F. started menstruating when she was 10. Unlike most girls, she started off with the pattern that she would follow for her entire reproductive life, her periods coming like clockwork every twenty-eight days. She never missed a period (except when she was pregnant or nursing) and never was either late or early. When she was 50 years old, her mother died. Natalie never had another period.

Often the traumatic event is not of such magnitude as the death of a parent. I have had women call me to say that they stopped menstruating after their dog died.

What are the reasons for early menopause?

Early menopause can of course be caused by surgical removal of the ovaries. But most women who have early natural menopause inherited a genetic predisposition for it. The exact reasons are unknown. Perhaps these women were born with fewer egg follicles, or perhaps their follicles simply had a shorter life span.

Factors other than inheritance also play a role. Smoking, as we have seen, shortens the number of years the ovaries continue to function. The ovarian function of women who have had chemotherapy and/or radiation as treatment for cancer often is either temporarily or permanently altered or destroyed. In some women ovarian function comes back fully after the therapy is completed; in some women it comes back partially; and in some women it does not come back at all. Although younger women, in their thirties for example, have a better chance of ovarian recovery than do older women, it is not easy to ascertain the final outcome ahead of time. With some diseases that require radiation therapy, for example Hodgkin's lymphoma, the surgeon can take protective measures, moving the ovaries out of the field of radiation, which makes damage and subsequent ovarian failure less likely.

Although there is no ironclad evidence, some data suggest that women who have had hysterectomies many years before menopause (but have retained their ovaries) may also have a somewhat earlier onset of menopausal signs. It has been suggested that surgery alters the blood supply to the ovaries, causing them to age more quickly. Some researchers have suggested that women who have had tubal ligations have earlier menopause, but there are no firm data supporting this observation.

Other reasons for early menopause include several rare conditions. In some autoimmune diseases a woman's immune system makes antibodies against her own ovaries. The situation is analogous to diabetes, where the immune system attacks the pancreas. Another rare condition that causes premature menopause is Turner's syndrome, a genetic disease that involves chromosomal abnormalities.

What problems are associated with early menopause?

Whatever its cause, a premature menopause, especially if it is abrupt, is associated with more symptoms and more serious medical consequences than the usual menopause. Early menopause leads to immediate inability to conceive children. It is also associated with increased rates of osteoporosis and coronary artery disease, and with incontinence. Of course, these problems respond favorably to ERT. It is just possible that there is a correlation between early menopause and other concerns of aging, such as Alzheimer's disease.

What signs or symptoms suggest the approach of menopause?

There is a classic group of physical signs that suggest menopause is approaching. These signs (they are not really symptoms in the pathological sense of the word, because menopause is not a disease but a normal condition of life) include hot flashes, night sweats, and changes in the frequency, length, and amount of flow of your periods. Many women experience sleeplessness or broken sleep, even if they do not have night sweats and hot flashes. Some women report psychological symptoms that include depression, mood swings, and irritability. Others comment on their poor memory or inability to focus mentally. Headaches, sometimes migraines, can be associated with menopause.

You may notice some of these changes, all of them, or none of them. You may have some of them occasionally but not all the time. Or, if you are lucky, you may be among the 15 to 20 percent of American women who simply stop menstruating one day without any noticeable evidence to suggest that they have just had their last period. If you are among the majority of American women, some 65 to 70 percent, you will find these perimenopausal changes troublesome in degrees that vary from mildly annoying to seriously disruptive. If you are very unlucky, you might be among the 10 percent who find the changes surrounding menopause overwhelmingly difficult to cope with. Fortunately, even if you are in the group with more severe menopausal signs, modern medicine should be able to help you.

There are also physical and psychological changes that simply go along with getting older. They come at about the same time as menopause and may (or may not) be associated with it. In fact, one of the problems associated with menopause is that it is sometimes very difficult to separate changes that are caused by growing older from changes that are caused by decreased hormone production. As we age, our hair (including pubic hair, eyebrows, and leg and arm hair as well as the hair on our head) gets sparser and may change in texture. In contrast, hair on the lower face increases. Skin becomes thinner and less elastic; we tend to accumulate fat around our middle and to gain weight on the upper arms, back, abdomen, and breasts. Studies show that a significant proportion of perimenopausal and postmenopausal women experience a decline in sexual interest, although it is not clear whether these changes in attitude come from menopause itself or simply from growing older.

Is there any way to predict whether menopause will be easy or difficult?

Unquestionably, some women pass through menopause with fewer symptoms and less discomfort than others. In the bad old days, it was generally believed that women brought discomfort on themselves by their neurotic responses to the physiological changes that were occurring.

Some older studies showed that married women were more distressed than single women, and that mothers were more distressed than women who had not had children, perhaps because married women and mothers were more likely to feel the pangs of loneliness and the "empty nest syndrome" when their children left home. But modern research has not really targeted any particular group of women as likely to experience extreme distress and any other group as likely to sail through menopause without any symptoms whatsoever.

Today many physicians are willing to acknowledge that the discomforts of menopause are caused physiologically rather than psychologically. It is true, however, that the mind shapes and refines our responses to the physiological changes that underlie menopausal discomforts. My own experience as a physician is that there does seem to be a kind of familial predictor, but one that results from conditioning rather than from inherited genetic traits or physiological problems. Women whose mothers described their own menopause as "terrible" and "really almost unbearable" are likely to experience more discomfort than women whose mothers did not complain of such severe symptoms. I find an analogue in menstrual discomfort: mothers who say they "nearly died" during their own periods are likely to condition their daughters to have uncomfortable periods.

I do tell menopausal women who are concerned because their mothers had such an unfortunate menopausal experience that in today's world we have therapies that can probably relieve discomfort completely. A woman who is 51 years old in the 1990s need not be overwhelmed with symptoms, as her mother was before her.

Are there laboratory tests for diagnosing menopause?

The answer to this question is a rousing yes and no. Yes, there are tests; no, they won't tell you absolutely whether you are menopausal or not; nor will they tell you how far along in the process you are.

What are these tests?

Physicians usually rely on one of two tests: the first measures estrogen in the bloodstream, the second measures blood levels of follicle-stimulating hormone (FSH). In general, the tests look for low estrogen levels in the bloodstream and high levels of FSH.

Of the several kinds of estrogen normally circulating in the bloodstream, estradiol tends to be the easiest to measure. The test for menopause looks for an estradiol level lower than 50 pg/ml (picograms per milliliter). During the normal premenopausal menstrual cycle estradiol varies widely, ranging between 50 and 400 pg/ml. (A picogram is one one-trillionth of a gram; a milliliter is one one-thousandth of a liter.) Physicians generally agree that an estradiol of 20 or 30 confirms menopause. Menopause happens because the ovaries no longer produce estrogen, so it is reasonable and indeed correct to assume that a menopausal woman will have lower blood estrogen levels than someone who is still menstruating regularly.

The other lab test for menopause is a blood test for follicle-stimulating hormone, which in a premenopausal woman is sent by the pituitary to stimulate the ovary to cause follicles to develop. The postmenopausal ovary cannot make estrogen in response to the FSH, so more and more FSH is produced by the pituitary in hopes of stimulating the ovary to its former function. Thus what physicians are looking for here as confirmation of menopause is a high level of FSH. Although the amount varies during the menstrual cycle of a premenopausal women, it generally remains below 30 (that is, 30 milli-international units per milliliter of blood). Menopausal women have FSH levels higher than 30, sometimes even in the 100s. So if your FSH level turns out to be 67 and you have other signs and symptoms, by laboratory indicators you are menopausal.

Why don't these lab tests always accurately diagnose menopause?

Women generally want to have blood estradiol levels and FSH levels taken for one of two reasons: they are partway through the menopausal process and want to know how far along they are, or they think they are menopausal and want to be sure. Unfortunately lab tests won't give a definitive answer to either question 100 percent of the time.

The problem with taking a blood estradiol level, and one of the reasons the utility of this test is controversial, is that during the menstrual cycle the normal estradiol level fluctuates anywhere between 50 and 400. Without knowing where a woman is in her cycle, the level alone does not mean much. Since a perimenopausal woman frequently has irregular ovulatory cycles and irregular periods, it is often very difficult to decide where she is in her cycle. Is she just about to ovulate? Or did she ovulate several weeks ago? Her low estradiol level may simply indicate that she is very early or very late in her cycle.

Louisa W., in her late forties, comes in to me experiencing occasional hot flashes, irregular periods, and some episodes of insomnia. A blood test shows that her estradiol level is 40 and her FSH is 67. Based on these tests, it looks as though Louisa is menopausal. I tell her and she feels relieved. Two months later she has a period. So she is not menopausal yet.

In fact, the tests didn't tell more than the history and the physical exam did. What did the numbers mean? Did that 40 represent a peak of estrogen for this cycle, or was it measured at a low point in the cycle? If she were ten years younger, would that 40 have been a 400? Was Louisa in the late part of her ovulatory cycle when the blood was drawn, in which case we would expect low estradiol levels, or was she just about to ovulate, in which case we would expect that 40 to be much higher? Since perimenopausal women have very irregular cycles, it is difficult from any one assessment to know just where Louisa is in her cycle.

If her estradiol level had come back at something like 20, we could have said yes, certainly this is low; premenopausal women do not normally have estradiol levels that low at any time during their cycles.

The same kinds of problems interfere with the accuracy of the FSH test. Like estradiol levels, FSH levels fluctuate both in premenopausal and in perimenopausal women, so the test is not necessarily conclusive. Louisa's FSH level is higher than we would expect in a premenopausal woman, whose normal FSH maximum is no more than 30.

Marian A. is 53 years old. She has gone almost a year without a period. She has hot flashes at regular intervals and wants to know whether she is fully menopausal. To my way of thinking, there doesn't seem much reason to do an estradiol or an FSH level to confirm that yes, Marian is menopausal. Her age, the length of time she has been without a period, and the presence of hot flashes all suggest that she is very nearly menopausal. These signs do not mean, however, that she will never have another menstrual period. Many women do have one or two after a significant amount of time without one.

In most cases, then, estradiol and FSH levels aren't really worth checking, because they will not tell you what you want to know any better than can be determined without the tests. Even if you do have an FSH level that is substantially elevated and an estradiol level that is very low, there is no guarantee that you are forever finished with your periods.

Many physicians will biopsy women like Marian if they go about a year without a period and then suddenly have one, because of concern about the possibility of cancer. What most biopsies show is normal, proliferative endometrial tissue, the type one sees in regularly menstruating women. A biopsy showed with certainty that what was happening to Marian was normal ovarian activity, not some pathological condition.

How much do FSH and estradiol tests cost?

These are expensive tests. In the area where I work they cost something like $200 apiece and are not always covered by insurance. Given the direction in which health care seems to be moving, they are unlikely to be covered in the future. So if your test is inconclusive and your doctor wants it repeated in six months, you will be faced with a bill for about $400, which is a substantial amount of money. Some women feel that it is definitely worth $200 or $400 to learn whether their estradiol and FSH levels are high or low. But at a time in history when many people are trying to keep down medical costs, it is worth thinking twice about drawing estradiols and FSHs.

What is the physiological explanation for these hormone levels?

We know that as a woman ages, her ovaries produce less and less estrogen, until at menopause they produce virtually none at all. It is this decline that results in the lower estradiol levels in the blood. Although levels fluctuate during a perimenopausal woman's cycle, rebounding upward now and again, the trend is definitely downward. Perimenopausal women produce less estrogen than women who have not begun the menopausal process.

The mechanism that accounts for the high levels of FSH in menopausal women is more complex. The ovaries do not independently decide how much FSH or estrogen to produce, or when, as we have seen; instead, they are driven and regulated by the pituitary gland through a process of feedback. When the pituitary senses low blood estrogen, it sends a message to the ovaries, in the form of a burst of follicle-stimulating hormone, to increase estrogen production. If the ovaries cannot make much estrogen because of their planned obsolescence, the pituitary continues to secrete more and more FSH signaling the ovaries to step up their estrogen production. Consequently the blood levels of FSH rise and rise, sometimes quite high. A newly discovered hormone called inhibin, which is secreted by follicles, has been shown to control FSH. So not having normal amounts of estrogen or inhibin in the blood is a kind of double whammy, giving a disproportionate increase in FSH in comparison to LH.

When do these perimenopausal changes appear?

Although ovarian function begins to decline when women are in their midthirties, signs of menopause usually become evident in the early to middle forties. But they can start as soon as the early thirties or appear as late as the midfifties. The age at which these changes begin does not necessarily indicate when menopause will actually take place, for the perimenopausal period in general lasts somewhere between five and eight years. Occasional women get their first hot flash at age 42 and are not fully menopausal until they are 55.

What variations in the menstrual cycle occur during the perimenopausal years?

One of the first things many women notice as they approach menopause is a variation in the pattern of their periods, a pattern established perhaps thirty years before in early adulthood. Periods may change in length, frequency, or amount of flow. The key word here is "change," because individuals vary widely. Menstrual periods can become heavier or lighter; they can be longer or shorter. Some women find themselves bleeding two or three weeks out of every month, while others notice that their periods are spaced further and further apart. Some women have light periods every couple of months, others have very heavy periods every couple of weeks. Some women skip periods for several months and then have very heavy flows. In short, there are many patterns of change and no one pattern seems to predominate.

Patterns may also change for a single individual. A woman may have very heavy periods for a while, which may then taper off and become more widely spaced. Conversely, after a period of light and infrequent periods, she may experience heavy, frequent bleeding. All these changes are normal. However, heavy and frequent bleeding, especially after intercourse, can raise the possibility of cancer and should trigger a visit to the doctor.

Are heavy periods a sign of approaching menopause?

Many women experience heavy bleeding, medically known as menorrhagia, during the perimenopausal period. For some women menorrhagia is merely an inconvenience, but others find that it can disrupt their everyday lives, interfere with their work schedules, or at the very least ruin their vacations. For some women loss of blood is itself worrisome.

How heavy is so-called heavy bleeding?

In general, women tend to overestimate the amount of blood they lose during a normal period. Dr. Ian Fraser, a researcher at the University of Sydney in Australia, weighed tampons and pads to determine blood loss during periods. He divided the test group into heavy and light bleeders and found that the women in the heavy group lost between 70 and 130 ml of blood each month. Thirty ml is one fluid ounce, so the average blood loss for the "heavy" group was about 4.5 oz of blood per cycle. In common household terms, the heavy bleeders in the study lost about a half-cup, or a quarter of the pint usually given at a blood-donation center.

You are unlikely to measure your blood loss this way, so doctors offer various ways to gauge how heavily you are bleeding. Some suggest that you can consider yourself to be bleeding heavily if you have to change a super tampon every hour for twenty-four hours; other physicians suggest a standard of every half-hour for six hours. While this rate of loss could be considered "heavy," it is not life threatening.

A relatively small proportion of perimenopausal women really do experience worrisome blood loss. On rare occasions women have come into my office with a towel between their legs because they were hemorrhaging so badly.

Cathy H., 48 years old, called me from the grocery store in the next town one Saturday morning. She was having a heavy period and had gone to buy tampons; while she was standing in the feminine products aisle, she suddenly started to hemorrhage, quickly soaking through her clothes. I told her to get to the emergency room immediately. We performed an emergency D&C (dilatation and curettage), the only measure that would control her flow. This kind of bleeding, however, is uncommon.

Is heavy bleeding dangerous?

Heavy bleeding is apt to be more of a nuisance and a concern to the women who experience it than it is a serious threat. On rare occasions, however, heavy periodic bleeding can be dangerous because it leads to significant anemia, in which the red-blood-cell count falls drastically. And strangely enough, women who become anemic tend to bleed more heavily with their periods, which creates a vicious cycle. Most of the time we think of the body as being "smart," that is, responsive to its own needs; but in this case, for reasons that are not understood, the body is "dumb."

For women the normal hematocrit (a measure of the percentage of red blood cells in the blood) is about 40; for men it is in the mid to high 40s. A small percentage of women bleed so heavily that their hematocrit drops two or three points every time they have a period, but if the hematocrit remains somewhere in the range of 35 or 36, that level does not interfere with their health or curtail their activities.

A significant degree of anemia does occur in the woman who gets her hematocrit down to the high 20s or low 30s. Her symptoms might include fatigue, light-headedness, and even shortness of breath with exercise. One of my patients, a woman in her midforties, bled so much that she lowered her hematocrit to 16, which means that she has only a little more than one-third of her normal measure of red blood cells. She obviously needs some kind of treatment, first because she will feel better, second because if she has a sudden very heavy bleed, she is not well supplied with hemoglobin. If someone who has plenty of hemoglobin loses a pint or two of blood, the situation is not life threatening. But if she starts with a borderline hematocrit, she has a serious problem. So women who have very heavy periods should have their hematocrits checked periodically.

Does heavy bleeding have any pathological or dangerous causes?

While much of the heavy bleeding women experience at midlife has hormonal causes, other factors, both anatomical and psychological, can be involved. Psychological stress, which can interfere with regular ovulation, may cause heavier bleeding. If the cause of stress is temporary or transient, then it stands to reason that the heavier bleeding should disappear along with the stress. But since this time of life is stressful for many women who are caught between aging parents and young adult children, or who are experiencing all kinds of changes personally and professionally, the stressful situations may be a long time resolving themselves.

Fibroids, which are fairly common, and endometriosis, which is less common, can also cause heavy bleeding and clotting even in women who are nowhere near menopause. Other causes are polyps and uterine cancer.

How can I distinguish between hormonally caused heavy bleeding and heavy flow caused by some pathological condition?

Unfortunately there is no simple answer; symptoms alone are not enough to tell you whether heavy bleeding is caused by changes in hormone levels or by something else. Women who are developing anatomical problems (for example, fibroids) that can cause heavy bleeding are likely to be in the same age group as women approaching menopause. Indeed, both fibroids and endometriosis, which are uncomfortable but not life threatening, often become symptomatic in women in their midforties, while uterine cancer seems to peak at about age 50. If you are concerned about heavy flow, you should talk to your gynecologist so that together you can determine if anything pathological or dangerous is involved.

Is any danger or risk associated with lighter periods as menopause approaches?

Many women experience lighter periods as they approach menopause, and most of them are pretty happy with this arrangement; but occasionally a patient comes in, worried about diminished flow. I assure her that if she wants heavy periods, medical science can give them to her. Most of the time, once a woman knows that lighter periods are simply a sign of approaching menopause, she is content with the situation. Certainly there is no medical reason to have periods identical to those she had earlier in life.

Are there problems associated with either frequent or infrequent menstrual periods?

While it obviously is inconvenient to be bleeding three weeks out of four, it is not necessarily dangerous—unless the periods are very heavy as well as frequent. In that case the danger, as we have seen, is anemia. In rare instances heavy flow can be associated with cancer, so it does need to be discussed with your caregiver.

The only difficulty associated with less frequent periods is that sometimes a woman's periods may space out for two, three, or four months and then, when a period does come, she will get very heavy bleeding, what I informally call Niagara Falls flooding. Usually such a woman is not far along in the menopausal process. Her ovaries are still producing estrogen, and in response the lining of her uterus is building up. If she is not ovulating, the lining will continue to build for a month or two; then suddenly, either she will ovulate spontaneously or her uterine lining will have built up so much that it reaches the saturation point and starts pouring out. The problem is that the bleeding is uncontrolled; there is no progesterone to make sure that the period tapers off and ends after an appropriate amount of time. Usually the blood count of such women drops several points and they may lose as much as a pint or two of blood with a period.

Is bleeding between periods dangerous?

We have seen that many women experience erratic menstrual periods as they approach menopause, and most of these irregularities can be considered normal. With perimenopausal women, changing levels of hormones are most often the culprit, but since spotting between periods is one of the indications of uterine cancer, it can be a cause for concern. Spotting can also be a manifestation of cervical cancer, though bleeding from the cervix generally takes place in the context of bleeding after intercourse, whereas bleeding from the uterus is apt to be spontaneous, unassociated with any particular activity.

How do I differentiate between the harmless spotting that is related to normal changes in my ovaries and the potentially dangerous spotting that might indicate something abnormal or pathological?

The answer is that in general you can't. If you spot once and the problem goes away, there is a good chance that nothing pathological is happening. One episode of spotting in a perimenopausal woman is usually nothing to worry about. But if you start spotting repeatedly or routinely, even though the spotting is just a little bit here and there, you should call your gynecologist and keep track of what is going on.

Many women are ovulatory spotters and bleed a few drops every time they ovulate. In most cases nothing is wrong. This bleeding will recur regularly, around day 14 in a woman who has a normal twenty-eight-day cycle and less predictably in a woman whose cycles are less regular.

But perimenopausal women who have irregular cycles cannot count on day 14 as being the time of ovulation. Thus, it is important to pay attention if you do spot. When in your cycle does the bleeding occur? How much bleeding is there? Does it happen after intercourse or is it spontaneous?

Spotting in postmenopausal women may well be a different matter. If you have gone for longer than a year without a period and suddenly begin to spot, you should inform your physician right away. I tell my patients that if something is wrong, if they have a polyp or uterine cancer, it will probably bleed more than once—so that, again, a single episode of postmenopausal bleeding usually does not indicate something terribly wrong. Nevertheless, many (but not all) gynecologists will perform a biopsy on the basis of just one episode of spotting in a postmenopausal woman in order to make sure that it doesn't represent something dangerous.

Gynecologists who choose to biopsy the lining of the uterus make that decision because a routine pelvic exam is not particularly helpful in revealing what is happening inside the uterus. Even a Pap smear, which gives information about the condition of the cervix, does not tell enough about the lining of the uterus itself to rule out cancerous changes. New techniques used to assess the uterine lining are relatively noninvasive and can give helpful information.

Are blood clots in the menstrual flow a sign of trouble?

Another thing that concerns many women is clotting. It is generally more troubling to the perimenopausal woman than to her doctor, for clotting is just a manifestation of heaviness of flow. Clots may be startling if you have never had them before; they may be unpleasant and messy, but they are a medical concern only because clots signal a greater blood loss and because they sometimes can cause pain. If a clot forms in the uterus, the uterus may try to expel it by contracting as if the clot were a fetus; these contractions can cause strong cramps.

Do perimenopausal women suffer from menstrual cramps?

Cramping is not a classic menopausal phenomenon. The kind of cramping that women sometimes experience with their periods, the ordinary garden-variety primary dysmenorrhea (menstrual pain that begins early in life), is actually caused by the manufacture of prostaglandins by the lining of the uterus.

Prostaglandins are chemical substances that serve as messengers and, like the hormones to which they are related, act in a number of ways. They cause the uterus to contract; this action restricts blood flow to the uterine muscle, thus causing pain. Prostaglandin production is highest in those cycles in which ovulation occurs, so if a woman is not ovulating, she doesn't usually make much prostaglandin and tends not to feel much or any discomfort.

This process explains why at the beginning of the menstrual spectrum young girls just getting their periods seldom have cramps. Perhaps after they have been menstruating for a year or so they will begin to have cramps, because they are then beginning to ovulate regularly. The dysmenorrhea is a result of the ovulatory cycles. Just the opposite is happening in a woman at the other end of the menstrual spectrum. As she approaches menopause, some of her cycles are ovulatory but many of her periods occur without ovulation.

I get a phone call on this subject about once a day. A perimenopausal patient will tell me that she had her regular period two weeks ago, a normal period with her customary cramps. Two weeks later she finds herself again bleeding heavily but with no cramps. She wants to know what's going on. Because she is not ovulating, she is not making prostaglandins. The lining of her uterus has built up in response to the estrogen she is producing, but what she is experiencing in the second, cramp-free period is a kind of breakthrough bleeding uncontrolled by progesterone, which would have been produced in larger amounts after ovulation. Loss of cramping is more characteristic of menopause than cramping.

Still, if you find yourself having cramps, especially when you have not had them regularly before, you should pay attention and alert your gynecologist. Cramps are not necessarily worrisome, but they may be an indication of some other condition such as fibroids or endometriosis.

What causes all these irregularities in the menstrual cycle?

The menstrual changes that women notice at midlife are basically related to changes in ovulatory patterns, which vary as ovarian function decreases. A woman in her late thirties or in her forties does not ovulate as well, and often not as frequently, as she did ten years earlier. While her ovaries are still making a significant amount of estrogen, her production of progesterone after ovulation is not as copious as it was when she was, say, aged 25.

Progesterone, a vital hormone in preparing the lining of the uterus to receive a fertilized egg, functions in three ways. It limits the buildup of the lining of the uterus, it stabilizes the lining until fertilization can take place, and if fertilization does not occur, the rapid drop in level triggers the shedding of the lining. When a woman in her twenties has a normal cycle, she produces an adequate amount of estrogen followed by an adequate amount of progesterone. The progesterone stabilizes the lining of the uterus; but if the egg that leaves the ovary that month is not fertilized, then the part of the ovary that makes progesterone (the corpus luteum) dies. When progesterone levels fall, the lining of the uterus (the endometrium) is shed in a nice, controlled way.

If your ovaries are not making progesterone at all, there is no hormone to trigger the shedding of the uterine lining, so you don't have a period. If you are making small amounts of progesterone, you may have an early period because your hormone level is too low to keep the endometrium intact. If you are making some progesterone but not enough to limit the growth of the endometrium or prevent excessive buildup, then you may bleed heavily.

What are hot flashes?

Hot flashes, which in England are called hot flushes, are one of the most common features of menopause. About 70 to 75 percent of women get them to some degree. Classically the hot flash is a feeling of heat over the face, shoulders, head, and upper torso; it is usually accompanied by sweating. Often hot flashes are preceded by a premonition that a flash is on the way. Women describe this feeling as one of anxiety or illness, or a tingling sensation or pressure in the head.

What happens in a hot flash is much like what happens whenever the body feels overheated, whether from strenuous exercise on a hot day or from fever. Overheating triggers the body to respond with vasomotor changes, changes in blood vessels that in turn cause changes in blood flow. This process is intended to cool the body to its normal resting state. The blood vessels near the surface of the skin dilate and blood flow to the skin increases, which makes the skin feel hotter and look flushed. Then the skin begins to perspire, and the evaporation from sweating cools the body. This is exactly what happens in a hot flash, although the trigger is not heavy exercise or elevated body temperature.

The classic hot flash is restricted to the face, neck, and upper torso, yet the feelings of flushing and heat can occur in any part of the body. One of my patients says that hot flashes affect only her ears, which turn bright red and feel as if they are on fire. Other women feel hot all over.

Often hot flashes are accompanied by profuse sweating, classically from the neck up, though some people sweat all over and some do not sweat at all. Some women have "cold sweats" instead of hot flashes. They feel chilled or clammy but sweat profusely and often shake and shiver. Many women alternate between hot and cold. The pattern of feeling hot, sweating, and then feeling cold is so predictable for many women that their husbands have been known to ask them, a few minutes after they have thrown back the blankets at the beginning of a flash, whether they are ready yet to have the blanket back.

Hot flashes are not figments of the menopausal imagination. Scientific studies using sensors have shown that skin temperature actually rises one to four degrees, although internal body temperature does not. In a series of experiments published as early as 1975, researchers monitored physiological changes during hot flashes and discovered that they included increased heart rate and profuse sweating.

In addition to the flushing, sweating, and sense of heat, some women notice prickly skin sensations, a feeling that ants are crawling on their skin. The scientific name for this phenomenon is formication, from the Latin word for "ant." Some women experience other odd vasomotor symptoms including palpitations; that is, fluttering or racing sensations of the heart. Others feel tingling sensations like "pins and needles" in their hands or fingers.

Other women have hypotensive sensations, as if their blood pressure had suddenly plummeted; they feel dizzy and light-headed and fear they are going to faint. An occasional woman has showed up in the emergency room feeling that she is about to pass out, because her hot flashes have made her weak and giddy; these women get so vasodilated from the flushing that their blood pressure really does fall. Some, especially small, slim women with low blood pressure, do pass out from hot flashes if they get overheated or dehydrated.

Hot flashes will not kill you; they will not even harm you seriously, but they can be extremely uncomfortable. They are also one of the most dreaded indications of approaching menopause, perhaps because they are so visible. No one knows, unless you tell them, that your period is heavy to the point of flooding or that your skin feels as if it is crawling with ants; but everyone, at least so it seems, can notice your dripping red face. The professional women I see in my practice, especially those in situations where dress and grooming are very important, are particularly embarrassed by this feature of menopause.

In some ways the stigma attached to hot flashes is like the shame a generation or two ago of being visibly pregnant. If you were pregnant, obviously you had engaged in sex. If you have hot flashes, obviously you are menopausal and are getting to be an old lady—not an admirable status in a society that idealizes and cultivates youth. While modern medicine cannot reverse the clock or change societal outlooks, it can at least make women more comfortable during the period when they are experiencing hot flashes. In most cases it can get rid of the hot flashes altogether, so that no one will know you are menopausal.

What factors trigger hot flashes?

The most obvious culprit is external heat, which can range from torrid weather (especially with high humidity) to a warm room, heavy clothing, a hot shower, or a scorching hair dryer. Women notice that they get hot flashes more frequently in the summer than in the winter; they also notice that the insomnia that often accompanies hot flashes is worse in the summer.

Drinking hot beverages, especially tea and coffee which contain caffeine, can bring on hot flashes. And alcohol is a well-known inducer of hot flashes.

Patty L. is director of nursing at a major hospital and as a medically educated person is very aware of changes in her body. She is 52 years old and takes estrogen replacement therapy, 0.625 mg of Premarin, to control her hot flashes. The other day she came to me and said that she knew she had her estrogen dosage right, because if she had one glass of wine she was fine. If she had two or three, she would turn bright red unless she took an extra Premarin the night before the occasion when alcohol was to be served.

Karen G., a nurse, activist in women's causes, and local officeholder, came home from the hospital after a total hysterectomy. Because her ovaries had been removed, she was surgically menopausal. She was taking ERT to control menopausal symptoms and generally getting along very well. Karen's housekeeper regularly cooked foods from her native country, a rich spicy cuisine that was heavy on black pepper and tomato sauce. Although Karen had enjoyed this food before her operation without any consequences, she discovered that the highly seasoned food now gave her hot flashes; lobster fra diablo in fact made her resemble a well-boiled lobster. To cope with the problem, Karen had to adopt a blander diet and increase the level of her ERT.

The relationship between hot flashes and eating is problematic. Often when you have a really large meal, the kind you indulge in at Thanksgiving, you may be in a stressful situation—for example, cooking dinner for twenty relatives. Or you may have wine with dinner and coffee or tea with dessert.

Certain medications are known to bring on hot flashes—for example, Sudafed and other over-the-counter sinus remedies that contain the chemical cousins of adrenaline. If you are taking sinus medications, you should not be alarmed if you start flashing.

Another cause is stress or nervousness. You are in a situation where you have to get up and give a speech, and suddenly you find yourself red in the face and sweating, thus doubling your anxiety. Or you start to worry about having a hot flash while you are giving the speech and, lo and behold, there you are with a red face, sweat dripping from the end of your nose, and anxiety beyond your wildest nightmares. Fatigue too can bring on hot flashes, just as fatigue heightens stress.

Are there other conditions that cause hot flashes?

Certain diseases, like hyperthyroidism, can look like menopause. Women with this condition have irregular periods, they get hot, their hair does strange things; in many ways they resemble perimenopausal women. Some other rare ailments can give you hot flashes; for example, a tumor of the adrenal glands called pheochromocytoma, or carcinoids, a tumor of the appendix.

Occasionally women experience hot flashes after childbirth. These women also have low blood estrogen levels, so it is not surprising that they have symptoms similar to those of menopause.

How long do individual hot flashes last?

Classically, hot flashes are said to last a few minutes, maybe as long as five minutes. But sometimes a woman comes into the office and describes what she has been feeling and says that the feelings of heat and flushing have gone on for two hours. Was it a two-hour hot flash? Probably it was. Was she maximally vasodilating for two hours? Probably not. But certainly it is possible that she was vasodilating enough so that those two hours were uncomfortable.

How frequent are hot flashes?

I have had people tell me that they get one a day. I have had people tell me that they get fifty a day. The answer to this question is that there is no simple answer, because women have such widely different experiences.

Hot flashes and other menopausal symptoms do seem to follow a bell-shaped curve for most women. As you enter the perimenopausal period, you may notice a few relatively mild hot flashes. They may increase in intensity and frequency, peaking in the year when menstruation ceases altogether. Most women at their peak experience no more than fifteen a day, though that may not be a comforting statistic. Gradually the flashes begin to taper off.

If your menopause is brought on suddenly, say by chemotherapy or by surgery that removes your ovaries, your hot flashes will probably begin immediately and be intense.

When do hot flashes start during the perimenopausal period and how long do they last?

Again, there is no one answer. Some women begin to experience hot flashes and the insomnia that sometimes accompanies them when they haven't even skipped a period. Perhaps they have noticed lighter flow and suspect that they are heading toward menopause; but perhaps they have noticed nothing different about their periods.

Hot flashes may be transient, lasting for perhaps a month and then disappearing, probably coinciding with temporary levels of ovarian function. Or they may continue at a significant level for several years. Classically, most women's hot flashes will subside within a year or two. In my clinical experience, five years is perhaps the outside limit for significant insomnia and hot flashes. Five years, however, is a long time. Whether you are vice president of a bank or have heavy responsibilities taking care of a sick parent or a couple of perfectly healthy but demanding teenaged children, five years is a long time to be flashing all day long and sleeping poorly at night.

I have had some women in their eighties report that they still get an occasional hot flash. But they also report that it doesn't really bother or incapacitate them; it simply reminds them of when they were going through menopause. The medical profession does not know exactly why this happens to women in this age group.

Do hot flashes cause insomnia?

While many women are aware of hot flashes as a sign of menopause, they are unaware that insomnia is another classic sign that menopause is on the way. Indeed, these two phenomena are physiologically linked, though the hot flashes do not necessarily cause the insomnia. Hot flashes plus insomnia probably also contribute to the mood swings and emotional instability that have been attributed to menopause.

Many women are awakened by their hot flashes, which often occur more frequently at night than during the day. In a classic example of a nocturnal hot flash, a woman wakes up sweating, often with the feeling that she can't breathe. Sometimes her nightgown feels too hot or else is so drenched with sweat that she has to change into a fresh one. She may sweat on the sheets or the pillowcases and have to change the bedclothes. Her hair may be wet. If she shares the bed, she and her partner may have real temperature wars. Unless they have a dual-control electric blanket, she throws off the covers and opens the windows while he complains that he is freezing.

Some women can toss off their covers, take a deep breath of fresh air at the window, and go right back to sleep. Others wake up but cannot fall back to sleep. A third group goes back to sleep, only to wake again in half an hour and continue that routine for the rest of the night. These women clearly become deficient in REM sleep, the kind that researchers feel is necessary for satisfactory rest.

If you can organize your schedule so that you can nap or rest during the day, perhaps nighttime sleep disruption is not so punishing. But if you must work according to someone else's schedule, you may have real difficulty in coping with the demands of your life.

What causes menopausal sleep disruption and hot flashes?

Unfortunately, the answer is that we don't really know. Neuroendocrinologists have discovered that the activity of the pituitary gland and the hypothalamus, and almost every endocrinologic hormonal system for that matter, peaks between one o'clock and three o'clock in the morning, which probably has something to do with the fact that many women have their worst or most frequent hot flashes at night. Researchers have not been able to show that high or low levels of particular hormones trigger hot flashes; nor have they been able to demonstrate that fluctuation in hormone level is responsible.

If I am having hot flashes and other perimenopausal symptoms, can I still get pregnant?

Although at the age when hot flashes and menstrual irregularities start appearing fertility is very much diminished, someone who is aged 45 can still become pregnant. Women who are trying to get pregnant at this time of life may find it difficult, but I have brought a few "cabooses" into this world.

Martha D. was 47 years old. She had been getting hot flashes and putting on weight, but since she had always been on the chubby side, she thought she was just getting a little thicker. She also attributed the weight gain to approaching menopause. Martha's elder daughter was getting married, and Martha figured that the additional weight came along too because of extra eating caused by the stress of planning a wedding. When she came into my office, she was five months pregnant.

So while fertility is greatly diminished at this time of life, it is not absolutely zero.

Is emotional instability a characteristic of perimenopause?

In former times menopausal women were thought to go through a period of extreme instability that in some cases resulted in mental derangement. Even today, women come to me feeling extremely anxious about what will happen to them psychologically when they hit menopause. They are afraid of turning into someone like Great-Aunt Tilly who, according to family mythology, became a virtual lunatic when she reached the age of 51. Indeed, many people can recall close or distant family members or friends who have had psychological or psychosocial problems when they were perimenopausal, and while there is no way to know retrospectively just what did happen to Tilly, several factors might have contributed to her instability. Or she might have been afflicted with depression that was indeed caused by fluctuating hormone levels.

The majority of women going through menopause do not experience significant and lasting emotional changes. Some do have feelings of depression, anxiety, tearfulness (even when there is no real reason to feel like crying), low energy, and excessive worry. Other women have mood swings, feel irritable, and have trouble concentrating.

Is loss of short-term memory a menopausal symptom?

Many women in the perimenopausal period complain of loss of short-term memory. They suddenly start misplacing their eyeglasses, their pocketbooks, their car keys. According to their teenaged daughters, they repeat the same stories or remarks over and over. They can remember their own social security number and their husband's, but not their children's, which they memorized at a later time in life.

Others suffer from the "what am I here for?" syndrome. They walk into a room with a specific purpose, then stand there wondering why they have come to the living room or the kitchen or the supply closet at the office. One of my patients ruefully recalls leaping into her car and racing five miles from her home to the center of town on an urgent errand; when she got there, she could not remember why she was there. Upon returning home, she suddenly recalled that her mission had been to pick up her daughter at the town green.

Other women feel themselves falling victim to a kind of mental vagueness or fuzzy thinking, when in the past they have known themselves to be alert, rational, even witty.

Both men and women can have problems with short-term memory as they age, but there is certainly anecdotal evidence that these problems become more severe during perimenopause.

Can headaches be a sign of menopause?

Although headaches certainly can occur at any time of life, they can be a menopausal symptom. Headaches, sometimes migraines, seem to be connected with changing—and especially with low—estrogen levels. Many menstruating women have cyclic headaches, particularly during the part of their cycle when their estrogen is low premenstrually. As they approach menopause and their estrogen levels taper off anyhow, they can experience significant headaches. Philip Sarrel, a physician studying menopause at Yale University, treats these women with estrogen pills under their tongue, the method of delivery used with nitroglycerin tablets for heart patients. The advantage is that the estrogen gets into the bloodstream very quickly, and some of the women who get these estrogen deprivation headaches have reported relief in as little as twenty minutes.

3 Perimenopause and PMS

Premenstrual Syndrome (PMS) is a wastebasket diagnosis: probably ten or twelve disorders are grouped under that title. Some of the symptoms categorized as PMS can also be associated with perimenopause, so that if you are in your forties it can be difficult to sort out which symptoms are attributable to PMS (which you may or may not have had before) and which are indicators of approaching menopause.

What are the symptoms of PMS? How can I differentiate between PMS and perimenopause?

The two most frequently reported symptoms of PMS are bloating and irritability. A close third is premenstrual sleeplessness. Women approaching menopause typically experience sleeplessness most of the time, not just before their periods, whereas women suffering from PMS report that they have difficulty sleeping a few days or perhaps a week before the onset of menstruation. Some women suffering with PMS have breast discomfort. Others report mental changes, such as lapses in memory and shortened attention span or difficulty in concentrating; others experience depression as well as irritability. These mental changes are also

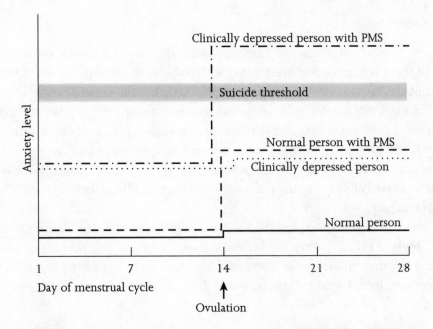

Figure 5. *Anxiety levels and PMS. Everyone has some baseline anxiety, but the level differs significantly from one individual to another. Premenstrually, most women experience some increase in their baseline level. A few women have a very significant increase.*

reported by women approaching menopause who do not consider themselves to be suffering from PMS. Some women have cravings for certain kinds of food, especially sweets (the chocolate bar phenomenon is well known), salty items such as potato chips, and caffeine.

The level of anxiety and emotional distress that women feel depends to some extent on what I call their baseline level of agitation. Some individuals are fairly calm most of the time; but if they have mild PMS they feel agitated or anxious premenstrually. Then there are more volatile women who are often agitated; when their baseline level of anxiety gets worse premenstrually, they feel really tense and overwrought. These are the people who are likely to go off the deep end and need significant intervention.

The pure PMS pattern, however, comprises women who are normally rather serene but spike wildly before their periods. For some of these women the emotional effects of PMS are intolerable.

What causes PMS?

No one knows, unfortunately. There are many theories and no real proof that any of them is correct. For every study which shows that one particular chemical imbalance causes PMS, another says no, that is not the cause. Leading theories include too much prolactin (a hormone secreted by the pituitary that stimulates milk secretion and is often produced in greater amounts during stress), too little progesterone, too much estrogen accompanied by too little progesterone, and changes in the levels of serotonin (a chemical messenger used by nerve cells to communicate with other nerve cells or their targets). The list is endless.

Since there is no accepted theory about which chemical imbalance causes PMS, there is no laboratory test for PMS. If someone tells you that if you give them $400 they will test your blood for PMS, don't do it. Use the money to buy a membership in a gym (or maybe a new dress or two or three or four).

What can I do to control PMS?

Since PMS is such a complex of symptoms and therefore difficult to treat, you are probably wise to start at the most basic level: take measures that may help you and certainly cannot hurt you.

Many women are helped merely by charting their lives and realizing when things happen. If you have the luxury of organizing your own time, you can set up your schedule so that on the days you know you are going to feel irritable or bloated, you will not be performing activities that increase stress. You can say, OK, I know I'm not going to be the most delightful person starting Tuesday, the 23rd, so I'm just going to stay home. If your life is not within your control to that degree, you can at least not schedule a potentially aggravating meeting with an unsatisfactory employee, or a job interview, or whatever, on those days. In this way charting can be therapeutic.

But charting can also be diagnostic. Suppose you are keeping track of your symptoms to observe cyclic changes. You notice that in fact you feel awful, depressed, irritable, and anxious every day. Because PMS is a popular ailment, because it's on the airwaves and therefore on everyone's mind, you automatically assume that your bad moods are cyclic. But when you begin charting, you may discover that there's nothing cyclic at all about your mental state. You may have garden-variety depression, which is socially a less acceptable disease than PMS.

Furthermore, the usual simple PMS measures are not going to make you feel any better.

We are fortunate in this day and age that a number of effective medications are available for depression; if you have charted your symptoms and find that you are depressed every day of the month, you can take an antidepressant. It will work a lot better than treating your depression as if it were PMS.

Can my diet help my PMS?

One major step to helping yourself get through PMS is controlling your diet. The closer anyone is to her ideal body weight, the better she will feel—whether she is perimenopausal, menopausal, or premenstrual. To achieve ideal body weight, I suggest a relatively low-fat, general weight-loss diet. Keep the calories adequate to maintain health, and lose weight gradually if you need to.

I encourage people to avoid concentrated carbohydrates, forget the chocolate bars, and keep their fat intake low. Cut down on salt and caffeine. Reducing salt intake decreases the bloating associated with fluid retention, and limiting caffeine helps both with breast discomfort and with caffeine-induced jitters.

If your body, like Audrey, the carnivorous plant in the *Little Shop of Horrors*, shouts "Feed me! Feed me!" you've got to respond negatively. If you eat the candy bar, you will feel worse with the extra sugar on board. If you eat the salty potato chips, you will increase your tendency to bloat.

Does exercise have any effect on PMS?

For any number of reasons, it is advisable to exercise regularly. Whether or not it helps your PMS, it is good for you. Researchers have discovered substances called endorphins, produced endogenously by the brain, that are natural opiates; they make you feel better, just as drugs do. Endorphins are produced in greater amounts during exercise and account for the phenomenon known as runner's high. Since premenstrual depression is an issue for many women who have PMS, the endorphins generated through exercise will probably help them to feel better. The goal is a half-hour of aerobic exercise intense enough to get your heart rate up to about 75 percent of its maximum capacity, three times a week. This is a goal, not a limit; if you feel like exercising more frequently, so much the better.

Lucy D. was 45 years old when she began feeling out of sorts premenstrually. She decided to start running to see if it would help her control her negative feelings. Lucy found that the more she ran, the better she felt. Eventually she became a marathoner and participated several times in the New York marathon. She then took up karate. But since she is so incredibly good-tempered from all that running, she has no intention of using the karate for violent purposes.

Lucy is an extreme case. Not every woman who takes up exercise to control PMS will become a marathoner, but her improvement does show very clearly what other patients of mine have also demonstrated, that exercise can have a real effect on PMS.

Do vitamins help with PMS?

Beyond the two simple approaches we've discussed, the management of PMS is very controversial. For every scientific paper that tells us something works, other papers say the same thing does not work. The next treatment I suggest is vitamin B6, at a dosage level of 100 to 200 mg daily. This dosage is much higher than the normal daily requirement, which is only about 2 mg; it is higher even than the amount in prenatal vitamins (which contain about 10 mg a day), but it is still safe. Although B6 taken in huge dosages, perhaps 1,500 to 2,000 mg daily, can be associated with neurotoxicity and produce symptoms such as tingling in the fingers, 100 to 200 mg daily is not a harmful amount. As with any kind of vitamin supplement, a lot is not necessarily better than a little. Just because B6 seems to make you feel better, don't take more than 100 to 200 mg daily.

How does vitamin B6 work? For one thing, it is a natural diuretic. For another, it seems to antagonize a couple of brain hormones, particularly one called prolactin, which may be involved in PMS (although researchers are not sure).

In my own practice I see a 60 to 70 percent response rate with vitamin B6, certainly much higher than the placebo effect. But as I have said, PMS treatment is controversial, and in some scientific research vitamin B6 has no greater effect than a placebo. All the same, because B6 is helpful for breast discomfort, because it is readily available, and because it is not harmful, it is worth trying.

A second substance useful in treating the breast discomfort that often accompanies PMS is vitamin E. I suggest supplementation at about 400 to 600 units a day. Even though vitamin E currently has a reputation as being useful in preventing cancer and promoting cardiac health, it is fat soluble and you have to be careful not to overdose on it. Vitamins that are soluble in fat can be stored easily in the body's fatty tissues and thus can readily accumulate to undesirable levels; water-soluble vitamins are more easily excreted.

Do herbal remedies help with PMS?

Therapies beyond diet, exercise, and vitamins B6 and E get a little esoteric and even more controversial. For many of my patients evening primrose oil seems to be useful. Evening primrose is a garden plant that happens to be very rich in an essential fatty acid called gammalinolenic acid—GLA in the health food business. Some women supposedly develop a deficiency in their fatty acid metabolism, a deficiency involving an enzyme called delta 6 desaturase. According to this theory, the women who develop such a defect cannot metabolize linoleic acid to gammalinolenic acid. By taking the gammalinolenic acid orally, they bypass the "deficient enzyme" and improve their fatty acid metabolism. What this has to do with PMS, no one is quite sure. However, I do get a 50 to 60 percent response with evening primrose oil, which is better than a placebo effect (generally about 30 percent). That is, in any drug trial the placebo helps about 30 percent of the people who try it, so to show that a medication is effective, you have to demonstrate an effect greater than 30 percent.

Evening primrose oil is expensive. You buy it at health food stores and, at least in my hometown, it costs about $26 for a two-month supply. Standard dosage is 500 units per capsule. The dose I recommend to women just starting is two capsules a day, though many of the practitioners who recommend evening primrose oil suggest up to six capsules daily.

One of the advantages of evening primrose oil is that it has no negative side effects. The only way it can hurt you is via your pocketbook, as it is more expensive than vitamin B6 or vitamin E or other common therapies.

Are hormones useful in treating PMS?

If someone has tried all the simple therapies—diet, exercise, vitamin B6 and vitamin E, evening primrose oil—and still feels awful, it may be time to consider hormonal intervention. The question is, what kind of hormonal intervention will work? Is estrogen a worthwhile consideration?

If sleep disorder is really becoming manifest as a prominent symptom, perhaps estrogen is a viable choice. I sometimes suggest trying it for a month to see whether it is effective.

Another option is progesterone. The initiative for using this drug comes from the work of a woman named Katharina Dalton, an English general practitioner who published her first articles in the 1940s and early 1950s. She was not a gynecologist, nor did she do laboratory research or basic science; yet her work has been quite influential. Dalton's theory on PMS was that it is a progesterone deficiency disorder, an idea that makes sense intellectually, especially with premenopausal women who also have bleeding disorders. Since, as a woman approaches menopause, progesterone production often falls before estrogen production does, and since progesterone is important in controlling the heaviness of the menstrual flow, Dalton's idea was to prescribe exogenous progesterone to replace what a woman was not producing on her own.

In clinical trials Dalton treated thousands of women and got very good responses; that is, her patients improved. Her approach was to give women afflicted with PMS supplements of natural progesterone for ten days or two weeks before their periods, to see whether they responded.

To be well absorbed by the digestive system, progesterone must be specially processed, broken down into very tiny particles. When Dr. Dalton first started using natural progesterone, this process had not yet been invented. She recommended vaginal suppositories, because natural progesterone can be easily absorbed across the mucous membranes.

Although according to Dalton's published results, her patients got better, no one has been able to replicate her work. Researchers have tried, but most of the studies from this country show no significant difference in response between placebo and progesterone.

Even though American research does not corroborate Dalton's work, gynecologists in the United States do use progesterone supplements as a therapy for PMS. Progesterone supplementation in appropriate doses is completely safe and it seems to help some people. I have patients who have been taking it for years and find it very useful. Other patients have been responsive to synthetic progesterones such as Provera, which are more readily accessible. Some people who have "flunked" synthetic progesterones do well with the natural progesterone. So there are many variations from one individual to another.

Progesterone as a therapy for PMS is also available in a long-lasting injectable form, something like Depo-Provera (a drug that incidentally has been re-approved by the Food and Drug Administration for contraceptive usage). The drawback to injecting progesterone (aside from the inconvenience) is that it is deposited in body fat; once it is on board it remains there for three months. Because some people do not do well with it, injected progesterone is not a treatment to rush into; nor should it be used without supervision.

Progesterone does have side effects. While Depo-Provera obliterates most women's periods, many women get breakthrough bleeding, spotting, or staining. Some people taking it get depressed. Some gain weight; women who remain on Depo-Provera for years often put on an unwanted, permanent ten pounds. Other women, however, respond well. They are happy with the loss of periods. Because progesterone can act as a sedative, it calms many women who suffer anxiety premenstrually.

Do birth control pills help?

It stands to reason that birth control pills might help with PMS. If PMS is a disorder of ovulation, then if you wipe out ovulation (as birth control pills do), won't you wipe out PMS?

For some women birth control pills do suppress PMS. If a woman comes to me with PMS symptoms, and she needs contraception, and perhaps she gets severe menstrual cramps, I suggest that she try the pill for a month or so and see how she feels. She may find that for her the pill is very effective.

So I do have women in their forties taking birth control pills because the pill solves several problems: it provides contraception, it helps with menstrual cramps, and it lessens bleeding problems caused by irregular or inadequate ovulation. Women who are approaching menopause will also find that the estrogen in birth control pills, though it is a low dose, serves as adequate ERT. Furthermore, as I have mentioned elsewhere, the kind of low-dose birth control pills used nowadays are considered safe for women in their thirties and forties, as long as they are not smokers.

But birth control pills do not work for all women with PMS. For reasons that are not at all understood, they make some women feel much worse. A doctor prescribing birth control pills for PMS should always suggest trying them to see what happens. If you feel worse, stop taking them and try something else.

If none of these therapies relieves the PMS symptoms, it is possible to think in terms of estrogen replacement therapy (or, as it is often called, hormone replacement therapy), even for women who have not done well on birth control pills. The amount of estrogen used in ERT (or HRT) is considerably smaller, only about one-sixth the amount of the estrogen in birth control pills.

If someone comes to me, menopausally or perimenopausally, and we start talking about estrogen, she may point out that she did poorly on birth control pills many years ago. First of all, if it was many years ago, she was taking high-dose birth control pills. Even if she couldn't tolerate a 30- or 35-mg low-dose pill, the estrogen in ERT is much less. Furthermore, the estrogens we use for ERT are naturally occurring estrogens. All those in birth control pills are synthetic.

To control ovulation, which is what birth control pills do, you need a goodly amount of estrogen and a goodly amount of progesterone in order to shut down the hypothalamus. But with estrogen replacement therapy you need only a small dose, because you are not shutting down ovulation.

If I am treating a woman who is perimenopausal, as opposed to post-menopausal, I still have to give her contraception protection with ERT. A woman 46 or 47 years old may be skipping periods, perhaps having a few hot flashes, perhaps not feeling well in general. But unless she has gone a full year without a period, she should still be thinking of contraception. If she goes on ERT, she must realize that it will not provide contraceptive protection, and she should still be sure she is protected some other way.

Are there other hormonal ways of controlling PMS?

If neither birth control pills nor ERT controls your PMS, certain hormonal medications will shut down your ovaries altogether, rendering you chemically menopausal. Lupron, one of the major drugs traditionally used to treat endometriosis, does this. Lupron is a very satisfactory diagnostic tool for PMS and is used for this purpose by a number of gynecologists throughout the country.

Suppose you are feeling really irritable and depressed. Is your problem PMS or is it clinical depression caused by something else? In order to distinguish between PMS and "something else," we can shut down your ovaries altogether for a month or two, give a little estrogen to prevent hot flashes and other discomfort, and see whether your PMS symptoms go away. If they do not, then clearly your problem is not PMS; if the symptoms disappear, at least you know what problem you are dealing with. Some physicians use Lupron plus estrogen, long term. The problem with this add-back therapy is that it is extraordinarily expensive, costing more than $300 a month.

How about treatments to reduce bloating?

Among the people I treat are women who gain ten pounds during their menstrual cycles. This is certainly not the norm, but it happens to some people and they are quite uncomfortable. I have patients who own one set of clothes for their follicular phase and another set for their luteal phase. Controlling the bloat is really important to them. I think vitamin B6 helps, and I think evening primrose oil helps. When these aids are inadequate, a diuretic, taken premenstrually for a week or two, may provide relief.

The diuretic that is recommended for PMS is a medication called spironolactone, sold under the trade name Aldactone. It seems to have other effects too on the symptoms of PMS, perhaps lessening irritability. Aldactone is a relatively mild diuretic that is potassium sparing, that is, it does not deplete your body of potassium as certain other diuretics do. It is relatively safe both because of its potassium-sparing nature and because, not being superstrong, it will not lower your blood pressure so much that you pass out.

No diuretic is totally safe, however, and there is a danger of becoming addicted. If you have mild bloating and take a diuretic regularly, then suddenly you stop taking it, you may get much more severe bloating. Yet some people, for example those with hypertension, have to take diuretics every day for long periods of time. If someone comes to my office with mild hypertension and some bloating, a diuretic can take care of everything. But patients should be fully cognizant of the fact that they are going to be on this medication for a long time, that they cannot stop and start whenever they like.

Diuretics are not intended as weight-control pills. Their use has to be carefully monitored.

Susanna Y., a very attractive woman in her early forties, was deeply concerned about her appearance and particularly about her weight. Her story is very sad and a dramatic example of how not to approach weight control. She came to me as a patient needing a hysterectomy for fibroids and pain.

One day, years after she had recovered from her hysterectomy, she called me complaining of belly pain. I happened to be at the hospital and saw her in the emergency room. I examined her and found nothing, though her abdomen was clearly sore. Although I might not normally do so under these circumstances, I asked for a round of blood tests.

Blood tests requested routinely from the emergency room often include tests for the amount of sodium and potassium. Her potassium, which normally would be in the 3.5 to 5.5 range, came back at 1.8, which is exceptionally low. Certainly that level could give her plenty of belly pain. It also could give her significant cardiac arrhythmias, which she was also experiencing.

We admitted her immediately into the intensive care unit and put her on a heart monitor. Initially we thought that she had a rare metabolic illness, because a potassium level this low is very unusual. I had never prescribed diuretics for her, so she had no prescription to purchase them. Still, someone on the staff did ask her whether she was taking diuretics and she said no, that she knew it was wrong and could be dangerous. But in fact, she was lying. We ran tests to screen her blood and urine for diuretics, and they turned out positive for Lasix, a diuretic that had been prescribed for her mother, who was taking it for a heart condition.

Susanna had apparently been taking the Lasix for a reasonably long period, though of course we couldn't tell exactly how long. Only a few weeks of it will bring your potassium way down. Susanna was even taking it in the hospital; she had it in her handbag, it turned out. Confronted with the fact, she denied it strenuously and signed out of the hospital against medical advice.

She came back to me several years later, for a routine gynecological checkup. As we were chatting, I asked whom she was seeing as an internist. She mentioned a friend of mine who works in a town nearby. Although gossip about patients is usually unacceptable, I felt that in this case the internist should know that she had done something that could have killed her, so I called and informed him.

When I told him about the episode in the hospital, he replied, "Oh no! She's doing it again."

I said, "What are you talking about?"

"I haven't been able to figure out why she has these very abnormal thyroid function tests." She was overdosing, getting thyroid extract somewhere, and taking it to try to make herself skinny. She even had tremors. Thyroid is available only on prescription, so she couldn't just walk into the drugstore and buy it, but somehow she had found a source. (She believed, incorrectly, that it would slim her down; it has this effect only on people with hypothyroidism.)

I never saw her again. Two or three years after her last visit to my office, however, I read her obituary in one of the local papers. Obviously I don't know what caused her death (the obituary wasn't specific), but she was a woman in her late forties. She had no medical problems that were life threatening. So I assume that she died of some medication that she was surreptitiously taking. Whether she got back on Lasix and managed to kill herself with that, or whether she put herself into a toxic condition by taking extra thyroid medication, I don't know. The sad part is that she wasn't even obese; in fact, she was slender.

So while diuretic therapy may be helpful in controlling bloating and the breast discomfort related to bloating, it must not be regarded lightly. It is not a magic bullet for instant weight loss; diuretic abuse can be life threatening.

Can PMS be treated with antidepressants?

Like injected progesterone, drugs such as Prozac are sometimes helpful for people, even those not necessarily depressed, who are totally resistant to all the other PMS treatments mentioned. Scientists know that Prozac and drugs like it affect brain chemistry, particularly serotonin levels, although they do not know the precise nature of the effects. Nor do they know precisely what changes in brain chemistry cause PMS. Although physicians may be treating symptoms such as depression when they put a patient on Prozac, they may also be getting at the root of the problem, the changes in brain chemistry that cause PMS.

In recent years a lot of negative talk about Prozac has suggested that people who take it have an increased likelihood of committing suicide or, less commonly, committing violence against others. Most psychiatrists of my acquaintance believe that Prozac is basically a safe drug, that its bad reputation arises from poorly designed studies and from excessive media attention. People taking Prozac are often depressed or disturbed individuals to start with. So a study that compares suicidal or aggressive behavior in a group of generally depressed and disturbed people who are not treated, with a group of depressed and disturbed people who are being treated may find little or no difference. In fact large-scale studies show that the individuals being treated with Prozac commit fewer violent crimes against themselves and against others. Because people being treated with Prozac are already in trouble, it is their baseline illness, not the Prozac therapy, that makes them behave violently. The worst that can be said is that Prozac is not effective in curing these people of their underlying illness.

As an antidepressant, Prozac is safe when its use is monitored by a physician. Some of the older antidepressants can have cardiac side effects, but Prozac does not. It is not addictive. It may depress your libido or sexual desire, but only during the period in which you take it. When you stop taking Prozac, your libido will return to normal.

4 Menopause and Your Body

The most obvious effect of menopause on your body is that because your ovaries are no longer producing significant amounts of estrogen, you stop having menstrual periods. Most women are aware of estrogen as a female sex hormone and associate its action with the development of female sex characteristics during adolescence and with the regulation of menstrual periods during their fertile years. But estrogen does more than regulate female sexuality. It is a very potent hormone whose effects are far-reaching and whose actions are only partly understood. Its presence affects the heart and cardiovascular system, the bones, the skin, the bladder, the breasts, the uterus, even the brain. Researchers can count hundreds of different actions of this hormone.

Since estrogen is so sweeping in its effects and plays a role in so many body systems and functions, it is not surprising that menopause, whose prime component is the loss of ovarian function, affects your body in lots of different ways.

Other physical changes come with aging and are not specifically related to estrogen loss or to menopause. For example, the gradual lowering of basal metabolic rate that can contribute to weight gain as people age occurs in both men and women. It is important to remember that while loss of estrogen causes many

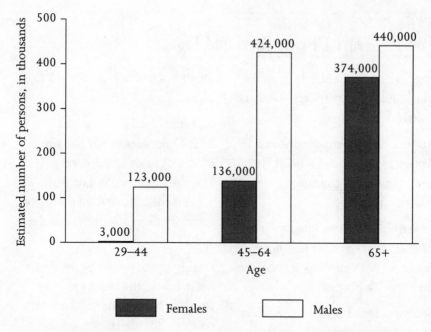

Figure 6. *The estimated annual number of Americans, by age and sex, who experience heart attack. Clearly, older women "catch up" with men in terms of vulnerability to heart attack. Source: Framingham Heart Study, 26-year follow-up. Reproduced with permission.* Heart and Stroke Facts: 1995 Statistical Supplement, 1994. *Copyright American Heart Association.*

changes, it does not cause them all. You cannot blame every negative effect on menopause.

What is the effect of menopause on my heart?

Estrogen, it appears, is good for your heart. It seems obvious, just from observation of our friends and acquaintances, that men (at least young men) are more prone to heart disease than women (at least young women). Probably everyone can recall at least one male friend or family member under the age of 50 who has suffered a heart attack.

Scientific studies bear out this informal observation. In 1948 researchers started following a group of 5,209 men and women in Framingham, Massachusetts, to assess their risks for heart disease. Since the 1970s the study has followed the children of the original participants. According to estimates made by the epidemiologists conducting the Framingham Heart Study, each year in the United States about 123,000 men but only 3,000 women between the ages of 29 and 44

Box 1. Heart Disease Facts and Figures

Heart attack is the single most frequent killer of American males and females.

About every twenty seconds an American will suffer a heart attack, and about every minute someone will die from one.

At least 250,000 people a year die of heart attack within one hour of the onset of symptoms and before they reach a hospital.

Many studies show that the risk of death from heart disease is much greater for the least-educated than for the most-educated people.

From 1982 to 1992 the death rate from heart attack declined 31.4 percent.

Based on the Framingham Heart Study, 5 percent of all heart attacks occur in people under age 40, and 45 percent occur in people under age 65.

Roughly four of five people who die of heart attack are age 65 or older.

An estimated 57,100 males and 20,800 females under the age of 65 die of heart attack each year. More than 37 percent of males and 29 percent of females who die of coronary heart disease are under age 55.

During the first four years after a heart attack, the rate of second attack is 20 percent for women, compared with 16 percent for men.

At older ages women who have heart attacks are twice as likely as men to die from them within a few weeks.

Within one year of having a heart attack 27 percent of men and 44 percent of women will die.

Source: Adapted from American Heart Association, *Heart and Stroke Facts: 1995 Statistical Supplement,* 1994.

have heart attacks. During the next twenty years of life, the decades that normally bracket menopause (age 45 to 64) an estimated 424,000 men have heart attacks while only 136,000 women do. But in the 65-plus age group, women almost catch up to men; the figures are 440,000 men and 374,000 women each year who suffer heart attacks.

What is the difference between men and women in terms of cardiac risk? Over the last few years a great deal of research has been directed toward this particular issue. The answer apparently is that estrogen does protect women against coronary artery disease and may protect against strokes. Not only does it seem to protect women against fatal heart attacks, but it also seems to lower the morbidity of heart disease (that is, lessen the severity of disease and reduce complications) in women who do have some form of cardiac disease. Menopause, then, increases a woman's risk of heart disease.

How does estrogen protect against heart disease?

Although the final answers are not yet in, estrogen seems to provide a safeguard for women in two ways: by increasing the level of HDL cholesterol in their blood and by relaxing their blood vessels.

Estrogen and cholesterol. Cholesterol is a fatty compound present in meat and dairy products in the diet. It is also manufactured by the body. Even though you may be a strict vegetarian and avoid all animal foods including milk and eggs, you do make your own cholesterol.

Cholesterol has a reputation these days as a contributing factor to coronary artery disease, yet it plays a significant role in producing certain hormones; it is a building block of cell membranes and other body structures, and it is necessary for the digestion of fats.

While cholesterol is made of several different components, LDL (low-density lipoprotein) and HDL (high-density lipoprotein) are the most important in determining risk of heart disease. LDL is often dubbed "bad" cholesterol because it seems to play a role in forming fatty deposits inside the arteries, whereas HDL is called "good" cholesterol because it appears to help clean out deposits from the artery walls and carry them off to be excreted from the body. Thus high levels of LDL increase the risk of heart disease; high levels of HDL appear to protect against it.

Researchers believe that the presence of estrogen probably stimulates the liver to produce more HDL. Studies show that women on ERT experience a rise of up to 20 percent of HDL in their blood. Exercise also has protective action and can increase HDL in the blood up to about 20 percent, so that women on ERT who also exercise can expect a significant boost in their HDL levels.

Estrogen and blood circulation. It is well known that elevated blood pressure contributes to heart disease and stroke. Today many people believe that estrogen has an even more important role in lowering the risk of coronary artery disease. Many women, both premenopausal and postmenopausal, have angina (chest pain caused by reduced blood flow to the heart muscle) even though their arteries are not clogged and narrowed with fatty deposits. Instead, the reduction of blood flow seems to come from spasm or constriction of the blood vessels. Researchers have shown that estrogen relaxes and dilates both the peripheral circulation (the blood vessels in your arms, legs, trunk, and the rest of your body) and the coronary arteries that bring oxygen to the heart muscle. A small amount of estrogen will significantly vasodilate the constricted area, just as nitroglycerin does.

Blood estrogen levels fluctuate significantly during the normal menstrual cycle, and episodes of angina occur in many premenopausal women when their estrogen levels are lowest, just before their period begins. Incidentally, women who have cyclic migraine headaches classically experience them at the same time of the month. When these women with angina are checked by cardiac catherization, it turns out that their blood vessels are not narrowed by plaque; they are constricted by spasm. They do not have obstructive disease; they have unusual responses to their own blood hormone levels. It is possible that there are many more women than men with angina because men do not have these odd responses to estrogen levels.

Menstruation and heart disease. A Finnish study published in 1993 in the *New England Journal of Medicine* suggests that one of the reasons premenopausal women have lower risk of heart disease is that they have lower hematocrits because of their monthly bleeds. This study has not found complete acceptance in the United States and it has not yet been backed by supporting studies. Since most women don't lose more than a couple of ounces of blood during each menstrual cycle, and since during the five or six days following a menstrual period women's bodies replenish the blood loss, it seems unlikely that this is the major reason women have fewer heart attacks than men.

But certainly it fuels the argument that continuing to have periods, one of the side effects of ERT that many women do not enjoy, cannot do any harm and may lower the risk of heart attack.

Do women who have had their ovaries removed have a higher rate of heart disease?

When women go through menopause the ordinary way, whereby estrogen declines gradually over a period of years, their risk of heart attack increases gradually. If they have their ovaries removed surgically as part of a hysterectomy procedure and their estrogen declines swiftly, their risk rises quickly. However, if they take ERT, their risk returns to normal.

What effect does menopause have on breast tissue?

Breast tissue is very responsive to estrogen as well as to other hormones. When estrogen levels fall off, the amount of glandular tissue in your breasts decreases. For most women this means a change in the contour of the breast, which tends to sag with age, and some very old women have flat breasts. Many women notice a decrease in breast size, but some notice an *increase* in breast size as they age, perhaps because body fat tends to gather around the middle section of the body. Women who have had tender and lumpy breasts during the premenopausal years may notice an improvement in these conditions.

What is the effect of menopause on bone?

Menopause is not helpful to your bones. Both men and women lose bone as they age, but women are at increased risk for osteoporosis, a disease of bone loss, because at menopause they lose the protective effect of estrogen. To understand this, you must understand something about bone.

Although we think of bone as stable, it is in fact constantly changing. Bone is made of a framework or matrix of organic molecules; crystals of calcium are deposited on this framework, giving it strength and rigidity. Everyone is aware that broken bone heals, that the broken area knits together in a process known as remodeling. But even bone that has not been injured is constantly being remodeled—broken down or resorbed and built up again.

While the scientific picture is complex, basically certain bone cells called osteoclasts break down bone, while other specialized cells called osteoblasts constantly build it up again. If the two activities, osteoclastic breaking down and osteoblastic building up, are balanced, then the amount of bone remains constant. If osteoblastic activity dominates, as it does during adolescence, then bone mass increases. If osteoclastic activity gets the upper hand, as it does after about the midthirties, then bone mass gradually decreases. Peak bone mass is attained somewhere between the ages of 30 and 35, after which it declines gradually.

Estrogen plays a role in keeping this constant construction and destruction of bone in balance. It seems to act on parathyroid hormone, a hormone that increases osteoclastic activity, speeding the breakdown of bone. Estrogen pro

A.

Micro damage

B.

Osteoclasts

C.

Excavation

D.

Osteoblasts

E.

Fresh, new bone

Figure 7. The bone remodeling cycle. All bone is constantly being broken down and rebuilt (remodeled). Osteoclasts are the cells that break it down; osteoblasts rebuild it.

hibits some of the effects of parathyroid hormone. Without estrogen, bone is resorbed, or broken down, faster than osteoblastic activity can rebuild, and so bone mass decreases.

It is in the first few years after menopause that the rate of bone loss rises dramatically. Researchers believe that a kind of bone thermostat is reset during this period, that eventually the body senses the increased rate of bone loss and resets the thermostat downward to compensate. For this reason women who are considering ERT should begin it within four years of menopause, during the period when the thermostat is getting reset.

What is osteoporosis?

It is a disease of bone in which bone mass decreases and the bones lose their calcium, becoming weak and prone to fracture. The name quite accurately describes the condition, porous bones. The little old lady with a dowager's hump suffers from osteoporosis. So does the woman who falls and breaks her hip or blunts her fall with her hand and breaks her wrist.

Who is at risk for osteoporosis?

Although bone mass decreases in everyone as the years go by, not all women develop osteoporosis. The factors that increase risk are well known. Some are beyond your control; others can be minimized.

You are at higher risk if you are female. Bone size influences risk: if you are small boned and delicate, you are at higher risk than someone who has a large, strapping frame. Small-boned people simply have less bone to lose.

If you are slender, you are at greater risk than someone who carries around more fat. Although fat is not desirable in many respects, it does protect women from osteoporosis. People think of fat, like bone, as being inert, as just lying there around your waist and hips. But fat tissue takes hormones from the adrenal glands, particularly one called androstenedione, and converts these hormones into an estrogen called estrone. Although it is not the kind of estrogen produced by the ovaries, it still retards bone loss. So a slender, small woman who doesn't have much fat does not have as much peripheral conversion from androstenedione to estrone as her fatter friend.

The down side of being fatter is that the same women who are protecting their bones from osteoporosis are significantly increasing their risk for cancer of the uterus. Estrone from their fat factories constantly stimulates the uterus, which can lead to excessive growth of the uterine lining (hyperplasia) and sometimes eventually cancer of the uterus. Obesity is indeed the biggest risk factor for uterine cancer.

Another risk factor for osteoporosis is activity level. If you fail to get adequate weight-bearing exercise, you are at increased risk of osteoporosis. Weight-bearing exercise, such as walking or running, increases bone strength by increasing osteoblastic activity. There is also some indication that bone mass can be improved by strength training, for example weight lifting or working out on exercise machines. The more you exercise, the more bone you build, as a glance at the left arm of tennis player Martina Navratilova will suggest. Some types of exercise, swimming for instance, are great for your cardiovascular system, but because your bones are not bearing weight, they do not help prevent osteoporosis.

Family history affects risk in ways other than by influencing body type. If you are fair-skinned and of northern European, Chinese, or Japanese ancestry, you are at higher risk than a darker-skinned Mediterranean woman. African American women have a much lower risk of osteoporosis; their hip fracture rates in the United States are one-third the rates of white women. Black women in Africa have even lower rates. Some believe that this advantage has to do with absorption of the sun's rays, that darker-skinned people get improved vitamin D action and utilize calcium better from their diet than light-skinned people.

Calcium intake over your lifetime is another risk factor. If you have had several children, breast-fed them, and never drunk much milk or eaten many dairy products, your bones are probably not rich in calcium even before you reach menopause. If, in contrast, you have maintained your dietary calcium, you probably have not depleted your calcium store. One reason sometimes given for the high risk of Asian women is that the Asian diet traditionally is quite low in calcium.

Two other lifestyle choices profoundly influence osteoporosis risk. Smoking and heavy alcohol intake are harmful to your bones. Smokers are doubly damned: they go through early menopause, and once they are menopausal smoking destroys their bones much faster than normal aging destroys the bones of nonsmokers. While scientists believe that nicotine has some effect on bone metabolism, the mechanism is not well understood.

Although it is clear that alcoholics have more osteoporosis than people who do not drink heavily, the reasons again are imperfectly understood. It is possible, however, that part of the cause relates to nutrition: alcoholics, who tend to drink rather than eat, probably do not get adequate calcium in their diets. Other factors may also be at work.

Some specialists believe that caffeine has an adverse effect on calcium absorption and that excessive coffee drinking therefore exacerbates bone loss. The data are still controversial, however.

Since bone loss accelerates at menopause, you are at much greater risk if you have an early menopause, either naturally or surgically, because you start losing bone rapidly. If, for example, your ovarian function is knocked out by chemotherapy when you are 40, or you simply have an early natural menopause at that age, you will have ten more years of accelerated bone loss than a woman who goes through menopause at age 50.

If several of these risk factors are working against you, you might want to consider ERT.

Does menopause have any effect on dental health?

By the age of 60, perhaps 40 percent of otherwise healthy women will have lost all their teeth. Some researchers believe that tooth loss and periodontal disease increase at the time of menopause and that these problems are related to the same kind of accelerated bone loss that can lead to osteoporosis. If that is the case, then ERT is helpful because estrogen helps you to absorb calcium, which is good for the bones in which your teeth are implanted as well as the bones in the rest of your body. The mandible, or lower jaw, is especially susceptible to osteoporotic bone loss, because it is made of a kind of bone that is more porous than, for example, the harder bone in the long shaft of your thighbone. One of my patients, a dentist and mother of two, believes in the importance of ERT for the maintenance of bone, and of course she believes in adequate calcium intake; I have found her in my waiting room reading a cookbook with high-calcium recipes.

Because tooth loss and periodontal disease do increase with age, it is especially important to incorporate good dental hygiene into your daily routine. Daily flossing and fastidious brushing are essential.

What effect does menopause have on the vagina?

The vagina, which is richly endowed with estrogen receptors, is definitely affected by declining estrogen levels. With menopause the vaginal lining thins, and gradually the whole vagina becomes shorter and narrower.

Among the most common symptoms mentioned by women of this age group are vaginal dryness, irritation or itching, and discomfort with intercourse (technically known as dyspareunia). Some women bleed during or after intercourse. Sometimes this is the first symptom that a woman notices as she approaches menopause: her periods have not changed noticeably, nor is she having hot flashes, but discomfort with intercourse caused by vaginal dryness is beginning to be a problem.

Dryness and the subsequent irritation make these tissues vulnerable to infection. Perimenopausal and menopausal women often have vaginal infections, which may be caused by bacteria or by yeast.

What effect does menopause have on the bladder?

One of the most frequently overlooked actions of estrogen is its effect on the bladder. While it may be well known that many older women have urological problems—urinary tract infections, feelings of urinary urgency, incontinence, and other urinary tract dysfunction—few women realize that these difficulties are often related to estrogen deprivation.

The root of the problem starts before we are born, as the tissues of the human embryo—not yet even at the fetal state—begin to specialize. The same tissue that specializes to form the vagina also forms the bladder. Not surprisingly, this tissue has many estrogen receptors.

So when estrogen is absent, the changes that take place in the vagina also take place in the bladder and other structures of the urinary tract. Just as the walls of the vagina thin out after menopause, the walls of the bladder undergo similar changes. When estrogen is not present, the muscles that support the bladder sag and the bladder loses its muscle tone.

Is incontinence a common menopausal problem?

Incontinence, which is the involuntary loss or leakage of urine, is a common and distressing problem among women, especially as they get older. Surveys show that as many as 16 percent of young women occasionally have incontinence, and perhaps half of women of menopausal age.

There are several reasons why incontinence is more a female problem than a male problem. First, lack of estrogen after menopause means a loss of muscle tone in the structures supporting the bladder. Second, the female urethra is relatively short and has less total muscle with which to control urine flow. Third, the stresses and strains of vaginal delivery during childbearing often weaken or stretch the tissues supporting the bladder.

Stress incontinence, the most familiar variety of incontinence, is loss of small or moderate amounts of urine because of increased pressure in the abdomen—the kind of pressure created by laughing, coughing, or sneezing. It can also be brought on by jumping or running, and it is particularly common in women who have had several children. The causes are usually anatomical, that is, loss of muscle tone created by the stress of childbirth or by a decrease in estrogen. This form of incontinence is the most common in menopausal women. Cigarette smoking, which can cause earlier menopause as well as smoker's cough, can be a contributory factor.

Another kind of incontinence, urge incontinence, is discussed in Chapter 10.

What is the effect of menopause on skin?

As we grow older, our skin ages along with the rest of us, becoming less elastic, less firm; it also becomes thinner, drier, and more sensitive to the sun. Are these changes caused or hastened by loss of estrogen? The data here are ambiguous. Researchers have tried to find some relationship between estrogen and "youthful skin," which is after all a subjective assessment. A few papers have suggested that perhaps estrogen does protect skin from the effects of aging, but at present there is no solid, incontrovertible evidence.

Does menopause cause weight gain?

One concern of many women as they enter perimenopause is weight gain. Patients come to my office complaining that already they have gained five or ten pounds; they wonder what is happening physiologically or hormonally that is making them put on the extra weight, especially since they feel they have not particularly changed either their eating habits or their activity level. At times this concern can escalate to levels of extreme anxiety.

Recently I had four phone calls from a patient. It seems that in reading on her own she had discovered that some psychiatrists were experimenting with two amphetamine-type drugs that, when used in conjunction with each other, produced dramatic weight loss. The woman was very eager to try the drugs and kept phoning me back to see whether I had called the pharmacist yet to fill a prescription.

To her it was an emergency weight-loss issue. She weighed 144 pounds, which in a person of normal height is not a tragedy. But she felt that she had to take these medications because she had ten or fifteen extra pounds that she simply *had* to shed.

Now I have never considered losing ten or fifteen pounds a medical emergency. But I did call the pharmacy, because I wanted to talk to the pharmacist about the medications. He was busy and said he would return my call later. At five o'clock the patient called back, wondering whether the pharmacist had returned my call. This woman will probably have a very difficult time psychologically when she finds it easier to gain weight as she gets older.

While I cannot believe that the need to shed ten or fifteen pounds is a medical emergency, I do understand why many women feel real anxiety about their weight at this time in their life. We live in a society that says you can't be too rich or too thin or too young. Maybe there is no way you can improve your financial status, and you certainly can't reverse the clock and get younger, but you do have control over your weight.

The scientific community used to believe that menopause itself did not have any specific relation to weight gain, that extra pounds were simply the result of a person's metabolic clock slowing down as she aged, or perhaps of her becoming less active physically.

However, there is recent evidence that perimenopausal women do experience some weight gain that may be strictly related to menopause and that may be physiological. A study at the Massachusetts Institute of Technology followed a group of perimenopausal women who continued the eating and exercise habits that they had previously established in their daily lives. During the period they were studied (about two years) the women gained an average of five to eight pounds. This gain was independent of whether or not they started estrogen replacement therapy. It was not the gradual weight gain that both men and women experience as they age and their basal metabolism rates fall.

The good news associated with this bad news is that the weight gain tends to stabilize. The increase does not usually go beyond the initial five to eight pounds, so any further increase is probably not related to menopause. Some of my patients find this information comforting. These are apt to be women who have been making legitimate efforts to keep down their body weight, and while they aren't happy about the five pounds they have added, they aren't frantic either. So when I tell them that yes, most women put on five pounds perimenopausally, they feel better. If they are already running twenty miles a week and eating a normal diet, perhaps the five pounds are not disastrous.

If you think you have gained weight because you are taking ERT (though there is no scientific evidence to support this theory), it is perfectly all right to stop taking estrogen for a while and see whether the weight comes off more readily. I have a number of patients who have tried this and found that ERT was not the culprit.

Could weight gain at menopause be caused by thyroid problems?

Yes, it is possible but not likely. Many people in our society tend to look for a quick fix to their problems; they hope to take this pill or that pill and suddenly become slender and gorgeous. Patients frequently want me to check their thyroid function, and in some cases this request is justified. I do perhaps a hundred thyroid tests a year and find one or two people who are truly hypothyroid. It is one of the few times when I can call someone on the phone and say, "You have a disease," and she is thrilled; she can take a magic pill and feel better.

Rebecca K. is a patient whom I have known for about eighteen years, since I was an intern, and she has been putting on weight steadily over the whole period. Rebecca is now perimenopausal and has been having problems with heavy blood flow; she has a fibroid uterus, and she has been feeling tired and sluggish. She said to me, "Listen, I swear that I am not really changing my diet pattern, I am not really changing my exercise pattern." She is still having periods, which are not that erratic, so she is not fully into the menopausal process.

We were considering managing her periods, maybe putting her on progesterone to control her heavy flow, something she has taken well in the past when she needed it. Suddenly I thought, "Let's get a set of thyroid function tests." Because fatigue, tiredness, weight gain, heavy periods, can all be symptoms of thyroid dysfunction. Sure enough, she turned out to be one of the very few women I turn up each year with thyroid dysfunction. So she can go on thyroid replacement therapy, which is easy—a pill a day.

We will need to get some blood tests to make sure that her thyroid levels are just where they should be. Her periods should get lighter. She should lose weight maintaining the same diet. And she should achieve a sense of well-being.

Occasionally at this time of life you do have to think about hypothyroidism, but it is confusing because some of its symptoms are similar to the signs of approaching menopause. One difference, however, is that thyroid dysfunction is not like menopause with a waxing and waning, waxing and waning. Thyroid function tends to go down and stay down.

Hypothyroidism can be a significant problem. Thyroid replacement therapy is not to be taken lightly, nor is it purely cosmetic, to be used for weight control. It is a serious metabolic issue and physicians don't just experiment with thyroid medication. Giving estrogen and giving thyroid are very different matters; while you can give somebody estrogen for a month or two, you can't just give someone thyroid extract for a couple of months.

It is also very important to realize that if you have normal thyroid function, you can take all the thyroid pills in the world and you will not get thin. Thyroid medication you don't need may make your heart beat a little fast; it may make you sweat; it may even make you have a fever. But it will not make you thin.

Does menopause have any effect on allergies?

While there have been no significant scientific studies that document a relationship between menopause and allergies, many of my patients tell me that their response to allergens has changed at menopause. Some women note an improvement in long-standing allergy problems, while others notice a distinct increase in the severity of their symptoms. It is well known that stress and fatigue contribute to allergies, and insofar as menopause is a time of stress and a time when many women feel fatigued because they have difficulty sleeping, those factors can exacerbate their allergic symptoms.

5 Menopause and Your Mind

The effects on your body of menopause and falling estrogen levels have been quite fully documented. The same is not true of the effects on your mind and on your mental health. These are complex and involve the interaction of physical, biochemical, even social factors.

Although not many women come into my office every week and say with elation, "Hurrah, I think I'm menopausal," many women feel very positive about menopause. Some of their reasons are physical. There are women who are relieved not to have to worry about birth control. There are women who have elected for religious or other reasons not to use birth control and no longer have to worry about getting pregnant. There are women who strongly dislike menstruating, perhaps because their periods are miserably uncomfortable or perhaps because they just don't like having them. There are women who are debilitated by endometriosis, for whom hormonal therapy has not worked, who don't want surgical intervention, for whom menopause is a great relief. There are women who have large fibroids or fibroids that bleed, and for them menopause is a positive event because they will no longer bleed, their fibroids are probably going to shrink, and life will be easier. Women who have undergone surgical menopause because of total hysterectomy often feel grateful that the health problems that made them seek surgery are over.

There are also women for whom menopause is a positive event for other reasons. For many, menopause symbolizes the end of the time when they are bound to family concerns, at least as primary caretaker of their children, and they feel liberated to pursue their own interests and activities. For these women menopause often brings a sense of selfhood and freedom from binding obligations.

Other women speak of a freedom from the expectations of others. Women are perhaps more strongly than men the creatures of other people's expectations. If we have always been "good girls," we may feel the need to conform less strongly at age 45 or 50 than we did when we were 20 or 30. We may have found that living up to the standard expectations of what women "ought" to be has not yielded the rewards we were led to expect. And the overt recognition of middle age that menopause forces on us gives us a chance to reevaluate what we want and how we want to act.

Despite the fact that many women feel positive about menopause, there are many myths and (one hesitates to say) "old wives' tales" to the contrary. One persistent and unfortunate myth is that menopause hits with a full barrage of distressing emotional signs: mood swings, irritability, anxiety and panic attacks, and serious depression. The myth of menopausal depression is so strong and so enduring that 80 percent of women who are not yet perimenopausal believe that when they do approach menopause they will become depressed. My own practice bears out not the prevalence of menopausal depression, but the level of concern. Every week several people come to me, worried about their mental status—not because they are in fact depressed or anxious, but because they have heard that they will be.

In actuality most women do not get seriously depressed as they pass through menopause, although they may notice various emotional changes, which for a relative few include depression or anxiety or even both together. While statistical studies have long shown that women are at least twice as likely as men to become depressed (or to seek help for it), recent epidemiologic studies have suggested that women are no more depressed during their forties and fifties than they are at any other time in life. There is no increase in the number of women hospitalized for mental illness during these years, nor do suicide rates, generally taken as an index of severe depression, rise for women during these decades of life. As a group, women are much more likely to be depressed in their twenties and thirties, when the life stresses they face are entirely different. You can be comforted, then, that at least statistically you are not automatically doomed to depression or anxiety at menopause.

One reason for the persistence of the myth of inevitable depression is cultural. In the United States today, as the media will readily tell you, youth is in, experience is out. Young is beautiful, old is ugly. Our culture is full of unpleasant stereotypes of the menopausal woman, from the wrinkled humpbacked crone with a disposition like Snow White's wicked stepmother, to the impossible mother-in-law like Wilma Flintstone's mother, Pearl, to the gray-haired airhead, Edith Bunker, made famous by Jean Stapleton.

Nor has science, at least in the past, done women any favor. Around the turn of the century, physicians described a syndrome that they called involutional melancholia. "Involution" means shrinkage or biological deterioration, so the term "involutional melancholia" meant depression that occurred at the time of menopause and was caused by menopause. Although the phrase was quickly picked up to describe what was thought to be a common phenomenon, in recent years both the idea and the terminology have been rejected.

A second and equally destructive menopausal myth, one that should wane as science probes the mysteries of endocrinology, is the notion that the symptoms of menopause are "all in your mind." That is, if you are suffering from heavy-duty hot flashes, or if you are miserable because of lack of sleep, it is because you are basically a neurotic complainer. If you were more stoic and heroic, you would either smile at these inconveniences or perhaps you would not notice them at all.

Armed with what we know today about how the body works, we can say, yes, to a certain extent your flushes and sleep disturbances and other menopausal symptoms *are* all in your head. But, as we have seen, they originate in your hypothalamus and your pituitary gland, not in your attitude.

Is there such a thing as menopausal depression?

Right now no one really knows. While involutional melancholia is no longer accepted as a recognized disease by the psychiatric community and while, statistically, women are no more likely to become depressed in their fifties than they are in their thirties, the fact remains that many women do report symptoms of serious depression at menopause. Although the final answers are not yet in, many physicians believe that this depression is in some way caused by changes in hormonal levels.

What other kinds of emotional and psychological symptoms do women notice at menopause?

Although some fortunate women have no menopausal distress at all, psychological or physical, many individuals do notice emotional discomforts around the time of menopause. These include irritability, tearfulness that is not caused by a sad event, excessive worry, anxiety, diminished energy, problems in concentrating, feelings of low self-esteem, and loss of memory. Some women even find themselves craving certain foods such as those classic offenders chocolate and potato chips. If some of these symptoms sound like PMS, they are indeed similar. Many women develop PMS-type symptoms in their early forties and then just continue with them into menopause. These women have not had PMS at all earlier in their lives, but they start showing up at their gynecologist's office describing classic symptoms: premenstrual irritability, bloating, malaise, lack of concentration.

Lois G. is 48 years old and the mother of four children, the youngest of whom is 14. Most of her life she was easygoing and even-tempered. She had never had any PMS-type symptoms until after her youngest child was born, but during the past ten years she has had migraine headaches and mood swings, both of which intensified as time went by. We tried all sorts of nonhormonal medications for the migraines, but nothing worked. Finally I persuaded her to try estrogen. After a couple of weeks she said that she felt better than she had in about 13 years—no headaches, no mood swings, no irritability.

How can I differentiate between symptoms caused by PMS and symptoms caused by approaching menopause if I'm still having regular periods?

Unfortunately no simple test will say these behavioral changes are caused by PMS and these are caused by the approach of menopause. My approach in this situation is to use techniques of PMS management. If these do not relieve the discomfort, my next line of attack is estrogen therapy. Ultimately, many women do respond to estrogen as if they were menopausal, even though their ovaries are still making some estrogen and they are still having regular periods.

What causes emotional changes around the time of menopause?

The answer again is that no one knows. While we lack definitive answers, we are not lacking in theories. One hypothesis is that stressful events in life bring on the emotional changes surrounding menopause. A second theory is that changes in hormonal levels are the culprit. Finally, some observers believe that declining estrogen levels bring about sleeplessness and that sleep problems in turn cause depression and other psychological symptoms. All these formulations have something to recommend them, and all may play a part in a woman's emotional perspective at menopause. It is very difficult to separate the strands of the tangle.

Are there particular stresses during the menopausal years?

When I look at my patients as a group, I see very clearly that many women's lives change drastically when they are in their late forties and early fifties. Their children are leaving home, going off to college, dating people (whom their mothers may or may not like), getting married, and having children of their own. Many women who thought they were through raising a family find that they have inherited a whole new set of responsibilities as their children call on them to raise the next generation. Many of my patients tell me that grandmothering, the kind you can go home from when you've had enough, is wonderful. But returning to primary motherhood is another story altogether.

At the other end of the spectrum, elderly people are living well into their eighties, and many of my patients who are dealing with their grandchildren are also dealing with aging parents. Often these parents are becoming infirm or incompetent. They need someone to manage their taxes and sometimes even their checkbooks. Sometimes health issues are involved: finding a nursing home, seeing that someone comes in regularly to help with medications, or other care. In some cases, women in midlife must actually provide this care for their aging parents. Often they have to cope with financial issues, not only managing money but finding enough of it to cover necessities.

Personal issues, such as household management and transportation, arise as well. Women, who as a group have been designated society's caregivers, sometimes have to deal not only with their own parents but also with their in-laws. While you may have a warm relationship with your husband's parents, the burden of caring both for them and for your own parents can be heavy and easy to resent.

Sometimes while juggling the demands of parents and children, these same women are trying to go back to school, preparing to reenter the work force or reenter it in a different capacity.

Many a woman in her late forties or early fifties is the victim of her husband's midlife crisis. These seem to be prime years for divorce as men cling to the illusion of their own youthfulness, often in the company of younger women. The male midlife crisis has been quite thoroughly explored in the media, though the midlife crisis in women is more or less terra incognita.

The generation of women who are currently in their fifties often find themselves facing new and different expectations. A middle-class young woman in the 1950s assumed that she would find herself a man, get married, raise his children, support his career, and nurture and share his interests. She was expected to put aside any ambitions for herself, or fulfill them in the time she had left over from her responsibilities to husband and family; but she would eventually reap the benefits of her husband's financial success and shine in his reflected glory.

For better or for worse, those days are gone. The dramatic rise in the divorce rate, the convictions of the women's movement, and the changes in our national economy have virtually demolished that set of expectations. The woman in her fifties who has more or less lived by these standards finds herself having to cope with a world that expects different things of her. She may want to enter the working world but may feel that thirty years of housework is a formidable obstacle.

Even women who have worked throughout their adult lives face significant changes. Some of the women I see express the same kinds of dissatisfaction that men seem to experience at midlife. They question the choices they have made. Finding themselves at the zenith of their careers, they wonder whether it is in fact where they want to be. Was the game worth the candle? And where do they go from here?

Now, any one of these factors can be stressful. And all of them together would put a crimp in even the happiest outlook. So there are significant and stressful changes that come into focus around the time of menopause.

Do cultural factors influence a woman's outlook at menopause?

Even if you do not have to take care of your sick mother-in-law or your grandchildren or strain your own pocketbook to help your adult children financially or go job hunting when you have worked in your home for the past thirty years, as an older woman you will experience cultural stress. Because women are not accorded a place of esteem and respect in our society, their status sinks as they age. As a nation we are devotees of youth, especially in women. While the silver-haired male may be admired for his power or his financial prowess or even his wisdom, the silver-haired woman—no matter how competent or successful or knowledgeable—is less highly valued. Women who did not feel the brunt of discrimination while in their twenties and thirties—protected perhaps by their youth and physical attractiveness or perhaps because they were not yet near whatever glass ceiling exists in their profession—may begin to feel it more acutely as they age.

Among the women I see are any number of vibrant, handsome, intelligent, athletic, talented, and able women who are considered over the hill because they are more than fifty years of age. Other cultures are kinder to aging women. Marcha Flint, an anthropologist who is a former president of the North American Menopause Society, has performed cross-cultural studies in societies where older women are valued and has come up with some interesting observations. She points out that although all women have declining estrogen levels in their forties and fifties and presumably experience the same physical symptoms, women's perceptions of what they physically feel at menopause seem to be culturally influenced, and their symptoms conform in some ways to cultural expectations. For example, a group of Rajput women in India whom Flint studied had no symptoms whatsoever, nor did Mayan women of the Yucatan Peninsula. Nor did a group of Navajo women studied by the anthropologist Ann Wright; in the Navajo language there is not even a word for menopause.

Other researchers have pointed out that in many cultures the status of women changes at menopause, and that when it changes for the better, women understandably experience menopause as a positive event. Among the Meo people of Thailand, for example, another group studied by Flint, the condition of menopause is honored. A menopausal woman throws a big party at which she announces that she is no longer of childbearing age and that, having attained this status, she deserves new heightened respect. Pauline Bart, whose pioneering *Women in a Sexist Society* was published in 1971, pointed out that women in cultures where age is revered, or at least respected, suffer fewer symptoms of menopause than women in cultures where age is denigrated.

What is the role of sleeplessness in menopausal emotional changes?

It is evident that sleeplessness can cause emotional changes, including irritability and depression and loss of a general feeling of well-being. Sleep researchers have shown that REM sleep, the part of the sleep cycle in which dreaming occurs, is important to the feeling of well-being and to the rejuvenation that comes from a good night's sleep. It is also known that women with lower than usual blood levels of estrogen have less REM sleep, even though they may not actually be sleep deprived. Whether sleep deprivation is caused by hot flashes or hormonal changes or just plain stress, it still can interfere with your emotional health.

If you solve the problems of sleep deprivation and your emotional state does not improve, then you will know that other factors are contributing. Improving the quality and the amount of your sleep will not solve the difficulties caused by your family, your marriage, or your inability to get a job that pays a reasonable wage. Nor will it alter depression that is caused by your brain chemistry.

Do the mood swings, irritability, and other psychological symptoms of menopause go away by themselves over time?

Although real clinical depression will probably not go away with the passage of time, menopausal mood swings and irritability generally get better on their own.

What are the symptoms of clinical depression?

Probably everyone feels dejected and downhearted from time to time, and probably everyone responds with feelings of sadness to life's unhappy events. But depression as a clinical disease has a group of specific symptoms beyond these normal melancholy feelings. The classic symptoms include sleep disturbances, especially difficulty in falling asleep and early-morning awakening; these are different from the typical sleep problems of perimenopause, which involve waking up in the wee hours with or without night sweats. The perimenopausal woman finds herself staring at the ceiling at something like one in the morning, while the depressed person wakes at four or five in the morning.

Change in appetite is another classic symptom, as is significant gain or loss of weight. A major change in libido, usually decreased interest in sex, is another warning sign. A depressed person usually experiences feelings of guilt and worthlessness, which may culminate in suicidal feelings. When someone comes to my office complaining of depression and admits to suicidal thoughts, I always ask whether she has made a plan for ending her life. Does she know how she would kill herself? If her vague musings on the subject of suicide have coalesced into a plan for action, I believe that her situation is dangerous and I take immediate action—which on one occasion involved driving someone to the hospital for emergency therapy.

Some women who suffer emotional problems at menopause are afflicted by bipolar disorder, which is characterized by depression but also by periods of mania. During these emotional highs, women may become completely sleepless, spend money recklessly, and experience increased sexual appetite.

Is there an organic component to postmenopausal depression?

Organic depressions are negative states of mind that arise within an individual because of his or her brain chemistry. An old joke tells of two children, an optimist and a pessimist, confronted with a room full of horse manure. The huge heap simply makes the pessimistic child more depressed. But the optimist is delighted; with all that manure lying around, she knows that there has got to be a pony somewhere. The optimist has a brain chemistry that makes her organically cheerful. The pessimist, for reasons that are not yet understood, unfortunately has a brain chemistry that makes her baseline outlook on life less than positive.

Now, you could argue that the depressed child had good reason to be discouraged and pessimistic when faced with a roomful of manure. This is what is known as exogenous depression; it is caused by events outside oneself. A woman who feels terrible because her son is marrying someone she feels is unreliable and dishonest, or whose mother-in-law with Alzheimer's is moving into her household, unquestionably suffers from exogenous depression.

But there are entities known as organic or endogenous depressions. They are caused by events inside oneself, changes in the brain chemistry. They can happen at any time, and they can come and go; they can be triggered by stressful events. People can get depressed in their twenties or their thirties or their forties. Or they can become depressed when their hormone levels start changing dramatically. Or they can get depressed as they age. Bipolar depression certainly has a genetic component that is independent of external events, and many people who have bipolar disorder have relatives—parents or grandparents—who have had the same disease.

Brain chemistry can be altered, as many menstruating women know, by changes in hormone levels. The depression, listlessness, and irritability that many women experience just before the onset of their periods are caused by the sudden drop in hormones that occurs at this time. Since the years surrounding menopause are marked by wide fluctuations in estrogen and progesterone levels, it is not surprising that mood swings similar to premenstrual fluctuations do occur.

Other accompaniments of aging, factors that are not necessarily mediated by the change in sex hormone levels can cause alterations in mood. For example, as we get older the secretion of melatonin decreases. Melatonin is a chemical, a sort of natural sleep drug, that is produced in the brain by the pineal gland—a gland that people used to think was useless (though Descartes thought it was the home of the soul). The symptoms of fatigue and disorientation during jet lag may be attributable to changes in melatonin level. Because the brain produces less melatonin as we age, we no longer sleep as well as we used to.

Changes in mood can also be caused by certain diseases, for example chronic fatigue syndrome, Epstein-Barr virus, and Lyme disease. Unfortunately, these diseases are frequently often used as smoke screens to avoid facing up to depression. I have had patients attribute a perpetually depressed outlook to fibromyalgia, a disease that causes generalized muscle pain, a sort of "ache all over" feeling. Because mental illness is such a stigma in this society (a worse stigma even than menopause), some people will indulge in a lot of fancy footwork to avoid acknowledging their mental state.

Often women will report to me that they have chronic fatigue syndrome, which is one of today's catch-all terms for diseases that diagnosticians and clinicians have trouble pinpointing. Chronic fatigue syndrome is a real disease, it does exist, but it is probably overdiagnosed. Fibromyalgia, which some researchers believe is a much less serious cousin of lupus, and Epstein-Barr virus are also real diseases, which are probably also overdiagnosed. Even Lyme disease, which is currently on the upswing and a hot media topic in southern New England where I live, sometimes gets blamed for my patients' depression.

The advantage to confronting depression is that in most cases it is treatable. A colleague at the University of Connecticut, an expert on chronic fatigue syndrome, tells his patients that no, they really do not want to have chronic fatigue syndrome; there are no effective treatments for it. But if they are clinically depressed, however unfashionable that may be, drugs are available that can really help. Other approaches, such as biofeedback therapy and self-hypnosis, can alleviate depression. Between effective psychotherapy and appropriate medical drug therapy, most depressed people can feel much better.

The analogy with diabetes is helpful. While people may resent having diabetes and wish not to have it, they are not ashamed of being diabetic in the way they are ashamed of being depressed. Yet diabetes is a chemical imbalance that affects millions of people worldwide. When the doctor tells diabetics to take insulin, in general they take it. In general they don't feel stigmatized by doing so and, fortunately, most diabetics don't believe that by right thinking they can cure their insulin deficiencies.

Many people have an organic chemical depression, which is a real disease, for which we fortunately have effective medicine. If you have a chemical imbalance, then you treat a chemical imbalance. It is not your fault that you have baseline organic depression. You will not feel better by calling it PMS, or fibromyalgia, or Epstein-Barr virus, and trying a lot of different approaches that don't work. But you will feel better if you take the appropriate antidepressant and follow a carefully managed regimen.

How can one tell whether depression is caused by hormones, endogenous brain chemistry, or external events?

The answer is that you can't always distinguish the cause of depression. Sometimes a patient says, "You know, I have gained (or lost) a lot of weight. I am tired all the time. I am not sleeping well at night. I have no interest in activities any more and I am bored with my life." These are pretty standard symptoms of depression, but we need to decide whether this depression is environmental, or caused by brain chemistry, or brought on by menopause.

I think the only way to rule out menopause as a factor is to try hormonal replacement, if only briefly. If the rapidly changing hormone levels that are characteristic of menopause are at the root of the problem, then ERT should help. Occasionally the additional administration of testosterone will help enhance mood and give a sense of well-being.

Do men experience depression and mood changes related to sex hormone changes?

Probably they do. However, the production of testosterone in men decreases very gradually over a long period; because men experience no sudden swings in hormonal level, their moods are probably less drastically affected. Another reason for the apparent stability in their moods as they age is that men in our society are trained not to exhibit their feelings outwardly. If their moods are affected by their hormones, they are less likely to show it.

What are the remedies for menopausal anxiety, depression, and mood swings?

There are several lines of approach, which include hormonal and nonhormonal therapies. If your emotional symptoms are mild and transient, commonsense approaches are in order. Exercise has well-known, positive effects on mood. Support groups bring comfort and relief to many women. If you know that what you are going through emotionally is not unique to you, that you are not alone, you may find yourself better able to cope. Education is a valuable tool that can give women higher self-esteem and enable them to communicate more fully with their caregivers.

If your symptoms are more severe and do not respond to these measures, there are other approaches. Among them are antidepressant drugs and ERT, and occasionally testosterone. Estrogen has a well-documented positive effect on mood in women with low levels of this hormone; and ERT relieves mood swings, depression, and anxiety for many perimenopausal and menopausal women.

Annette L., now about 81 years old, was depressed for years. She had been to her doctor. She had tried the usual antidepressants but remained down and depressed. When she was about 75, her son, who had worked with me for quite a while, persuaded her to come to my office. We talked about estrogen and, although she is a very conservative French Canadian lady, she agreed to try it. After she started the ERT, she really took off. She has become a demon housekeeper, filled with energy and a true zest for life.

How long do I have to take ERT to find out whether it helps my mood swings and psychological outlook?

Within one or two months you will know whether hormonal replacement is helping. Once you have started taking estrogen, blood tests can measure the amount of estrogen in your blood. If you continue to feel depressed and the hormonal replacement therapy does not help, you will know that your depression is not caused by lack of estrogen. I have treated many women who feel much better with estrogen, whose moods really change, and it is clear that the hormonal swings of menopause were making them feel psychologically miserable.

How do you determine the correct dosage of estrogen to help with these psychological symptoms?

In this as in other areas, I am a sort of biotitrater. If someone comes to me with mood swings or what seems to be hormonally mediated depression, I start out prescribing just a small amount of estrogen. If she feels better, but maybe not perfect, I try a little more. Some doctors would take blood estradiol levels, but I personally do not believe these are entirely helpful. If my patient with the mood swings feels a little better when her blood estradiol level is 75, would she feel a lot better at 175? I don't know. So I tend to juggle dosages according to their results.

The menopause expert Leon Speroff, of the University of Oregon Medical School, notes that levels above 200 pg/ml probably will not further alleviate symptoms that are caused by menopause. So if someone has a blood estradiol level somewhere around 200 and still feels bad, it is important to pay attention to nonmenopausal causes of her distress. If she finds out after a month or so that the estrogen doesn't make her feel any different than she did before, we need to try to find out what is causing her depressed feelings. If the root of the problem is organic depression or external events, I refer her to someone in the health care profession who can help with biofeedback technique or psychotherapy.

Can antidepressant drugs help in depressions that are caused by external events?

Fortunately, the answer is yes. No one knows exactly by what pathways the brain interacts with the external world. But many people who have very good reasons to feel depressed find help with antidepressant drugs. The drugs obviously cannot resolve the troubling situations, but they can help people cope with them.

What kinds of drugs are used to treat depression?

Among the advances in medicine in the two decades since I was in medical school has been the development of a whole new range of psychogenic drugs, drugs that affect a person's state of mind. Twenty years ago the only available antidepressants were tricyclics, among which were Elavil (amitriptyline) and Tofranil (imipramine). Modern derivatives of these early tricyclics have been developed and include drugs such as desipramine.

These drugs, which work at the level of the neurotransmitter in the brain, are

effective and still do the job for many people. In recent years they have been successfully used in treating fibromyalgia and chronic fatigue syndrome. They seem
to alleviate muscle pain and also help insomnia, whether caused by menopausal
symptoms or something else.

Tricyclics, which increase the levels of neurotransmitters in the brain, do
have bothersome side effects. They cause dry mouth and sometimes constipation. Some people gain weight on them, though when people are depressed they
tend to gain weight anyhow because they exercise less. A more serious side
effect, especially when people overdose on tricyclics, is cardiac arrhythmia
(abnormal heart rhythm).

In the last decade we have seen the emergence of Prozac, another kind of
antidepressant, and its relatives. Zoloft is a newer medication similar to Prozac,
and today drugs that are derivatives of Zoloft, and hence grandchildren of Prozac,
are coming on the market. Prozac is a very effective antidepressant and helpful in
many situations (including PMS, which is felt to be a separate entity, different
from regular depression). Prozac and its descendants are serotonin reuptake
inhibitors, which means that they increase the levels of serotonin in the brain.
And although all the functions of serotonin are not understood, it seems to be
important in controlling mood.

Is Prozac dangerous?

Prozac's poor reputation has two principal causes. First, it is overprescribed, like
many other psychogenic drugs: there is no question that many people are taking
it who should not be. Yet a great many depressed people probably should be
taking it who are not, for it is a very effective antidepressant and really does make
many people feel better.

Second, Prozac has gotten a very bad press because a number of people who
were taking it have committed suicide. And a few people taking it have committed murder. Recognizing this, you have to recognize also the diseases you are
treating. Would these people have committed suicide or murder if they were not
taking Prozac? Was it the Prozac that caused the violence? These are people who
were seriously depressed or had serious mental illness. Blaming the Prozac is like
accusing an anticancer drug of killing a cancer patient.

Can my gynecologist prescribe antidepressants if my depression is caused by menopause?

Because mental illness carries such a burden of shame in this country, many people feel embarrassed to see a psychiatrist. Therefore, my gynecological patients sometimes want me to prescribe their antidepressants and oversee their therapy. Some of my colleagues feel comfortable doing this, but most of the time I do not. A psychiatrist whose specialty training includes experience with mind-altering and mood-altering drugs has greater competence in this area than I do. Furthermore, many patients will do better with a combination of psychotherapy and medication. A specialist can best judge what psychotherapy is needed. I do feel comfortable prescribing ERT. Because I am experienced in observing its effects and side effects, I feel competent to oversee therapy, adjusting dosages and dealing with occasional small glitches.

What is the relationship between estrogen or progesterone and mood?

Although the exact relationship between sex hormones and mood is still ambiguous, some facts are beginning to emerge. Estrogen does have a positive effect on mood in some people, though neither the mechanism nor the reason behind it is understood. David Keefe, a researcher at Yale trained in both psychiatry and gynecology, believes that changes in hormone levels trigger certain depressive symptoms, rather than an absolute low level or an absolute high level of estrogen or progesterone. This theory might explain why women taking exogenous estrogen, and thereby keeping their estrogen levels fairly stable, tend to be a little less depressed than women whose estrogen levels are less stable. Keefe has concluded that the same kind of fluctuation in estrogen levels triggers the emotional swings of PMS.

Is there such a thing as postmenopausal zest?

Many years ago the anthropologist Margaret Mead coined the term "postmenopausal zest" (PMZ)—a sort of positive PMS—to describe the surge of physical and psychological energy that certain women feel after menopause. There is no scientific explanation, no hormonal or endocrinological evidence, to suggest why women should feel this way.

Does everyone experience it? No, I don't think so. But many women feel very positive about menopause. For many, it releases energies that have been bound up in other things; these women say things to me that suggest that at menopause they are happy to be finished with the part of their life they have lived. They feel that they have succeeded, that they have done well, that they are getting on with their lives.

Some feminist psychologists believe that PMZ is sort of a large-scale equivalent of the positive energy that many women feel after their menstrual periods. If you take as your baseline mood or attitude the kinds of feelings that you have before your period—those sometimes blue or blah or negative emotional states—then what you feel after your period is a kind of high, a sort of postmenstrual zest. Similarly, what you may feel after the hormonal ups and downs of the perimenopausal period can be thought of as a kind of postmenopausal zest.

6 Coping with the Symptoms

If you are bleeding heavily and irregularly, or suffering the discomfort of hot flushes that drench you with sweat at the most inappropriate moments, or you are becoming irritable and hard to get along with because you haven't had a good night's sleep, or your mood is swinging back and forth like Tarzan on a vine, plenty of help is available. Medical science and feminine experience have developed the tools for dealing with most of these symptoms in the majority of women. And for many of these annoyances, you can find therapies that fit your own pattern of health care preferences.

Some of the available therapies are nonhormonal. Others involve the use of hormones—estrogen, progesterone, and testosterone—either alone or in combination. Some have been scientifically proven in controlled clinical tests; others seem to help women with their symptoms, though no one knows quite why. No one treatment may be absolutely perfect for you, relieving your own personal symptoms and at the same time fitting your pattern of expectations and tolerances. If you do not want or cannot use hormonal treatments, you still have options; but you may have to work harder to achieve your desired goal. The choice of whether or not to use long-term estrogen replacement therapy, which is a very effective way to alleviate common menopausal symptoms, is a controversial issue and merits its own chapter.

But declining to take ERT doesn't mean that you can't do anything to control perimenopausal and menopausal symptoms. The alternative therapies range from vitamins to herbal remedies to other nonhormonal medications. Some hormonal regimens are short term and directed at specific problems. The old standbys such as exercise and dietary change can go a long way toward relieving different kinds of discomfort.

What can be done to control heavy periods as menopause approaches?

Many women are content to live with heavier periods during their perimenopausal years, once they know these periods are not abnormal or dangerous. Women who find the heavy periods distressing or disruptive, or those who bleed heavily enough to lower their hematocrit or interfere with their lifestyle, have the option of either hormonal or nonhormonal therapy. There are basically two avenues of treatment: replacing the iron that is lost during heavy periods, and controlling the heavy flow so that the iron loss does not have a chance to occur.

Nonhormonal therapies begin with *iron replacement*. If you are in danger of becoming anemic because of blood loss during heavy periods, but you do not want to try hormonal therapy to regulate the flow, you must maintain your blood count by taking supplementary iron. You can get additional iron either through your diet and through iron pills.

Iron is available in tablets. You can start with 325 mg of iron sulfate daily, an amount far higher than that recommended for pregnant women, and enough in many cases to maintain a hematocrit of 38 to 40. If you choose this route, you should have your physician check your hematocrit after a month or two just to make sure that it is within the acceptable range. If the hematocrit is still low, you'll probably need more iron; most women can't absorb much more than three 325-mg iron sulfate tablets a day.

In order to maximize the amount of iron absorbed from the tablets, you should take them on an empty stomach, an hour before a meal or several hours afterward. Taking this much iron every day is not difficult or seriously inconvenient, though some women do not tolerate it well and become constipated. Constipation in general seems to be more of a problem for women than for men, and one that increases with age for a number of reasons including decreased physical activity. Sensible measures to counter constipation include drinking plenty of fluids, getting a lot of exercise, and eating foods that are rich in fiber. A few people find that supplementary iron tablets upset their stomach. These people may need to take the pills with food.

Because of these side effects, some women prefer not to take iron supplements and wish to obtain the required iron through dietary sources. While a woman who is not afflicted with heavy bleeding should have no trouble getting enough iron in her diet, a woman who is trying to maintain her hematocrit by increasing her dietary iron does have to pay careful attention to what she eats.

Many foods contain iron, but not all iron is absorbed equally. There are two kinds of iron, heme iron and nonheme iron. Heme iron, which makes up about 40 percent of the iron in animal tissues, is more easily absorbed by the body and is found in meat (particularly liver and red meat) and to a lesser extent in fish. Nonheme iron, the other form found in animal tissues as well as in dairy products, eggs, certain vegetables, grains, and fruits, is less readily absorbed by the body. Nonheme iron is also used to enrich flour and cereals. "Total" cereal, for example, has 15 to 18 mg of iron per serving. As people eat less and less red meat, it becomes increasingly difficult to get enough iron through diet alone if you have to increase your intake to maintain your hematocrit.

For menopausal women and adult men, the requirement is 10 mg daily. For menstruating women, the requirement is 15 mg. The level previously was set at 18 mg daily, but in 1989 a committee of the National Academy of Sciences lowered the requirement—in part because women were having difficulty achieving the 18-mg level, and in part because the lower requirement was deemed sufficient.

About 30 percent of the heme iron from meat or fish is actually absorbed by the body, in contrast to only about 5 percent of the nonheme iron content of fruits, vegetables, grains, and eggs. Cooked broccoli, for example, contains 1.8 mg of iron per cup, so six cups of cooked broccoli contain 10.8 mg of iron, just about what you need if you are a menopausal woman. But since only 5 percent of the iron you consume with food is actually absorbed, you would have to increase your daily broccoli consumption twentyfold, to a whopping 120 cups of cooked broccoli a day, if you intended to get your recommended daily requirement of iron solely by eating that vegetable. This example is extreme, because probably no one intends to get her entire iron requirement by eating broccoli, but it does show how attentive you have to be if you do want to get enough iron without eating red meat or taking iron supplements.

As the broccoli example illustrates, foods do have iron content that is not easily absorbed; but there are several tricks for improving absorption. Eating something rich in vitamin C at the time you are eating something rich in iron improves absorption of nonheme iron. If you were to drink a 5-oz glass of orange juice while eating your broccoli, you would absorb three to seven times the amount of iron. Eating a food with heme iron at the same meal you are eating foods rich in nonheme iron (chili beans and meat, for example) makes more of the nonheme iron available to your body. Cooking in nonenameled cast-iron pots also increases the iron content of foods, especially acidic foods.

Is there a way to keep perimenopausal periods from being so heavy?

If instead of replacing lost iron, your concern is lessening the heavy flow of your perimenopausal periods, you can look at either surgical or hormonal options.

One long-standing approach to occasional episodes of heavy, uncontrolled bleeding is the D&C (dilatation and curettage), a surgical procedure that involves scraping the lining of the uterus. It can usually be done on an outpatient basis and often helps to control bleeding for up to two or three years. No one knows exactly why.

A hormonal treatment that helps many women with uncomfortably heavy bleeding or very frequent menses is the use of progesterone, which can be administered in several different ways. Oral contraceptives, which are a combination of estrogen and progesterone, can be used to manage irregular menstrual periods and to lessen heavy flow. The pills work in the same way as they do to prevent conception: they shut down your ovaries altogether and then reprogram the uterus according to the estrogen and progesterone content of the pills. With birth control pills, you can have a period regularly every month and avoid the kind of "Niagara Falls bleeding" that happens to some women when they have periods several months apart.

A second advantage of birth control pills is that they lessen other menopausal symptoms. A perimenopausal woman who is bleeding three times a month, having hot flashes, and feeling truly miserable, is likely to do very well on a low-dose birth control pill. It will put her ovaries out of commission and give her the estrogen that her body needs to control both the hot flashes and the frequent periods.

Marilyn B. is 45 years old. She has signs of approaching menopause, a mild and not especially bothersome hot flash now and then, and irregular periods. Her menses are coming further and further apart (three- or four-month intervals) and are very heavy. She wears tampons plus pads, but the frequency with which she must change this protection still keeps her near a bathroom all day long for several days.

Progesterone alone, without the addition of estrogen, is an important adjunctive therapy for women like Marilyn. By taking progesterone to challenge her uterus every three months, or more frequently if she desires, she can trigger a period that will clean out the endometrium she has built up.

If you are using progesterone to control your period, you can schedule it more or less at your convenience. When you plan your vacation, you can manage your progesterone so that when you arrive in Kenya or Boca Raton or wherever you are going, you probably won't start flooding with a very heavy period.

The therapeutic regimen is simple: you take one tablet, usually 10 mg, of medroxyprogesterone each day for ten days. When you withdraw the progesterone, you will usually get your period within a week of the day you take your last pill. Because progesterone is on board, this period should result in a controlled bleed as opposed to an extravagant flow.

Can women over 40 safely take birth control pills?

The attitude toward birth control pills has changed dramatically in the last five years here in the United States, both among gynecologists and among the general public. In years past, the Food and Drug Administration restricted birth control pills to women less than 40 years of age (35 if they were smokers), since the pills were associated with a higher incidence of cardiac disease. Then the FDA reviewed all the data on cardiac disease, thrombotic phenomena, and other complications of birth control pills. What they discovered was that in nonsmokers there is no increased risk at any age. Today most ob-gyns are very comfortable prescribing birth control pills to nonsmoking women over 40.

The story with smokers is very different, however. For them the risk of cardiac disease associated with birth control pills rises significantly at age 35 and dramatically at age 40. Occasionally I have a patient in her forties who would benefit overwhelmingly from birth control pills, but she smokes. I suggest that she try the pills for perhaps two months to see whether they help her heavy bleeding or her frequent periods. I use the two-month figure to represent an arbitrarily short period, short enough so that the effects of taking the pills will be apparent but the risks will be minimal. I advise her to call me immediately if she feels any uncomfortable side effects or symptoms such as chest or leg pains. And then I suggest that perhaps she will feel so much better being on the birth control pills that she will think seriously about giving up cigarettes.

Clearly, such a patient must be closely supervised, and some physicians will not prescribe birth control pills under any circumstances to a woman who smokes. But because the pills are available by prescription only, it follows that any woman who is taking them has to be under a physician's care and observation.

After the smoker has tried birth control pills for a couple of months, she will have to decide whether to continue them and give up smoking, or to give up the pills and continue smoking.

What therapy is available to reduce clotting?

If you are one of the women who does not need therapy to control heavy flow, but who finds clotting gross and offensive, you can benefit from anticlotting drugs. The most commonly used is Ponstel (generically, it is mefenamic acid), a cousin of Motrin (or ibuprofen). Like all prostaglandin inhibitors, Ponstel can upset your stomach, so always take it with food.

How can I reduce the discomfort of hot flashes?

There are many things you can do to reduce the intensity and frequency of hot flashes or to get rid of them altogether.

The temperature surrounding your body seems to be critical in bringing on hot flashes—so much so, that some women notice that hugging or other skin-to-skin contact with someone will trigger a flush. Try to sleep in a cool room (although battles between bed partners over the thermostat are not uncommon during menopause). While you can cannot control the temperature of every room in which you find yourself, you can control what you wear. Dressing for menopause can be like dressing for travel to a country with an unknown climate: think layers. Many women find that fabrics of natural fibers are more comfortable than synthetics.

There are some things to avoid. If you know that alcohol or hot coffee brings on hot flashes, you can sidestep them. If you notice that eating large meals brings on hot flashes, you can rearrange your eating schedule.

Some women find that relaxation techniques, meditation, or other spiritual exercises help relieve the stress that causes or intensifies hot flashes, and there is scientific evidence that these approaches may work. One study, for example, showed that breathing techniques reduced the frequency of hot flashes.

Beyond these simple, commonsense measures, which may not alleviate all your hot flashes, other steps are possible. Therapy for hot flashes can be directed toward the lowered estrogen levels that stimulate the activity of the pituitary and the hypothalamus; or it can work to stabilize the blood vessels, whose inconsiderate constriction and dilation cause the flushing and sensations of heat that constitute a hot flash.

Estrogen replacement therapy (ERT) raises the level of estrogen in the blood so that the pituitary and hypothalamus glands do not release into the bloodstream the hormone FSH whose vasodilating action can trigger a hot flash. You can take estrogen alone, estrogen with cyclic progesterone, or you can take oral contraceptives—which, as we have seen, contain both estrogen and progesterone. Androgens are sometimes effective. Any of these regimens, calibrated for your own body's needs, will in almost every case take care of hot flashes.

Nonhormonal approaches include the use of vitamins or drugs that stabilize the blood vessels.

Finding just the right way of controlling hot flashes can be a process of trial and error. Certainly no solution is perfect for everyone, and there may not be an absolutely perfect solution for you. Still, you and your physician together eventually should be able to find a solution that works for you.

Which vitamins help to control hot flashes?

While estrogen replacement therapy can almost certainly reduce the flushes, therapies are available for women who cannot or do not want to try ERT. Vitamin E works well for some, both in reducing the intensity of their hot flashes and in easing the sleep disturbances that are secondary to the flashes. Research is beginning to suggest that vitamin E may be useful in other medical conditions, for example in lowering the risk of atherosclerotic heart disease and as an antioxidant in soaking up free radicals and secondarily lowering cancer risk. Since cancer and heart disease are both associated with aging, vitamin E certainly cannot hurt; and it may help.

The dosage generally recommended is 400 to 600 units daily. If you skip a day, nothing untoward will happen. If vitamin E helps your hot flashes, they will probably return if you forget to take it, but there is no danger in starting and stopping vitamin therapy. Usually you will notice an improvement in about two weeks.

Some women report anecdotally that vitamins B and C help suppress hot flashes. Although there have been no supporting scientific studies, these vitamins may help and won't hurt if you use them in moderation. Try 500 mg daily of vitamin C and see whether it helps. The standard dosage of B-complex vitamins is contained in one B-50 tablet.

Will herbs reduce hot flashes?

Women who are interested in herbal medicine believe that ginseng helps with hot flashes, certainly for good reason. Ginseng and various other plants contain plant estrogens, also called phytoestrogens. Estrace, one of the most commonly used brands of estrogen used in ERT, in fact is derived from phytoestrogens, from South American yams.

In traditional and folk medicine, plant estrogens have long been used to treat a wide range of female complaints involving menstrual disorders as well as the discomforts of menopause. Ginseng comes in tablets, capsules, powder, tea, or elixir.

Of the several different types of ginseng, Korean ginseng is known botanically as *Panax ginseng*. Dong quai, also called tan kwai or Chinese ginseng, is *Angelica sinensis*. Other herbs said to have estrogenic qualities are black cohosh (*Cimicifuga racemosa*), licorice (*Glycyrrhiza glabra*), unicorn root (*Aletris farinosa*), and fennel (*Foeniculum vulgare*).

The problem with these herbal medicines is that dosages are not standardized. When you are taking 0.625 mg of Premarin, you know exactly how much estrogen you are getting. When you drink three cups of ginseng tea, you have no idea how much estrogen you are getting. So it is a lot easier to overdose on ginseng tea than on Premarin. Plant estrogens, just like estrogens synthesized in the laboratory or developed from natural animal sources, have effects on the body other than the ones primarily intended. Plant estrogens may well help to control hot flashes, but they can cause excessive growth of the uterine lining, just as other estrogens can. If you decide to try ginseng or other plant medicines, you should do so under the guidance of a naturopathic physician. Very few M.D.'s are familiar with herbal medicines.

What medications can control hot flashes by preventing the blood vessels from dilating?

Medicines that stabilize the blood vessels are effective in preventing hot flashes for many, but not all, women. A host of these drugs exists, from old standards to more modern medications.

The archetypical drug of this sort is Bellergal, which has been around for years. It is a standard combination of several drugs including belladonna, atropine, and barbiturates, and the usual dosage is one to two tablets daily. Bellergal is a prescription medication, but you take it as you need it, that is, when your hot flashes are troublesome. It is not like estrogen, which you take on a daily basis to prevent hot flashes, although some people do take Bellergal daily until their hot flashes have disappeared.

Like all other drugs, Bellergal has side effects. The main one is drowsiness; so if you are going to be driving or operating heavy machinery, or doing anything where your safety demands alertness, Bellergal may not be an appropriate drug for you. If you can take it at night and not wake with a hangover, then the drowsiness should not be a problem. The other side effect that many women experience is dry mouth.

Bellergal does not help everyone; among my patients I find about a 50 percent success rate. But if you are really bothered by hot flashes and have decided against hormonal therapy, Bellergal is relatively safe and certainly worth a try.

Other nonhormonal mainstays of hot flash treatment are the beta-blockers, drugs such as propranolol (brand name Inderal) and the newer versions of these drugs that have been developed over the last twenty years. Beta-blockers work on the principle of vascular stability, preventing your blood vessels from going through the massive dilation-constriction-dilation-constriction routine that typifies hot flashes.

Beta-blockers can work effectively to prevent hot flashes in small dosages, about 40 to 80 mg of Inderal daily. By comparison, cardiac patients who use a beta-blocker such as Inderal take up to 800 mg daily—ten to twenty times the dosage for hot flash prevention.

Although beta-blockers work for some women, they are not universally effective. They do have side effects and they are extremely dose dependent, which means that the dosage can really differ from one person to another. Some people who are quite sensitive to this kind of drug report that they get depressed from beta-blockers; others report a fatigue or drowsiness that is not the sleepiness people feel when they take Demerol or Halcion or an antihistamine.

A second side effect is that some people, both men and women, find that beta-blockers interfere with sexual function by dulling sexual responsiveness. Men may have difficulty getting or maintaining an erection; women may have difficulty reaching orgasm.

Beta-blockers can also lower blood pressure; people taking them should have their blood pressure checked regularly. (Light-headedness is a symptom that might indicate low blood pressure.)

One of the beneficial effects of beta-blockers is that they tend to make people calmer, to take the edge off stage fright or general nervousness. People who perform in public, everyone from concert violinists to doctors presenting papers at scientific meetings, occasionally take beta-blockers to blunt the physical symptoms of nervousness—the shaking knees or trembling voices that interfere with successful performance.

Another drug that provides vascular stability is clonidine, which is marketed under the name Catapres; it is an antihypertensive drug, used normally to lower blood pressure, but may be useful in suppressing hot flashes. Again, since clonidine lowers blood pressure, you have to be sure that the dosage you are taking doesn't reduce your pressure to the point where you feel faint or dizzy. I cannot say that I have had overwhelming success with clonidine, but if other efforts have failed, it is worth a try.

Are there women who are resistant to all these therapies and still have hot flashes? Yes. Almost everyone responds to estrogen, and most women respond to one or more of these other therapies, but a small fraction still report some hot flashes. Since the amount of discomfort experienced with hot flashes is quite subjective, it is hard to know just how uncomfortable these people are.

If you are one of these women, it is worthwhile to check your blood levels of FSH and estradiol, because hot flashes can have causes other than lack of estrogen. If your estradiol and FSH levels are premenopausal and should not be giving you hot flashes, then you will know to look for something else.

Will acupuncture help control hot flashes?

Right now it is hard to say. One research project, still in the preliminary stages, has suggested that acupuncture decreases the number of hot flashes.

What help is there for insomnia?

Some old-fashioned commonsense approaches to sleeplessness are good starting points, especially for women who prefer not to take hormones. Cut down on caffeine or cut it out altogether, especially later in the day. Alcohol may make you feel sleepy, but it can cause you to wake up in the middle of the night.

Try exercising in the evening and taking a tepid bath before bedtime. Drink a glass of warm milk before you go to bed; milk contains tryptophan, an amino acid that has mild sedative properties. (To be honest, I am not sure why people always suggest that the milk be warm, but it certainly is the standard recommendation.) If you practice yoga, you may find that controlled breathing helps you get to sleep, or go back to sleep if you have wakened in the middle of the night. Some women find that herbal teas or ginseng promote relaxation. Remember that ginseng has hormonal properties and like other herbal preparations should be used with care because you never know how much (or sometimes what) you are taking.

If these remedies don't work for you, there are other approaches. Because insomnia is often a by-product of hot flashes, the first line of attack is to relieve the hot flashes (by any of the methods we have already discussed). The second is to deal with the sleeplessness as a separate entity.

Remember that hot flashes and the sleeplessness that accompanies them tend to be worse in summer. If you are taking ERT, you may have been completely comfortable with your dosage in January and suddenly find in July that you are awake in the wee hours, awaiting the dawn. You should check with your gynecologist and have your dose adjusted if your symptoms change in this way. Estrogen therapy is also effective in relieving insomnia caused by hormonal changes, even though that insomnia may not be accompanied by hot flashes.

Many women wake up at two in the morning and can't get back to sleep though they don't have hot flashes. And there are women who don't mind the hot flashes but can't live with the insomnia and the fatigue that follows it. Using traditional sleep medications is one obvious approach.

Sleep medicines belong to a variety of chemical families, including benzodiazepines and barbiturates, and almost all of them can be addictive. Some people get habituated to a certain dosage level and have to increase the dose or switch from one medication to another. While most people know that barbiturates (which include phenobarbital, Nembutal, and Seconal) can cause chemical dependencies, benzodiazepines can also be addictive. Valium, for example, along with its cousins Xanax, Ativan, and others, is sometimes prescribed as a sedative and sometimes as an antianxiety drug. While Valium is now recognized as addictive, it is still prescribed too freely in many parts of the country.

Sleep medications can also cause a hangover, making you tired or sluggish the next day, and possibly giving you a headache. If you must be fully alert, for example when driving or negotiating a contract for your company, we have indicated that you should be very cautious about sleep medications. Most physicians do not encourage nightly use of sleeping pills, but they can be used judiciously. Be sure to discuss the subject thoroughly with your physician.

What kinds of therapy are available for hot flashes and sleep disturbances?

Therapy to deal with hot flashes and insomnia can take one of three general directions: it can be directed toward the lowered estrogen levels that stimulate the activity of the pituitary and the hypothalamus; it can work on the sleep centers of the brain; or it can be directed at stabilizing the blood vessels.

What therapy exists for insomnia and hot flashes together?

Estrogen replacement is the one major therapy for insomnia that also controls hot flashes. To speak simplistically, ERT tells the brain to go to bed. There is a constant feedback loop between the brain and the ovaries, and the brain continuously responds to the levels of estrogen that it senses being produced. But the brain is "dumb"; if it sees an elevated estrogen level in the blood, it doesn't know whether the estrogen is coming from the ovary or entering the body by mouth and being absorbed by the intestines. It merely recognizes the estrogen and allows the pituitary and hypothalamus to remain quiescent; they are not urged on to greater nocturnal activity. Increased quantities of FSH are not secreted into the bloodstream. Since estrogen replacement short-circuits the whole hypothalamus-pituitary cycle, and FSH with its vasodilating activity is not released into the blood, ERT also controls hot flashes and decreases the component of insomnia caused by the flashes themselves.

Estrogen therapy works very quickly. Women who have been troubled with sleep disturbances and insomnia usually find relief within a week of beginning ERT.

With ERT it is possible to adjust dosages from the outside in much the same way your ovaries do it from the inside when they are functioning at peak levels, say in your twenties and thirties. Some women who are perfectly comfortable with a certain dosage in the winter might start flashing in the summertime, and it is acceptable to increase the dosage during the hot months. If one of my patients for some reason wants her dosage reduced during the summer, I prefer to wait until autumn; it can be confusing to decide whether they are getting more hot flashes because their estrogen dosage is too low or because the temperature is ninety degrees and they need more estrogen anyhow.

What are the remedies for breast discomfort?

Strictly speaking, breast discomfort is not a perimenopausal problem. Many women have it throughout their reproductive years, but many report that their breasts feel more sensitive as menopause approaches. Although researchers have not discovered the causes of fibrocystic breast condition, as tender, lumpy breasts are called, many doctors have noticed that certain foods can stimulate the breasts and make breast tissue lumpier or more painful. Anything that contains caffeine (coffee, tea, cola, chocolate) can have this effect. Although drinking coffee won't give you breast cancer and there is no association between the amount of caffeine you ingest and your risk of cancer, some women are very sensitive to even small amounts of caffeine. Obviously it makes sense to avoid foods and beverages containing caffeine, if they make you uncomfortable.

A second approach is to take vitamin E and vitamin B6. The standard recommendation is 400 to 800 units of vitamin E a day, and 100 to 200 mg of vitamin B6. The literature contains no conclusive evidence that taking vitamins or cutting out caffeine will improve lumpy or uncomfortable breasts, but many women do notice a distinct improvement. In my experience, about 70 to 90 percent of women are helped by taking vitamin B6 and vitamin E and cutting down on caffeine consumption.

One of my colleagues recommends kelp to her patients with breast discomfort. Available at health food stores, kelp contains iodine, but it is not understood why this treatment should be helpful for breast discomfort.

Testosterone also seems to have a positive effect in reducing breast tenderness. Indeed, young women who have tried reducing caffeine, taking vitamin E and vitamin B6, and so on, often do better on Danocrine, a medication that decreases estrogen production and has some effects similar to those of testosterone.

Must I give up caffeine if I am not bothered by the lumpiness in my breasts?

As long as you are not uncomfortable (or nervous and jittery) and the lumpiness does not interfere with self-examination or examination by a doctor, it is not necessary to give up caffeine.

7 What ERT Can and Cannot Do for You

Probably the biggest issue today for women approaching menopause is the choice of whether or not to use estrogen replacement therapy (ERT)—or, as it is sometimes called, hormone replacement therapy (HRT). What are the benefits of estrogen replacement therapy? What are the risks? What will happen ten or fifteen years down the line if you do elect to undergo ERT?

Like most important questions, this one does not have a simple answer that is appropriate for every woman. Women must decide whether they wish to take ERT on a short-term basis, to help them cope with the acute symptoms of menopause; whether they wish to take it long term for health reasons, to help reduce the risk of certain diseases whose likelihood increases with age; or whether they want to take ERT long term to improve quality of life, by preventing conditions such as frequent vaginal and urinary tract infections, incontinence, or vaginal changes that can make intercourse painful or impossible.

We do not have many conclusive studies involving large numbers of women who have used ERT for a long time. This lack of data arises partly because menopause, along with other health issues that affect women, has not received enough coordinated attention. And partly because long-term use of estrogen replacement therapy, with or without added progestins, is relatively new. However, risk-benefit studies are beginning to be available. In 1992 Deborah Grady of the University of California at San Francisco and her colleagues published an important broad-based study. Grady, an epidemiologist with degrees in medicine and public health, looked at the data from all the major research published in the English language since 1970 on the effect of estrogen therapy and estrogen plus progestin therapy. In particular, she looked at how ERT influenced the risk for endometrial cancer, breast cancer, coronary heart disease, osteoporosis, and stroke to determine relative risks and benefits of the use of hormones postmenopausally. Her conclusions were that ERT definitely reduces the risk of coronary heart disease and hip fracture (a consequence of osteoporosis). The combined effect of estrogen replacement plus progesterone did not increase the risk for endometrial cancer, but the effect of progesterone added to estrogen in replacement therapy in other respects is not known.

Two important long-term studies are under way now. The Women's Health Initiative, sponsored by the federal government, is a thirteen-year project that will monitor the health of some 140,000 women 50 years of age and older. A second important study is the Postmenopausal Estrogen/Progestin Interventions Trial of the National Institutes of Health, which has been conducted at seven centers in the United States to answer questions about the effect of progestins added to an estrogen replacement regime.

The question of the risk-benefit relationship, not a simple issue in itself, is complicated by society's attitudes toward menopause, by feelings about taking medication in general, and by our attitudes about taking hormones in particular.

Feelings toward the medical profession make the decision still more complex. In the past decade or so the women's movement has encouraged women to question the authority of their physicians (who until very recently have been predominantly male). Most women do not want to be passive receptacles for the advice dispensed by an authoritative and authoritarian physician; they want instead to be an active partner of their caregivers, taking a significant role in their own health and well-being.

To make an intelligent decision, one that you will be comfortable with, you must understand the general risks and benefits of ERT and then weigh your own attitudes, your medical and family history, and your personal risk profile as determined by your lifestyle as well as by your genetic inheritance. Your decision should reflect your own psychic makeup, your feelings about taking medication on either a short-term or long-term basis, your relative fears about different diseases (for example, cancer and heart disease), and your willingness or unwillingness to put up with the annoyances of continued menstrual periods.

Sally N. is 50 years old, generally healthy, and very athletic. She has cycled, run, played golf and tennis, and hiked for recreation all her adult life. Sally has red hair, but not the pale skin that normally goes with it; she has big bones. About fifteen years ago she had a hysterectomy for a precancerous condition, but her ovaries were left intact. She takes care of her health, runs a couple of miles several times a week, and pushes herself to improve her conditioning. She is proud of her energy and the fitness level she has maintained, and in her heart of hearts (like most well-conditioned people) she is a little intolerant of people who cannot push themselves as she can. Sally maintains good dietary habits and has real preferences for healthy foods. She is the kind of person who, without even thinking about it, prefers a couple of slices of seven-grain bread and sprouts to a Big Mac.

Sally drinks very little alcohol and no coffee (because caffeine makes her nervous and edgy), and she prefers herbal tea to nonherbal. She has never smoked. Her politics are liberal; she is concerned about world hunger, pollution, women's rights, and other such issues. There is no history of breast cancer or heart disease in her family.

Sally obviously has an enviably healthy lifestyle and she is fortunate in her genetic endowment. She does not seem to be at risk for osteoporosis, in that she is very active and large boned. Her low alcohol consumption, her status as a non-smoker, and her general fitness level lower her risk for both osteoporosis and cardiac disease. Her liking for natural foods and a healthy diet, and her general political outlook, suggest that for psychological reasons Sally might feel uncomfortable with ERT. Her pride in accomplishment and endurance, which are apparent in her level of fitness and conditioning, suggest that Sally is a person who can tolerate discomfort fairly easily. Since she is not at risk for either heart disease or osteoporosis, there is no reason for her to try ERT if she does not feel so inclined.

Priscilla F. is 51 years old, blonde, attractive, and the mother of four children. Only 24 when her first baby was born, she breast-fed all four. These days she is slender to the point of being skinny. She is a highly excitable and nervous person, who smokes to calm herself and cannot break the habit. Although Priscilla has plenty of energy, she does not enjoy exercise, saying that she is too nervous even to play tennis. Obviously she doesn't need exercise to help control weight because she tips the scales at about 98 pounds, and although she admits she should exercise for other reasons, she cannot bring herself to do so. Her mother had significant osteoporosis and in fact died of the complications of a hip fracture. Her family has no history of breast cancer.

Priscilla is an obvious candidate for ERT. Her fair hair and skin, her smoking and slenderness, and her family history all put her at high risk for osteoporosis. She is a low-risk candidate for breast cancer, in part because of her family history, in part because of her youth at the time her first child was born, in part because of her breast-feeding. Priscilla seems, to some extent, to be the victim of her habits—smoking and low exercise tolerance—so there is little chance that she can change her lifestyle to adjust her risk for osteoporosis. She has no psychological objections to ERT.

Nancy C. is 50 years old, a pleasant, very capable woman with two children. She is blonde and fair-skinned, but not particularly thin—about average in both height and weight. She does not smoke. She works on an assembly line in a factory, where her job involves a certain amount of lifting and moving, so that she is quite active physically even though she does not follow a specific exercise program.

Nancy has an unfortunate genetic heritage. Her mother had a mastectomy while she was still young, but died of coronary artery disease at age 55. Her aunt had premenopausal breast cancer. One brother had coronary artery bypass surgery eight months ago; another brother died in his forties of coronary artery disease. Nancy herself has angina and a high level of LDL (bad cholesterol). She has decided to take ERT.

Nancy, like most of us, was not a clear-cut yes or no with regard to ERT. It could definitely benefit her because of her cardiovascular problems—her high LDL cholesterol, her symptoms of coronary artery disease, and her family history of heart problems. There is also a strong history of breast cancer in her family, with both her mother and her maternal aunt developing the disease before menopause. Clearly, Nancy has risk factors in both directions. Her decision was a difficult one, which she made after considerable thought. She will be sure to have an annual mammogram and to perform monthly breast self-examinations.

As Nancy's decision suggests, another important psychological consideration in a woman's choice are her fears about disease. Most women are concerned about the possibility of getting breast cancer and, realistically, it is a worrisome disease. In some women this concern reaches the level of phobia. If you are taking ERT and read about a study that links breast cancer with estrogen and if that study unravels you emotionally, then you are probably not an appropriate candidate for ERT; an affirmative decision would compromise your outlook on life and your psychological well-being.

Both heart disease and breast cancer are serious, life-threatening and life-compromising diseases. Breast cancer also suffers from a stigma that is indepen-

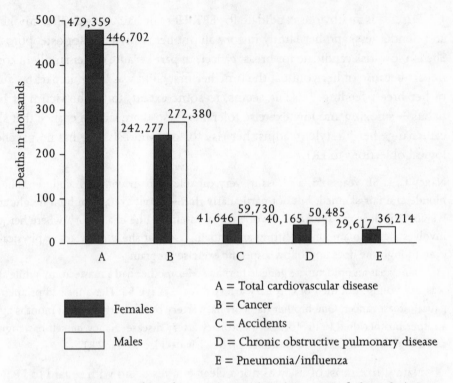

A = Total cardiovascular disease
B = Cancer
C = Accidents
D = Chronic obstructive pulmonary disease
E = Pneumonia/influenza

Figure 8. *The leading causes of death for men and women (United States: 1991 final mortality). Contrary to popular belief, more women than men die of cardiovascular diseases; more men than women die
of cancer. Almost twice as many women die of cardiovascular disease as of all kinds of cancer combined.
Source: National Center for Health Statistics and the American Heart Association. Reproduced with
permission.* Heart and Stroke Facts: 1995 Statistical Supplement, *1994. Copyright
American Heart Association.*

dent of its seriousness as a disease. That stigma puts an additional burden on
many women who have it and adds to the fear of women who do not have it.

Although no one goes out and asks for heart disease, it does not have the
fearsome reputation that breast cancer does. Nevertheless, heart disease is serious
business and can end your life abruptly or compromise your life to the point
where you cannot move from your bed without serious pain. Perhaps Americans
think of heart disease as a man's disease, although half of the nearly one million
people who die yearly of heart attacks are women. In the popular imagery, heart
disease has a macho connotation: it fells hard-driving business executives or
basketball superstars, not carpool-driving mothers or underpaid office workers.
Furthermore, the heart is a socially acceptable organ, unlike the bowel or the
breast. People don't make denigrating jokes about the heart. You can talk publicly

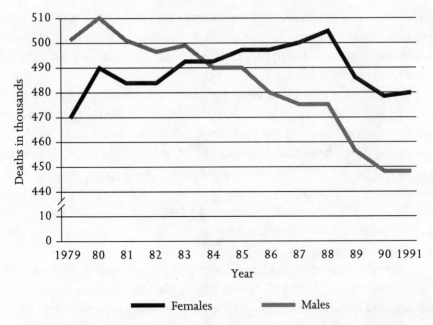

Figure 9. Trends in mortality from cardiovascular disease, for men and women (United States). While men are doing better in reducing their mortality from cardiovascular disease, women apparently are doing less well. Source: National Center for Health Statistics and the American Heart Association. Reproduced with permission. Heart and Stroke Facts: 1995 Statistical Supplement, 1994. Copyright American Heart Association.

about your heart and its infirmities, as you cannot about your colon, or your vagina, or your breast. So, for several reasons, breast cancer is a disease that carries heavy emotional baggage.

If you are one of the numerous women who feel extremely anxious about breast cancer and would blame yourself if you got the disease because you elected to take ERT, then you are probably better off psychologically not taking it.

Many women feel more comfortable about taking "medicine," let's say aspirin for a headache or an antihistamine for allergies, than they do about taking hormones for menopausal discomforts. Our attitudes toward taking hormones have flip-flopped several times in the past generation.

Laboratory researchers isolated estrogen and progesterone in the 1920s and estrogen became commercially available in the 1930s. During the 1950s and 1960s, hormones had very good press: birth control pills appeared and began to be used widely in the 1960s. The media applauded this new liberation of women. And certainly many young women found themselves more in control of their reproductive processes than ever before. They did not have to use contraceptives at the last minute, or plan ahead in order to be ready with the appropriate contraceptive at the appropriate moment. Nor did they have to leave contraception to their partner.

A 1966 book entitled *Feminine Forever* claimed that with estrogen you could remain young, healthy, and vibrant always. Written by a physician named Robert Wilson, who was born in 1895, this book reflected cultural attitudes that had been filtered through the consciousness of a 71-year-old physician. The assumptions were that the only woman worth having, so to speak, was a youthful, unlined, and therefore sexually desirable creature—someone indistinguishable from, let us say, Jeannie with the magical powers, or Lucy (the one loved by Ricky Ricardo), or June Cleaver, who were served up for our entertainment by the television of the period.

From the time of the book's publication, use of estrogen postmenopausally increased considerably. In 1975, however, an important article was published in the *New England Journal of Medicine*, one of the most prestigious journals read by practicing physicians. The article showed a relationship between the use of estrogen therapy (which at that time was given without the balancing action of progesterone) and endometrial cancer.

At about the same time, it was discovered that DES (diethylstilbestrol), a synthetic estrogen once routinely given to help prevent miscarriage, was associated with cancers of the genital tract of the *children* of women who had taken the hormone. By that time close to a million women had been exposed to DES from the late 1940s or early 1950s through the early 1970s. Here was a new situation: a drug we had thought capable of doing a lot of good twenty years later turned out to have had unforeseen risks.

The association between DES and estrogen therapy and cancer started the pendulum swinging in the other direction. The bad press began to affect other drugs. Birth control pills became suspect in the late 1970s and early 1980s. At the same time, the controversy prodded researchers to study the effects of taking hormones over the long term and stimulated more research about menopause in general. As people begin discussing the subject openly, as they have over the last few years, hormones are beginning to get a more balanced press than formerly. So it is worth realizing that our attitudes toward them are determined by complex factors, some of them cultural, others scientific.

Yet another component of your decision about ERT is the way you feel about menstrual periods. If you look forward to menopause as a release from periods or dread having those periods continue, you may well not be a candidate for ERT. In fact, one of the main reasons that women advance for giving up their therapy is their annoyance with menstrual periods.

Once you have analyzed all these factors in your personal psychological makeup, you should give careful attention to your profile of health risk and your family history. Are you a high-risk candidate for coronary artery disease? Has your mother or your grandmother gotten hunchbacked or significantly shorter as she aged, which suggests that you may be at risk for osteoporosis? Do you have a family history of breast cancer? All of these factors should enter into your decision about ERT. Essentially the choice is one that you must make for yourself, although you certainly should seek help from your physician or caregiver.

What are the short-term benefits of ERT?

Estrogen replacement therapy is the best, most effective way known to medical science to relieve the discomfort of hot flashes and other vasomotor symptoms such as sweating and clamminess, crawly skin, tingling fingers, and palpitations.

Researchers do not yet know exactly what mechanism triggers an individual hot flash. Scientists do have some understanding of the mechanism by which falling estrogen levels at menopause lead to hot flashes and other vasomotor symptoms, but it is still a mystery why 20 percent of American women (all of whom have falling estrogen levels at menopause) never have any menopausal discomfort at all. So while areas of mystery still exist, numerous scientific studies as well as mountains of anecdotal evidence show that ERT does work for practically everyone.

Hormone therapy is also very effective in preventing the sleeplessness and frequent awakening that are among the most distressing symptoms of menopause. Some women say they wake in response to feelings of being overheated, or the sweating and cooling of hot flashes; others do not notice hot flashes or heavy perspiration, but they wake anyhow, sometimes several times a night. Even if you are not aware of having a hot flash before you wake, estrogen can still be a big help in giving you a solid night's rest. If, on the other hand, you can't sleep because your children are in trouble, or your husband is out of a job, or your boss is driving you crazy, then ERT won't help.

What are the long-term benefits of ERT?

Used long term, ERT has benefits that can affect the quality of your life and can lower your risk for heart disease and osteoporosis. First of all, ERT can greatly lessen those degenerative or atrophic changes to the vagina and urinary tract that can make sex uncomfortable and lead to incontinence and frequent vaginal or urinary tract infections. These degenerative changes are often accompanied by urinary incontinence. The rapid bone loss that results in osteoporosis can be prevented or slowed by ERT. And, perhaps most important, ERT protects against heart disease and coronary artery disease, which are significant killers of post-menopausal women.

A host of other benefits, some of them cosmetic, have been reported anecdotally but not scientifically proved. Among them are improvement in mood or outlook, better skin, enhanced memory, and heightened sex drive.

Which menopausal symptoms eventually go away by themselves?

In general, hot flashes will resolve themselves eventually, but a few women have them throughout their life. Other vasomotor disturbances also will probably disappear in time. Sleeplessness, if caused by vasomotor disturbances, improves with time, although both men and women may have increased trouble sleeping as they age. The acute mood changes and feelings of anxiety or even panic that are brought on by hormonal changes at menopause tend to get better with time, peaking early in perimenopause and then gradually fading away.

Which menopausal symptoms don't go away with time or get worse as time goes on?

Vaginal dryness and atrophic changes get progressively worse with time. Incontinence gradually increases. Bone loss starts when we are in our thirties, apparently accelerates just after menopause, and continues more slowly throughout life. Cardiovascular risk increases gradually with age. Menopausal short-term memory loss and its companion, difficulty in concentrating, probably do not get better spontaneously, though so far the evidence is not conclusive.

How long do I have to take ERT before I notice improvement in hot flashes, sleep disturbances, and other vasomotor symptoms?

Usually women notice that their symptoms are abating within a week or two.

If I start on ERT, do I have to take it forever?

No, you can stop any time you want. If you are taking ERT to control your hot flashes or your sleeplessness, two symptoms that will probably get better on their own as time passes, then you can stop the ERT for a while and see what happens. If the symptoms return, you can go back to ERT; if they don't, you can assume that you are probably in the clear. But if you have chosen ERT to protect you against cardiovascular disease or osteoporosis, you will lose the protection estrogen provides when you stop taking it. Since the years right after menopause are those of most rapid bone loss, you should consider taking estrogen for five to ten years postmenopausally.

If I decide to stop ERT, can I stop "cold turkey," all at once?

Gradual withdrawal by cutting down on your dosage will probably produce fewer symptoms. We know that women who have a sudden menopause—women whose ovaries are removed surgically or shut down in response to chemotherapy—often have severe hot flashes. But many women can just stop their therapy and not be uncomfortable.

Will ERT give me contraceptive protection?

In the doses normally given, ERT will not give you contraceptive protection. If you take low-dose birth control pills as a form of ERT during your perimenopausal years, then of course you will be protected against unwanted pregnancy.

Will ERT increase my fertility?

No, it will not. Nor will it postpone the time when your natural menopause will occur.

Will ERT prevent Alzheimer's disease?

This topic is currently of significant interest to scientists and physicians. We know that there are estrogen receptors in the brain and that blood flow to the brain is intensified when estrogen levels are high. Statistical studies show that older women on hormone replacement are less likely to develop Alzheimer's disease than women who are not. Researchers have also suggested that estrogen has a positive effect on nerve cell growth and functioning. Although the evidence is tantalizing, it is too early to tell whether ERT will prevent Alzheimer's disease or even arrest its growth.

Will ERT prevent osteoporosis?

Currently, ERT is the best known way of preventing osteoporosis, a progressive loss of bone that affects many older women. Estrogen plays a role in balancing the breakdown and rebuilding of bone that goes on throughout our lifetime, and it doesn't seem to matter to our bones whether this estrogen is produced by our own ovaries or by a pharmaceutical company. Nor does it matter by what route the estrogen reaches your bones. ERT can be delivered either orally or through a patch placed on the skin. We know that 0.625 mg daily of conjugated estrogen (Premarin or its cousins) or 1 mg daily of 17-beta estradiol (which is Estrace, the same basic dosage as the 0.05 estrogen patch) all give excellent protection against osteoporosis.

Does adding progesterone to ERT decrease protection against osteoporosis?

No, estrogen plus progestin prevents fractures just as well as estrogen alone. Indeed, although the subject is very controversial, some studies suggest that natural progesterone alone may stimulate bone production.

Will starting ERT later in life bring back bone that has been lost through osteoporosis?

Probably not. That is why women who plan to take ERT to prevent osteoporosis should begin early, not wait several years after menopause. Starting ERT will prevent loss of more bone, but it will probably not bring back bone that you have already lost.

How serious is osteoporosis?

Obviously no one wants to lose height or to be hunched over; but that, after all, seems at first glance to be merely a cosmetic problem. Nor does anyone hope for a broken hip or wrist, but those injuries also seem tolerable: many people have suffered from broken bones and recovered by the time they are adults. So it is easy to make light of this disease.

In actuality, its consequences in terms of human suffering are often extremely serious. One in three American women fractures a hip before she reaches age 80; more than 250,000 women in this country do so every year. Of these, 30,000 die of complications from the fracture. Another 100,000, almost a third, need to enter a nursing home or some other facility for long-term care, which means losing precious independence. A broken hip, then, can permanently alter the shape of your life.

Osteoporosis also causes very small fractures in the spinal column and elsewhere that account for chronic severe backaches and other pain. These micro-fractures often go undetected.

What is my risk of getting osteoporosis?

According to the statistics developed by Deborah Grady and her colleagues, if you are a 50-year-old white woman not taking ERT, the relative risk of sometime in your life having a hip fracture (generally taken to mean your risk for osteoporosis) is 36.2 percent. In other words, of any 1,000 white women who are now 50 years old, 362 will at some time fracture a hip. The risk is less for black women.

How effective is exercise alone in maintaining bone mass?

Many women at risk for osteoporosis wonder whether they should take estrogen or exercise. The answer is that to maximize bone health throughout life, you should do both. There is no question that if you are not taking estrogen post-menopausally, you will lose bone. Exercise helps, but studies have shown that moderate exercise alone, for example brisk walking, is not sufficient to prevent osteoporosis.

The ideal preventive is a combination of estrogen and exercise, plus adequate calcium intake in your diet. While estrogen alone may prevent significant postmenopausal bone loss, estrogen plus exercise may even help you build back bone that has been lost.

Can I prevent bone loss by increasing my intake of calcium?

While studies have shown that you can increase bone mass by exercise at any time during your life, if you are not taking estrogen the effect of drinking even a gallon of milk a day is debatable. Remember that women in their thirties and forties should be sure they are getting enough calcium (about 1,000 mg) in their diet, because they still have enough estrogen to absorb it; in terms of building healthy bones, now is better than later. Physicians recommend 1,500 mg of calcium daily for postmenopausal women, but researchers have not yet completed the clinical trials that will demonstrate the effects of increased calcium intake.

Are there drugs other than estrogen for osteoporosis?

Yes, but their value is really unknown. The medication most commonly considered nowadays is Etidronate, or Didronel, a drug that has been used since the 1960s for a rare bone affliction called Paget's disease and more recently for postmenopausal osteoporosis. Fosamax, a drug introduced in 1995, seems more effective than Didronel in rebuilding lost bone. It has minimal side effects and, unlike Didronel, seems to produce bone comparable to the bone that has been lost; it can be used in conjunction with estrogen. Like Didronel it is a treatment for established osteoporosis, and is not used in preventing the disease.

What is the relationship between ERT and heart disease?

Probably the greatest single benefit of ERT to the greatest number of women is that ERT will reduce your chances of having a heart attack. We have seen that women are protected from heart disease during their reproductive years, but that women's risk rises gradually after menopause so that by age 65 their chances of having a heart attack are almost equal to those of men in the same age group.

Several studies have shown that women on ERT have better cardiovascular health than women who do not take estrogen postmenopausally. One of the most important of these is the Nurses' Health Study, which provides solid evidence to support the cardiovascular benefits of ERT. In 1976 a group of researchers in the Boston area began a study of 122,000 married female registered nurses. The nurses, between 30 and 55 years of age when the study started, were followed up every two years. The women on estrogen were taking oral "natural" estrogen, that is, the kind of estrogen in Premarin or Estrace. They did not take progesterone along with it. Statistical results on heart disease, first published in 1989 and based on the first ten years of data, showed that the 48,470 postmenopausal women who were taking ERT had significantly fewer heart attacks than the women who were not.

Who is at high risk for heart disease?

Risk factors for heart disease include age, heredity, diet (high fat, heavy salt consumption), high alcohol consumption (generally defined for women as more than two drinks a day), stress, obesity, and smoking. Some of these factors— diet, smoking, alcohol consumption, obesity—are controllable. Others are not.

The single most lethal controllable factor is smoking. Many women say they continue to smoke in order to keep their weight down. While obesity is certainly a risk factor for heart disease, smoking is even riskier: according to the American Heart Association and the American Cancer Society, to offset the health benefits of quitting smoking, the average smoker would have to gain 75 pounds.

Smoking seems particularly deadly in women because in addition to accelerating the hardening of the arteries, it weakens women's two best defenders against cardiac disease, estrogen and HDL.

How important a threat for women is coronary heart disease?

According to Grady and her colleagues, a 50-year-old white woman has a 46 percent lifetime probability of getting coronary heart disease, the leading cause of death among postmenopausal women. In a sample of one hundred of these women, then, forty-six of them can be predicted to get coronary heart disease. The average 50-year-old white woman's chances of dying of this disease are 31 percent. The median age at which women die of coronary heart disease is 74 years, which means that half of the women are older and half are younger at the time of death.

Strong evidence suggests, however, that ERT will lower your risk. Further data imply that this risk reduction will be even greater in women who already have coronary heart disease.

Does adding progesterone to ERT have any effect on risk for heart disease?

When American physicians prescribe ERT, they usually prescribe a progestin (synthetic progesterone) as well as estrogen in order to protect women from uterine cancer. Unfortunately, progestins tend to increase the LDL (bad cholesterol) or decrease the HDL (good cholesterol) levels in blood, so that some of the positive effect of the estrogen is lost. Many researchers believe that natural progesterone does not have this negative impact on blood cholesterol levels, and in fact preliminary data suggest that natural progesterone has almost no adverse effect on blood lipids.

Overall it is highly likely that the benefit of estrogen outweighs the risk of progestins. If you are taking estrogen and progestins in the appropriate dosages, you are still better off than you would be if you were not taking either, but you are less well off, as far as cardiac disease goes, than you would be taking estrogen alone. Since women generally did not start taking progestins until the late 1970s, there are no definitive long-term studies on the relationship of estrogen, progestins and cardiac disease.

Does ERT raise blood pressure?

It was formerly believed that ERT did raise blood pressure but more recent research shows that blood pressure generally doesn't change much with estrogen therapy. However, a small proportion of women, about one in twenty, responds to ERT with higher blood pressure.

Does ERT raise the risk of blood clots?

Unless you have a history of clotting problems (for example, thrombophlebitis), ERT is not dangerous to you. It is usually safe for women with varicose veins. The reasons for its safety are that ERT contains quite small amounts of estrogen and that the type of estrogen used is different from that incorporated in birth control pills.

In the years after "the pill" was introduced, evidence mounted that the estrogen in oral contraceptives encouraged blood clots, heart attacks, and strokes. Although there were several different brands of oral contraceptives with different configurations of estrogen and progesterone, all contained high doses of synthetic estrogen, which decreased the anticlotting factors in the blood and therefore made clots more likely. But times have changed and so has the pill. In the early 1960s when the pill was first introduced, oral contraceptives contained what would now be considered huge doses of hormones, sometimes up to three times the amount in today's low-dose oral contraceptives. Even today's contraceptive pills contain about six times the amount of estrogen per day in the standard ERT dosage prescribed for postmenopausal women.

Furthermore, contraceptive pills contain a different kind of estrogen from that used in ERT. Birth control pills contain synthetic estrogen, whereas the estrogen in ERT is "natural," which means that it is identical or very similar in its chemical structure to estrogen produced in nature. The estrogen in Premarin, for example, is isolated from the urine of pregnant mares. The estrogen in Estrace is also "natural" estrogen. Though manufactured in the laboratory, it is still a kind of estrogen called 17-beta estradiol, which is made by the ovaries of female mammals. So while early birth control pills did have their hazards, the estrogen in ERT is not dangerous—first because of the extremely small dosage, second because it is natural estrogen.

Researchers also point out that while synthetic estrogen might well affect clotting factors, which in turn might have a negative impact on cardiovascular problems, it also relaxes the blood vessels, which has a positive impact on cardiovascular problems.

Does ERT increase my risk of gallbladder disease?

Women, particularly overweight older women, are already at increased risk for gallbladder disease. Estrogen, taken orally, does approximately double the risk. However, risk does not increase if you use a patch instead of taking the estrogen orally.

Does ERT protect against stroke?

Again, this is an area in which more research needs to be done. Studies up to now show contradictory results. Deborah Grady and her colleagues, after reviewing some fifteen scientific studies, concluded that statistically the risk for stroke among estrogen users is about the same as for women who do not use estrogen. Their study shows that a 50-year-old white woman has a 20 percent probability of developing a stroke. The median age of death from stroke is 83, which means that half the women who die of strokes are older and half are younger than 83.

How effective is ERT in reducing vaginal dryness?

It is the most effective known way to prevent postmenopausal vaginal problems. After menopause, vaginal dryness tends to increase progressively with age unless you do something about it. Without estrogen the walls of the vagina will continue to thin out and become less elastic, a condition known as vaginal atrophy. Dryness and the subsequent irritation make these tissues vulnerable to infection, so that women of this age group often have significant bacterial and yeast infections of the vagina.

Fortunately, these discomforts are easily treated and no one should have to endure them. Women taking ERT do not experience vaginal atrophy comparable to that which occurs in the absence of estrogen. Estrogen creams, applied directly to the vagina, also help with problems of vaginal atrophy. The benefits last as long as you take the estrogen.

Do I have to use vaginal estrogen cream constantly from the onset of menopause, or can I use it as I need it?

Some women approaching menopause who are not currently sexually active anticipate becoming active at some time in the future. They wonder whether they can start using estrogen cream at that point. The answer is yes; it will help at any time and there is no harm in starting later. While it is perfectly all right to use it in an ongoing, continuous way, it is also fine to start and stop.

One of my patients is a nun who left the convent in midlife and got married postmenopausally. She started using estrogen cream and is enjoying a normal sex life. Unlike bone loss, vaginal atrophy or dryness is almost 100 percent reversible.

Can I use commercial lubricants for sexual intercourse instead of ERT?

The products that provide on-the-spot lubrication for intercourse may work for their intended purpose, but they do not help the vaginal walls provide their own lubrication, as estrogen does. The only commercial product that seems to have somewhat the same effect as ERT is Replens; still, it is not as effective, generally, as estrogen cream.

Will ERT keep my skin youthful?

Is it loss of estrogen or just the process of aging that makes skin lose its youthful elasticity and smoothness? No one knows for sure, and we lack incontrovertible data that estrogen will protect your skin as it will protect your heart and your bones. While nothing known to modern science will make 70-year-old skin look like 20-year-old skin, estrogen does seem to have positive effects. The informal observation that plump middle-aged women often have more youthful skin than slender middle-aged women supports this belief. After all, plumper women make more estrogen because their fat manufactures it.

Some researchers also believe that estrogen improves skin tone, perhaps by causing water retention, or by stimulating the production of subcutaneous fat, or by causing collagen to be built up in layers beneath the skin. Well-designed experiments have shown that the skin of women taking ERT is thicker than the skin of women not getting estrogen replacement.

On an anecdotal level, many of the women I talk to say that taking estrogen has helped their skin. They notice that their skin retains moisture better and feels less itchy and less irritated. A few say that estrogen makes their skin oily, so that in one respect they feel like teenagers again. I even have one patient who complains of getting pimples from her estrogen. She is a slender little woman and is worried about osteoporosis. When we measure levels of estradiol in her blood, we find that at an estradiol of 50, which is low-normal for a menstruating woman, she gets pimples. We have tried different sorts of estrogen preparations, but they all seem to affect her the same way. Her reaction is rare, however.

Does estrogen cream rubbed into the skin convey any benefits?

Since some of the estrogen in the cream is bound to be absorbed through the skin, the benefits will be those of ERT taken orally. But remember that estrogen taken by any route carries with it the danger of causing excessive growth of the uterine lining. And if you are rubbing estrogen cream into your skin, you cannot be sure exactly how much estrogen is reaching your uterine lining.

Will ERT prevent hair loss?

One of the unpleasant facts of growing older is thinning hair—on the head, in the pubic area, under the arms, and elsewhere on the body. No one knows with certainty whether this is strictly a menopausal problem, that is, caused by decreased production of estrogen, or whether it is caused by aging and just happens to become noticeable at about the time of menopause.

Estrogen replacement therapy will not keep your hair from graying and it probably will not prevent it from gradually thinning, though some women tell me that their hair seems to thicken up a little when they start ERT. Nor will ERT necessarily improve the texture of your hair, which may have changed for the worse as you have grown older.

Will ERT prevent unwanted facial hair?

Although ERT will not keep your hair as thick as it was when you were 21 years old, it may help with that other menopausal hair problem, unwanted facial hair. Since the ovaries continue to produce androgens (hormones associated with male characteristics) even after their production of estrogen has dropped off, the premenopausal balance between these hormones changes. There is no circulating estrogen to block the action of the androgens, and many women notice that their hair tends to grow in a more masculine pattern after menopause. This can mean increased facial hair and changes in the texture of this hair, which typically becomes darker and coarser. The ERT may help reverse this process, but its benefits will continue only as long as you continue to take it.

Will ERT prevent weight gain?

Unfortunately, no. Nor will it prevent the redistribution of fat on the body, which tends, as we get older, to rush to the area between our thighs and shoulders.

Some evidence suggests that on a cyclic basis estrogen does influence weight. Very few women are the same weight all through the month, as their hormone cycle changes the amount of fluid their bodies retain. The same is true of women whom I put on ERT; they often report a weight gain of two to three pounds of retained water, which they generally maintain as long as they are taking estrogen. Although we say "never say never" in medicine, it is possible, but highly unlikely, that a person will gain fifteen to twenty pounds from estrogen alone.

Sometimes a patient will call me and say, "Look, I started ERT and I have gained ten pounds, and I really think that it is that darned estrogen." So I suggest that she stop the estrogen for a couple of months and see whether the unwanted pounds melt away. (Contrary to popular opinion, it is not dangerous to go on and off estrogen, though you may notice some symptoms.) Generally I get a phone call about two months later. The ten pounds have not miraculously disappeared, and the patient would like to go back on estrogen again.

Occasional patients lose dramatic amounts of weight when they go on estrogen therapy. These are usually people who felt awful, who weren't sleeping at night, and who didn't have the energy to exercise, so it is very possible that they just stayed home and did a little extra eating. When these women found new energy because they were sleeping better, they began running around again and started burning their calories better.

Of course you can certainly diet while you are on estrogen. There is no reason to say, "Well, I might as well not diet because I am on ERT and it is causing me to gain weight." That's equivalent to saying, "Well, I am on birth control pills, so I will gain weight and therefore I might just as well not diet." You can diet any time you want to diet.

Will ERT help with the mood swings, tearfulness, and irritability of menopause?

Many women say that ERT helps their psychological outlook, that they are less likely to become grouchy and angry when they are taking estrogen. Irritability and mood swings can be caused by sleeplessness, and insofar as ERT promotes a good night's sleep, it helps with these problems.

Will ERT help with memory lapses and lack of concentration?

Some women say that they are less susceptible to strange memory lapses and lack of concentration when they are on ERT. But these feelings are very subjective, and we all forget things from time to time, especially as we age.

Barbara Sherwin, a professor at McGill University in Montreal, recently undertook a study on the relationship between memory and estrogen deprivation. She and a group of coworkers gave several tests of memory and abstract reasoning to women whose ovaries had been removed surgically as part of a hysterectomy. The women were divided into two groups: one received estrogen therapy; the other received a placebo, a pill that looked like the estrogen pill but contained no active ingredients. Sherwin discovered that the women who were given estrogen therapy after the operation did better on the tests of short-term memory than did the women who were given a placebo, though long-term memory in the two groups was about equal.

Other research has suggested that estrogen plays an important role in maintaining short-term memory (like where you put down your reading glasses) but doesn't have much influence on long-term memory (like remembering the songs you learned in the third grade).

What are the side effects of ERT?

Most women tolerate estrogen very well, but 5 to 10 percent do experience side effects. The most common are breast tenderness and fluid retention or bloating—symptoms, incidentally, similar to those that many women feel just before their periods. A few women on ERT feel queasy or slightly nauseated. These symptoms may be caused by too much estrogen; changing the dosage usually controls the discomfort.

Some women, especially those who are prone to migraines, find that estrogen brings on headaches. This phenomenon is difficult to deal with, because headaches can be caused either by too much estrogen or by too little. I have patients who get headaches from too little estrogen, and when I put them on higher dosages the headaches disappear. I have one patient who gets an occasional hot flash when she takes the usual dosage of estrogen (0.625 mg of Premarin) but when I boost the dosage to 0.9 mg, she gets headaches. Some women who get headaches if they take their ERT orally do not do so if they use the transdermal patch.

Although many women feel that estrogen helps their skin, a few have pigmentation problems: they may develop a darkened area on the face, as some women do during pregnancy. Moles may get darker.

Most of these symptoms are mild and don't mean that you have to give up ERT. Occasionally, however, women are just plain allergic to estrogen and respond to ERT with skin rashes, itching, or other typical allergic symptoms. Sometimes changing the brand of medication will help.

Does ERT raise the risk of endometrial cancer?

If you have a uterus (that is, if you have not had a hysterectomy) and you take estrogen without taking progesterone to ensure periodic cleanout of the uterine lining, then you do increase your risk for endometrial cancer (cancer of the lining of the uterus). The longer you take the ERT, the greater your risk.

If you take progesterone along with the estrogen, however, either cyclically or as continuous therapy, you do not increase your risk for endometrial cancer. Several scientific studies have shown that the risk of endometrial cancer for women who take estrogen plus progesterone is not increased by the use of these hormones.

What are the side effects of progestins?

If you have your uterus, you will probably be taking progestin along with your ERT. Unfortunately, many women find that progestin gives them the kind of emotional outlook that they used to experience premenopausally, including irritability, jumpiness, anxiety, and mild depression. Others report bloating and breast tenderness. Some women report headaches. These side effects seem to be milder in women taking low-dose daily progestins and in women taking cyclic natural progesterone. Cyclic progestins such as Provera, seem to give slightly more severe side effects than either cyclic natural progesterone or progestins taken every day.

Does ERT cause fibrocystic breast changes?

Because one of the side effects of ERT can be breast tenderness, ERT may in some cases make fibrocystic breasts more tender.

Does ERT raise the risk of breast cancer?

This question poses today's most vexing dilemma for women who are making the choice of whether or not to use ERT. In the past two decades, numerous studies have attempted to determine whether breast cancer risk increases with estrogen use. They are, however, only a first step toward the knowledge we really need.

Early investigations, undertaken during the 1970s and 1980s, produced conflicting results. Some suggested no increased risk, some suggested slightly increased risk, and some suggested slightly decreased risk of breast cancer in women who took ERT. Long-term studies have been longer arriving, for obvious reasons. Use of ERT (without progestins) first became widespread during the late 1960s and the 1970s; after the discovery that the addition of a progestin protected against endometrial cancer (and that estrogen replacement alone without the opposing progestin increased the risk of endometrial cancer), use of estrogen dropped for a while; then the use of estrogen, now usually combined with progestin, began to increase. Thus not many women have undergone ERT for very long.

Newer studies are beginning to arrive. In 1989 researchers in Sweden published a large epidemiologic study that involved some 23,244 women, a study that made the front page of the *New York Times*. The research showed that women on long-term ERT (that is, women who had been on ERT for longer than nine years) had a slightly increased risk of breast cancer. Their risk factor was placed at 1.1, which means that if under normal circumstances 100 women per thousand would get breast cancer, then of a thousand women taking ERT for more than ten years, 110 of them would get breast cancer. Furthermore, the study showed that women who were taking combined therapy, estrogen plus progestin, had a higher risk than those taking estrogen alone.

These data made waves. However, scientists who reviewed the study found several significant differences from the way ERT is prescribed in this country. First of all, the estrogen used in the Swedish study was primarily estradiol, while in this country the most commonly prescribed estrogen, Premarin, is conjugated equine estrogen. Second, although the statistics were gathered for a period beginning in 1977, many of the women might have begun taking estrogen well before that. Furthermore, the dosage levels in the European study were much higher than those conventionally used here, as were the recorded blood estrogen levels of the women receiving these dosages.

In 1992 Deborah Grady's study concluded that ERT definitely reduces the risk of coronary heart disease and osteoporosis. She also found that while postmenopausal estrogen alone does increase the risk of endometrial cancer, that risk can be avoided by adding progestin to the estrogen regimen. From her review of the available studies, Grady suggested that long-term estrogen therapy may be associated with a small increase in risk for breast cancer, but that short-term ERT (less than five years) apparently does not increase the risk at all. Although scientific evidence is inconsistent about the effect of estrogen plus progestin on the risk for breast cancer, some evidence points to slightly increased risk for long-term users.

In 1995 a group of researchers at Harvard University published further statistics from the Nurses' Health Study, incorporating data from 1976 to 1992. Again the results hit the front page of the *New York Times*. These researchers found that women aged 55 to 59 who had been taking ERT for five or more years had a 40 percent higher risk of breast cancer than women who had never taken ERT. That is, if no women in this age group had taken ERT, the expected number of cases of breast cancer for 1,000 women would be something like 35. If all the women in the same age group did use ERT for five years or more, then statistically there would be 50 cases of breast cancer. The risk increase was higher in older women, who have a higher incidence of breast cancer under any conditions. In the 60 to 64 age group, long-term use of hormones was associated with a 70 percent increased risk. Again, this means that of 100,000 women in that age group, if 100 were expected to get breast cancer without taking hormones, then 170 cases would be expected among women who had taken hormones for five years or longer.

The researchers came to some other conclusions. Women who stop taking ERT revert to their original risk category within two years. Use longer than five years makes no difference in risk; that is, women who take ERT for ten years are not at higher risk than women who take it for five. The addition of progestins does not protect women against breast cancer, though it does protect against endometrial cancer.

Critics of this study, as of earlier ones, note that the increased risk of breast cancer must be weighed against the benefits of ERT, particularly its benefits in protecting against heart disease. Dr. Fred Naftolin of Yale University points to the irony that many older women on ERT who get breast cancer might well have died previously from heart attacks or their complications if they had not taken ERT; the estrogen they took kept them alive long enough to get breast cancer.

Other researchers, both clinical and epidemiological, question the validity of the study on the basis of estrogen's known tendency to speed the growth of some types of breast cancer. In an interview with the New York Times, Trudy Bush, an epidemiologist at Johns Hopkins University, pointed out that while estrogen may increase the growth of small tumors that are already present but not yet clinically detectable, it is doubtful that it stimulates the growth of new tumors. If ERT caused a true increase in tumors, she said, doctors would be seeing this increase clinically in their practices. The fact that the incidence of breast cancer does not increase with length of ERT use beyond five years, suggests the same thing. Leon Speroff, in a review published in the Journal of Obstetrics and Gynecology, concluded that on the evidence available so far, neither a protective nor detrimental effect on breast cancer has been convincingly shown.

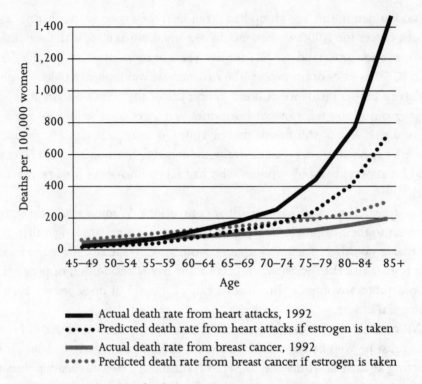

Figure 10. *The risks and benefits of estrogen replacement therapy. Although long-term use of ERT may somewhat increase the risk of breast cancer, especially as women age, heart disease remains by far the primary killer of older women.* New York Times, 15 June 1995, copyright © 1995 by the NewYork Times Company. Reprinted by permission.

What about estrogen and uterine cancer?

Today it is known that unopposed estrogen, that is, estrogen given without the countering action of progesterone, can increase the risk of cancer of the endometrium. Estrogen causes the lining of the uterus to grow. During your pre-menopausal years, you shed this lining every month during your menstrual cycle. After menopause, unless you take and withdraw progesterone to mimic the menstrual cycle, or limit its growth with a continuous small dose of progesterone, the endometrium just grows and grows, sometimes leading to a condition called hyperplasia.

Hyperplasia is not uterine cancer, but it can precede uterine cancer. Still, even with unopposed estrogen the risk of endometrial cancer is quite small. Not only is the risk statistically small, but uterine cancer associated with ERT is, as cancers go, very easy to treat. Uterine cancer associated with ERT is usually what is called well differentiated, which means that the cancerous cells don't look much different from the normal cells lining the uterus. There may be more of them (hyperplasia) but, to use the pathologist's term, they don't look "nasty."

Second, uterine cancer associated with ERT is usually diagnosed very early, because its first symptom in most women is bleeding at an abnormal time. Women bleed; they go to their gynecologist; and they get diagnosed early. Treatment is usually by hysterectomy, which in postreproductive women is not a tragic event.

A fascinating study about fifteen years ago investigated women with endometrial cancer. It compared women who had very early, noninvasive stages of endometrial cancer with women who did not have cancer. The two groups were matched by age and comparable medical histories. It turned out that essentially the women with the cancer had a better survival rate than the control group. Why? What the study showed is that the factors that put you at risk for endometrial cancer—obesity, hypertension, and diabetes—also put you at risk for other, potentially more serious problems. The reason that obese women are at high risk for endometrial carcinoma is that fat tissue converts adrenal-gland hormones to estrogen. Heavy women are walking around with a lot more than one tablet of Premarin a day in their bloodstreams; they have their own estrogen factories, which are constantly stimulating the uterus.

Fat women are also at high risk for other disorders, especially diabetes and high blood pressure. What probably happens is that women who have early, well-differentiated tumors of the endometrium go to their doctors because of their bleeding, and their other epidemiologic risk factors are taken care of. Their blood pressure will probably be checked. If their blood sugar is out of control from their diabetes, it will be taken care of. If they are obese, they will probably be reprimanded and perhaps they will take off a few pounds.

8 *A Practical Guide to ERT*

There are several approaches to ERT, and physicians have different attitudes about when to start therapy, what kinds of routines or schedules to establish, and whether to use pills, patches, or some other route of delivery. In most cases you can tailor the regimen to your own needs.

Starting ERT

Who cannot take ERT?

There are a few conditions under which it is unwise to take ERT. If you have active thrombophlebitis (that is, an inflammation of the veins involving a blood clot), or active gallbladder disease, or active breast cancer, you are not a candidate for estrogen therapy.

There are other conditions that you should discuss with your caregiver if you are interested in taking ERT, though these conditions will not necessarily rule it out. If you have a history of clotting problems, or a family history of breast or uterine cancer, you should certainly alert your caregiver. If you have had impaired liver function (that is, a history of hepatitis) or have had gallbladder disease, you may still be a candidate for a variant of ERT.

Can I take ERT if I have fibroids?

If you have fibroids, you can still take ERT; but since fibroids are estrogen sensitive, your caregiver will have to follow you carefully to see that the estrogen therapy does not cause them to grow.

Can I take ERT if my blood pressure is high?

High blood pressure was long thought to be a reason for not taking ERT. Recent research, however, actually seems to show some beneficial effects of estrogen on the walls of the blood vessels, so current thinking among many physicians is that ERT can possibly help women with elevated blood pressure. For a small percentage of women, however, blood pressure goes up on estrogen therapy.

What about ERT for women with fibrocystic breasts?

There is no reason, in terms of health risk, why women with fibrocystic breasts should not take ERT. But for some of these women ERT may introduce discomfort.

Probably half the women I see as patients have fibrocystic breasts; it is a very common condition. When menopause comes along, most women who were bothered by fibrocystic breast discomfort begin to feel better. Their breasts are no longer affected by the estrogen-progesterone cycle, so they have less lumpiness and less tenderness. If we reintroduce estrogen with ERT, many of these women get some discomfort back, though usually not as much as when they were having periods (because the dosage of estrogen in ERT is much lower than what the ovaries produce during the reproductive years). Many women can control the discomfort by eliminating caffeine and taking vitamins E and B6, but a very few women cannot tolerate estrogen even in small doses. For these individuals, ERT is probably not a therapy of choice.

Again, you must remember that ERT is an ongoing regimen. You should have a dialogue with your caregiver and know that things may change; the dosage that was appropriate at one point in your life may not be appropriate at all times.

Can women who have not done well on birth control pills take ERT?

For two reasons, many women do well with ERT even if they have had difficulty with birth control pills. First, the dosages in ERT are much smaller, only about one-sixth the amount of hormone in low-dose birth control pills. The amount of estrogen that your body makes during your premenopausal years is somewhere between what you get on ERT and what you get on birth control pills.

A second difference between the two preparations is that birth control pills all use synthetic estrogens, whereas in this country the estrogens used in ERT are chemically identical to estrogens occurring in nature. So if you have had unpleasant side effects from the synthetic estrogen in birth control pills, your body may respond differently to the naturally occurring estrogen in ERT.

When should ERT begin?

Although the benefits of ERT are clear, the issue of when to start is controversial. Many women begin having menopausal symptoms, especially hot flashes and sleeplessness, long before they stop having periods. These women definitely benefit from taking estrogen and indeed feel better on ERT even though they have not yet reached menopause.

One school of thought, however, holds that women should not take any estrogen at all until they have had no periods for one year, that is, until they are fully menopausal. The members of this group argue that adding further estrogen to what you may still be producing yourself could lead to hyperplasia; since you are probably not making as much progesterone as formerly, you may not be producing what you need to trigger a menstrual period when you withdraw the progesterone; therefore the uterine lining can continue to build. Physicians who recommend starting ERT before full menopause believe that as long as you achieve a withdrawal bleed at least every two months, hyperplasia is unlikely to be an issue.

Another school believes that women who are still having fairly regular periods should take a small dose of estrogen every day without added progesterone. Since your body is maintaining a schedule of cleanout bleeds, you don't need the progesterone to protect your uterus, and the tiny extra amount of estrogen taken exogenously will not give you hyperplasia.

Yet another group suggests administering some progesterone and synchronizing it with the woman's natural cycle. The approach seems particularly useful for the woman who is having problems with flow. Her heavy bleeding suggests that she is not ovulating properly, that her own ovaries are not making enough progesterone. Giving this woman progesterone roughly day 16 through day 25 of the menstrual cycle, which her ovaries are still more or less orchestrating, often helps to control the bleeding. Some physicians prescribe the progesterone for twelve days, others give it for ten.

If you are concerned about osteoporosis somewhere down the line, you should begin ERT during the first few years after menopause, because that is the time of most rapid bone loss. Timing is less crucial for those concerned about cardiovascular protective benefits, which will start as soon as you begin ERT and continue for as long as you take it.

If I start ERT before I'm completely menopausal, how do I know when I'm going through menopause?

You will not be able to pinpoint the date of your menopause precisely because you will never know when your last period (regulated by your own hormones) occurred—but you can certainly make some assumptions. Since the average age at menopause in this country is about 51 years, you can infer that if you are 55 you have passed through menopause.

If you really are curious to determine your status, you can stop the estrogen for a while (say about two weeks), then have your FSH measured. If you are menopausal, your FSH should be significantly elevated after this time, somewhere over 30.

What should I do about birth control if I don't know whether I'm menopausal or not?

For many women the issue is not simply knowing that menopause occurred at age 51 or 52, but dealing with contraception. The old-time attitude is that you should wait a year after your last menstrual period before you stop using contraception. But if you don't have a "last" menstrual period, it is difficult to decide when that year is over. Nevertheless, you can make a pretty good decision based on age: it is extremely unlikely that you will conceive when you are 51 or 52 years old.

The problem is similar with women who are on low-dose birth control pills, which some physicians recommend for heavy or irregular perimenopausal bleeding and other symptoms of approaching menopause. If that is your situation, you will not know precisely when you are menopausal and when you should stop the birth control pills and start using ERT instead. What many physicians do is stop the pill, wait two weeks, and do a blood test to check the FSH level. If it is elevated, you can switch over to ERT; if it is not elevated, you can go back on the birth control pills. Obviously the birth control pills will give you contraceptive protection. If you are starting ERT while you are still having periods, let's say when you are 46 years old, then you should continue to use some kind of birth control. Your options are condoms, a diaphragm, or an intrauterine device (IUD).

How long do I have to use ERT?

The issue is two pronged: ERT can be used short term for alleviating problems such as hot flushes and sleep disturbances that are associated with the perimenopausal years. Or it can be used long term, which conveys important health benefits but also has potential risks. The benefits have been well defined, but because we lack sufficient research on women taking estrogen long term, the risks are not yet completely understood.

The average length of treatment in this country is currently only nine months, which means that women are using estrogen to deal with perimenopausal symptoms rather than for its long-term benefits. No increased risk of any disease seems to be associated with short-term estrogen therapy, as long as the woman taking the ERT had no medical reason not to start the therapy in the first place.

Routes of Delivery

All the estrogen used for ERT in this country is natural estrogen. Natural estrogens are those found in nature, or those made in laboratories whose chemical forms are identical to the estrogens occurring in nature. Among the natural estrogens are conjugated equine estrogens, 17 beta-estradiol (usually written 17 β-estradiol), estropipate, esterified estrogens, and estradiol valerate.

Synthetic estrogens are estrogens whose action may resemble that of natural estrogens, but whose chemical structure is different. Examples of synthetic estrogens are ethinyl estradiol and diethylstilbestrol (DES). These are never found in nature.

In what forms is estrogen available for ERT?

In this country estrogen is available in pills, on transdermal patches, and in vaginal creams. Most commonly, estrogen is taken orally, in the form of tablets. The dosages vary from brand to brand, but the usual routine is to take one tablet daily or half the dose twice daily, whichever is easier to remember.

Of the pills or tablets, one widely used brand is Premarin, generically known as conjugated equine estrogen. Premarin, derived from the urine of pregnant mares, has been sold since 1941, so most scientific studies on ERT have looked at this brand. A second widely prescribed brand is Estrace, which is micronized estradiol, a natural estrogen based on plant estrogens but produced in the laboratory. Estradiol is the main form of estrogen produced by the ovary during the reproductive years. Micronizing reduces the estradiol to particles small enough to be broken down by the digestive system. Ogen, Ortho-Est, and Estratab are other brands of natural estrogen tablets.

Estrogen can also be administered through the skin, by means of a transdermal patch. The original transdermal patch, sold as Estraderm, is a small plastic disk on which estradiol has been dissolved in a jellylike solution, which is contained in a little reservoir on the surface of the patch. You pull off the backing and stick the patch on your skin, usually on your buttocks or abdomen. You should not place the patch on your breasts; because breast tissue is so sensitive to estrogen, it should not be exposed directly to the undiluted dose. The patch remains in place for three or four days. The estrogen is thereby absorbed in a gradual manner through the skin into the bloodstream.

In 1995 a new kind of transdermal patch was introduced, which needs changing only once a week. Marketed under the name Climara, this patch has the estradiol impregnated in the adhesive on the patch instead of dissolved in a solution on the surface, allowing the whole surface of the patch to adhere to the skin. It seems to deliver more constant levels of estrogen over its one-week lifetime than did the earlier patch. Preliminary tests also suggest that it stays on better.

For certain purposes estrogen can be used as a vaginal cream. Premarin, Estrace, Ogen, and Dienestrol are available in this form. The cream comes with an applicator, a plastic tube with a plunger (basically the same kind you get with contraceptive foams), which you use to insert the cream into the vagina. Vaginal estrogen is used solely for atrophic vaginal symptoms and for urinary problems, since only a small amount is absorbed into the body. Most people devise a regimen that keeps them comfortable and use it perhaps two or three times a week.

The cream is best applied at bedtime, because it tends to leak out when you are standing or sitting.

Estrogen is also available in injectable form, as estradiol valerate. Before the introduction of the transdermal patch, injectable estrogen was used quite widely for people who did not tolerate oral estrogen well, but since patches have become available, injectable estrogen is used much less frequently. Nonetheless, it is still manufactured in the United States and is still available. To maintain satisfactory levels you need fairly frequent injections (unlike Depo-Provera, which lasts a long time) and most women are not anxious to have a lot of shots.

In England, but not in the United States, estrogen is available as an implant, a pellet that is placed under the skin by a physician. The implant slowly releases estrogen over a fairly long period and is replaced at intervals; the procedure is similar to that of Norplant, which is progesterone implanted under the skin for birth control. No particular danger is associated with these implants, and they have been extensively used in England for years. Although many women might find implants a convenient way to take estrogen, there is no apparent impetus toward introducing them in this country.

Other ways to take estrogen are available in England and Europe. A product called Oestrogel, which is absorbed through the skin, is used in Europe. The gel is rubbed on the arms, shoulders, and abdomen and dries in a few minutes without stickiness or odor. The skin acts as a reservoir for the estrogen in the gel, releasing it gradually into the bloodstream. Vaginal rings containing estrogen have also been developed overseas.

Which is better, patch or pill?

Sometimes people who do poorly on one form of estrogen, say oral Premarin, will do better on another type. If you get queasy on Premarin, you may feel better using transdermal patches, because by this delivery route the estrogen bypasses your digestive tract. If you get headaches from the oral estrogen, you may do better with the patches. Still, some women experience skin irritation from them and find the oral delivery route an improvement. Preliminary data suggest that the Climara patch is less likely to cause skin irritation than other patches.

The propatch people say that patches are better because estrogen that is absorbed gradually across the skin is not metabolized directly, at full strength, by the liver in what is called a first-pass effect. If estrogen can be injurious to the liver, the transdermal route is probably preferable. Women at risk for gallbladder disease and phlebitis might also be better served by the transdermal route. Clotting factors (substances that cause blood to clot) are manufactured by the liver. Since high levels of estrogen in the liver increase its production of these clotting factors, oral estrogen is not desirable for people with phlebitis.

Antipatch people point out that by bypassing the liver with the first-pass effect, you do not get as strong a rise in HDL, your good cholesterol; it is really metabolism of estrogen by the liver that affects the amount of HDL in your bloodstream. Research has not yet provided a definitive answer about the relative desirability of the patch and the pill.

What are the pros and cons of vaginal estrogen creams?

Although small amounts of estrogen do get absorbed through the tissues of the vagina, vaginal estrogen cream will not protect you from osteoporosis or coronary artery disease; nor will it relieve your hot flashes. Because the vagina and bladder are located so close to each other, the estrogen absorbed through the vagina does affect the urinary tract, and many women find that symptoms of urinary frequency and discomfort improve when they take vaginal estrogen.

Researchers are not in agreement on exactly how much estrogen is absorbed through the vagina; and studies show anything from zero absorption to complete absorption. In general, however, scientists agree that far less estrogen is absorbed from the vaginal cream than from the pill or the transdermal patch.

If you are worried about breast cancer, yet you still have problems of dryness and vaginal discomfort, this route is a reasonable solution for you. Women who have had chemotherapy for breast cancer that has shut down their ovarian function, either temporarily or permanently, often find vaginal estrogen helpful.

What are standard dosages and commercial brands of progesterone?

Most physicians try to start with the lowest dose of progesterone. The progesterone that most physicians prescribe is medroxyprogesterone, which comes under several brand names: Provera, Cycrin, and Amen. The standard dosage used to be 10 mg of medroxyprogesterone, but in the last five to eight years many physicians have begun to believe that 5 mg of progesterone for twelve days of the month will give virtually the same protection of the endometrium with fewer side effects. While you may get slightly better protection with 10 mg for the same time frame, the higher dosage may not be worth the side effects.

Researchers have looked at even smaller dosages, and their studies seem to confirm that 5 mg is the smallest amount (assuming standard estrogen dosages) that prevents hyperplasia when the progesterone is given cyclically. When progesterone is given throughout the month, the usual dosage is 2.5 mg.

In what forms is progesterone available for ERT?

Like estrogen, progesterone is available in synthetic and natural forms, but most of the progesterone used in this country for ERT is synthetic. Most commonly, progesterone is delivered as a pill or tablet. Common brands are Provera, which is medroxyprogesterone, and Aygestin, which is norethindrone acetate.

Researchers are currently testing progesterone rings, but these have not yet been released for general use. Made of plastic coated with progesterone, they are placed in the vagina rather like a diaphragm; over time the progesterone is absorbed up into the uterus. The concept behind these vaginal rings is protection of the uterine lining from hyperplasia without all the systemic side effects of progesterone.

Does progesterone have side effects?

Unlike estrogen, which generally seems to make people feel better, progesterone can have negative side effects. It can cause headaches. It can cause chest pain if people have reactive, sensitive coronary arteries. It can increase the levels of LDL (bad cholesterol) in the blood. It can make women irritable, so that they feel very much the way they do just before their menstrual periods. In fact, the side effects of progesterone are annoying enough that some women give up ERT.

Schedules and Regimens

On what days of the month do I take estrogen? What are the usual cycles?

The standard regimen used to be that you would take estrogen on days 1 to 25 of each month and add progesterone on days 16 to 25. For the last five or six days of the month you would take neither. During the week when you were taking neither estrogen nor progesterone, you would have a period. Then, starting the first day of the next month, you would begin the estrogen again. This regimen mimicked the body's action during the normal menstrual cycle.

What has changed over the past ten years is in response to the fact that a lot of women don't feel well on their days without estrogen. Women who have very sensitive coronary artery disease get chest pains; others experience hot flashes and insomnia. So during the past decade many physicians have switched to continuous ERT; the patient takes estrogen every single day of the month and adds progesterone for twelve days of the cycle.

Some women still prefer to have five days off all hormones at the end of the month, often because they get tender breasts and five days without estrogen relieves the soreness. Certainly skipping these five days causes no problems. All the same, more women seem comfortable using the estrogen straight through.

What are the usual routines for adding progesterone?

As we have seen, the major reason for taking progesterone is prevention of hyperplasia, and progesterone is very effective for this purpose. There are several schools of thought about when and how long to take progesterone, but the choices are basically between daily progesterone and cyclic progesterone. The notion of cyclic progesterone (estrogen on days 1 to 25 of the menstrual cycle with progesterone added on days 16 to 25) was inspired by the hormone sequence of the normal menstrual cycle. The ovaries make estrogen almost all the time, but the body makes progesterone only during the second half of the cycle, after ovulation.

Many physicians still use this method and most suggest using progesterone for twelve days, in order to get full protection of the lining of the uterus. Some actually recommend progesterone for fourteen days, which perfectly mimics the twenty-eight-day menstrual cycle in which ovulation occurs on the fourteenth day and progesterone is produced for the subsequent fourteen days.

Another school believes in continuous low-dose progesterone. Because many women objected to the periodic bleeding that cyclic progesterone withdrawal causes, physicians began experimenting with different regimens of progesterone usage. What would happen, for example, if a patient took a very small dose of progesterone every day instead of a larger amount for twelve or fourteen days each month? This continuous regimen turned out to be quite effective in preventing cancer of the endometrium; in fact, all the studies done today show basically equivalent protection from the two approaches.

If I take progesterone, will I have periods even though my own have stopped?

If you are taking cyclic progesterone, you will probably have periods. Even though you are fully menopausal and your own ovaries are not producing enough estrogen for your uterine lining to build up, the estrogen in ERT will stimulate your endometrium. When you take progesterone and then withdraw it at the end of the month, that withdrawal will cause the lining to shed.

A small percentage of women do not bleed when the progesterone is withdrawn. For them the lack of withdrawal bleeding is normal and nothing to worry about.

Women who have been taking progesterone and estrogen for some time after menopause often find that their bleeding becomes progressively less. Some skip a period from time to time. Indeed, many women who have been on estrogen with progesterone for a while have almost no bleeding; a few continue to have periods that seem fairly similar to the ones they had when they were younger.

If I have periods when I withdraw progesterone, will I have cramps?

Even if you have had heavy cramps during your periods, chances are that you will not have them on ERT.

How long after withdrawal of progesterone will I get my period?

Usually bleeding occurs right at the end of the progesterone regimen or within three or four days of withdrawing it. If this pattern changes (if, for example, your period comes very much later than expected), you should notify your caregiver.

If I start bleeding while I am taking progesterone, what should I do?

As with any unexpected postmenopausal bleeding, you should alert your physician. You should also keep on taking the progesterone. It is the progesterone that protects you against hyperplasia, not the bleeding, so you must keep taking it for the length of time your physician recommends. If you bleed while you are taking progesterone, it is possible that you are not taking enough, so you should also be able to discuss the pattern of bleeding when you talk to your caregiver. When did the bleeding begin, on the fourth day after you started the progesterone or the tenth? Is there any pattern to the bleeding? For example, have you occasionally started bleeding on day 10 after you started the progesterone, whereas this month you suddenly began to bleed on day 4?

If I have been taking cyclic estrogen and progesterone and don't get a period when I stop the progesterone, can it mean that I am pregnant?

If you have never skipped a period except when you were pregnant, it can be worrisome if suddenly you skip one even after withdrawing progesterone. If your ovaries have shut down and are no longer releasing their monthly follicles, you cannot be pregnant. But if you worry that you started ERT before you were fully menopausal, you can have a blood test to ascertain whether you are pregnant.

If I take progesterone cyclically, does it matter which twelve days I take it?

Obviously you should take your progesterone at the same time each month. Many women find it convenient, and easy to remember, to do so the first twelve days of the month, but there is no reason you can't start on the thirteenth or the twenty-seventh or any other day—as long as you are consistent.

Do I still get the protective action of progesterone, even though I don't have periods when it is withdrawn?

Yes. Even if you don't get the withdrawal bleed, progesterone is acting to flatten out the lining of the uterus, to control the growth of the endometrium. The situation is similar to that of many women who don't get much of a period on low-dose birth control pills. It's not the period, it's the progesterone that counts. So even if you stop getting periods when you withdraw the progesterone, you still need to keep taking it.

What happens if I forget to take a progesterone pill one day?

Nothing. You might have some bleeding, but continue with your regular progesterone schedule.

What happens if I forget to take my estrogen pill one day?

Again, nothing dangerous happens, since going on and off ERT is not hazardous to your health. You might have a hot flash or two as your body reminds you that you have forgotten your pill, or you may find yourself waking up in the middle of the night. Just take another pill the next day.

What are the lowest doses of estrogen that will protect me against coronary heart disease and osteoporosis?

Generally it is believed that 0.625 mg Premarin or 1 mg Estrace will protect you against coronary heart disease and osteoporosis. Most people are comfortable at up to twice that level.

Occasional women, even with the lower of these dosages, will experience breast discomfort, bloating, or queasiness. Tablets with smaller amounts of hormone are becoming available. Nowadays there is a 0.3 mg dose of Premarin and a 0.5 dose of Estrace, which you might consider "baby" dosages of these drugs, but there is no patch form available lower than the 0.5 patch.

These lower dosages, however, may not give you absolute protection against osteoporosis and coronary artery disease. Some research papers published in England have shown that 0.3 of Premarin is effective in preventing osteoporosis. However, these studies included women who were taking a great deal of calcium as well as the smaller amount of estrogen. Studies in this country generally do not focus on calcium intake, but instead examine only estrogen intake. Therefore, if you choose a lower estrogen dosage, you should be very vigilant about getting enough calcium in your diet or in supplements and about following a weight-bearing exercise program.

How can I lower my dose if I am taking ERT with the patch?

It is easy to lower your dosage if you are taking ERT orally, but since the smallest patch size delivers 0.5 mg of estradiol daily, you have to resort to ingenuity to lower your dosage. The best approach is to stretch out the time you use each patch. If you are using the Estroderm patch, you can change every four or five days instead of every three or four days. If you are using the Climara patch, change it at intervals somewhat longer than a week.

Do these dosages remain stable forever?

If you find that the dosage of estrogen that formerly worked for you is no longer appropriate, you might have to either increase or decrease the amount you are taking. Dosages change for a lot of reasons. Suppose you start taking ERT in your perimenopausal years. As you get further into the menopausal process, you may find that you need to increase your dose to relieve menopausal discomforts because your ovaries are making less estrogen. Some women, on the other hand, find that after they have been on estrogen for a while, they can cut back on their dose and taper off.

Many individuals find that in hot weather they need more estrogen. If it's 95 degrees outdoors and you are hot and sweating, and then you start flashing, you might want to take extra estrogen to help regulate your temperature. If you are going on vacation to a tropical climate, you might want to take a slightly higher amount. There is nothing wrong or dangerous about doubling your dose periodically. So just because in August 1995 you are taking a certain dosage, it doesn't mean that you will be taking that amount forever.

How do I find the dosage that is right for me?

Physicians tend to start with the smallest dose of estrogen that will prevent osteoporosis and use that as a baseline. That is my own approach. From that point I continue to be something of an empiricist and adjust the dose upward or downward until it relieves menopausal symptoms without causing side effects.

Some physicians believe in taking estradiol levels or FSH levels to determine the appropriateness of a given dose, but problems arise in determining what the tests mean. Let's start with the estradiol levels. The Premarin or Estrace that you are taking in your ERT is converted by the body to several different kinds of estrogen, estradiol being just one of them. Even 17-beta estradiol (the main ingredient of Estrace) is converted to other forms of estrogen in the blood. So if the lab test measures only the estradiol in your blood, it is ignoring the other estrogens that are present and may be contributing to the total level of estrogen circulating in your blood. Maybe your estradiol level is low, but you are still comfortable. Do you need to change your dose? Probably not.

Or look at the other extreme. An estradiol level of 100 is, by general consensus, an adequate level. But suppose you are still not sleeping. Suppose you are still getting hot flashes. Is there danger in taking larger doses and reaching a blood level of 150? Probably not.

A problem with using laboratory tests for FSH to determine dose level is that even women who are being adequately replaced on ERT will have slightly elevated FSH levels. You may be comfortable, able to sleep, and undisturbed by hot flashes, you may be getting good osteoporosis protection and adequate protection against coronary artery disease, but your FSH level will still be high. So the FSH test will not tell you that the dosage is appropriate.

What are the concerns about taking too much estrogen?

The major concerns are the effect on the breasts of increased estrogen levels and the side effects of too much estrogen. So far, researchers have not documented the effects of different blood estrogen levels on the breasts and do not know whether the risk of breast cancer is dose related. The main side effects of too much estrogen are breast discomfort, bloating, headaches, and queasiness.

Can each of us find a dosage that is comfortable?

As in the rest of life, there are trade-offs. For some people it is very difficult to find just the right amount of estrogen. One patient whom I see gets occasional, though not frequent, hot flashes when she takes 0.625 mg of Premarin. When I raise her dose to 0.9 mg, the hot flashes go away but she gets headaches.

What should she do? There are no pills that come in dosages between 0.625 and 0.9 mg, but she could alternate a 0.625 one day with a 0.9 the next. She could break a 0.3 mg pill in half and take that plus a 0.625 mg pill. Beyond that, the decision is up to her. Is it worse to get the headache or is it worse to get the hot flash?

What are the advantages and disadvantages of continuous progesterone?

The main advantage is that you do not get the regular withdrawal bleeds you get with cyclic progesterone. Unfortunately, some women—not all, but a fairly large number—do get some spotting, staining, or light flow on an erratic basis when they take these small doses of progesterone. The bad news is that this spotting is irregular. It may come on day 2 of the cycle, or it may come on day 16, or on day 25.

Any unpredictable spotting or staining can be worrisome, and many physi-

cians will biopsy women who have begun spotting after taking daily progesterone, just to be sure that nothing is wrong.

Most of the time this staining or goes away within three months. If it is persistent, it can become a major annoyance. Women who would prefer a light
period at a predictable time to unpredictable spotting and staining probably
would do better on cyclic progesterone, but it is an individual decision.

Must I have a period every month to protect my uterus?

One of the main reasons that women stop ERT is that they don't like the inconvenience of bleeding, even though these periods may be considerably lighter
than the ones they were getting before therapy began. If you are planning a
camping trip in the mountains or a vacation to the Virgin Islands or China, or
you are going to be involved in some activity where it would seriously inconvenience you to have a period, don't take your progesterone that month. You will
not get uterine hyperplasia from skipping one month of Provera. The next
month, just start again.

If you are one of the people who is seriously and significantly troubled by
taking progesterone, but you want to remain on ERT, you can probably get away
with taking the progesterone every other month. Although there are no scientifically documented, rigorously controlled studies to verify this hypothesis, the
clinical experience of many menopause experts suggests that taking progesterone
every other month provides adequate protection.

In general, the older you are, the less important it is to produce a withdrawal
bleed each month. If you are in your fifties or sixties, you should withdraw the
progesterone at least every other month; if you are in your seventies or eighties,
probably every third month is all right. Dr. Philip M. Sarrel, head of the
Menopause Clinic at Yale, has 90-year-olds on ERT. He withdraws all these
elderly women from Provera on January 1 each year and gives them one period
per year. And sometimes they do not get a withdrawal bleed.

Do women who have had hysterectomies need progesterone?

Because the sole reason for taking progesterone postmenopausally is to protect
the uterus, there is no reason whatsoever for anyone who has had a hysterectomy
to take it. It used to be thought that progesterone had a protective effect on the
breast, but most physicians no longer believe that to be true. Progesterone does

not have an effect on the breast similar to its action on the uterus. In the last five years physicians have certainly gotten away from routine use of progesterone in women who have had hysterectomies.

What can I do if I am someone who does not tolerate progesterone well?

There are a few strategies for women who don't tolerate progesterone well but need it to prevent hyperplasia. First, you can try using the minimal dose. Many women still take the old-style 10 mg of Provera for twelve days of every month. These women can try 5 mg, and many will feel better.

Second, there are substitutes for Provera, Amen, or Cycrin, all of which contain the synthetic progesterone, medroxyprogesterone. Aygestin, whose generic name is norethindrone, is just as effective in preventing hyperplasia, and some women tolerate it better than they tolerate medroxyprogesterone. Micronor, another synthetic progestin based on norethindrone and used in birth control pills, is a different option.

Women who tolerate neither of these progestins can try natural progesterone. Oral natural progesterone must be micronized, that is, prepared specially so that it is not inactivated by the digestive tract but can be absorbed orally. The equivalent dose is 200 mg a day. Recent studies have shown natural progesterone to be safe, and many people tolerate it better than synthetics. Because it has a relatively short half-life in the body, it really should be taken twice a day.

The problem with natural progesterone is that it is not available at every corner drugstore because it is difficult to synthesize. None of the major pharmaceutical companies make it. Still, some pharmacies in the United States will make it up if you ask, and it is available at some mail-order pharmacies (for example, the Women's International Pharmacy in Madison, Wisconsin: tel. 800-279-5708). Natural progesterone is a bit more expensive than synthetic progesterone.

Natural progesterone, available in the form of yam extract creams, is recommended by many naturopaths. It is well absorbed through the skin, but the amount absorbed varies from woman to woman and the preparations themselves are not usually standardized. Thus you do not always know exactly how much you are getting.

A handful of women don't do well on any progesterone at all, natural or synthetic. For them there are several options. If they want to take estrogen postmenopausally, they can do so—realizing that their risk of uterine cancer does increase without progesterone. Statistically, you are better off taking estrogen even without progesterone than you are not taking estrogen at all, because your risk of coronary artery disease goes down, as does your risk of osteoporosis.

If I am taking estrogen alone, are there ways to check for possible excessive growth of the uterine lining?

First of all, if you experience any type of bleeding, you should report it to your caregiver. Beyond that, many physicians recommend either an annual ultrasound of the pelvis or a yearly routine biopsy for women who are taking estrogen but not countering it with progesterone.

Ultrasound technology makes the lining of the uterus visible as a kind of stripe along the muscular inner wall of the uterus. By measuring the width of the endometrial stripe, as it is called in the technological jargon, a doctor can get some information about whether or not there is hyperplasia. If the endometrial stripe measures 7 mm or less, you can be reasonably sure that there is no hyperplasia. This does not mean that if the stripe is wider than 7 mm, hyperplasia is definitely present, but it does mean that a biopsy may be in order.

This application of ultrasound technology is relatively new and may not be available in smaller population centers. Instead of just performing routine biopsies, which can be uncomfortable, physicians who have access to the technology are using ultrasound, in part to distinguish those who are bleeding from normal atrophic changes in the uterus from those with hyperplasia.

The traditional way of checking for endometrial hyperplasia is with a biopsy, during which a sample of the endometrial tissue is taken for checking.

What if I have hyperplasia and still want to continue with ERT?

If women on estrogen replacement therapy who cannot tolerate progesterone develop hyperplasia, the only alternative to stopping the estrogen is a hysterectomy. This significant decision should be made only after careful thought. Some of my own patients feel strongly enough about ERT that they have preferred hysterectomy to withdrawing the therapy.

Grace Q. is 59 years old. She has significant arthritis but keeps it under control by exercising daily, so she is quite mobile. When she doesn't exercise, she stiffens up and has increased pain. Grace has taken estrogen since menopause and does well on it. However, she cannot tolerate progesterone, which gives her headaches. Without the progesterone

Figure 11. *The endometrial stripe. Ultrasound can be used to measure the thickness of the lining of the uterus, which shows up on the scan as a stripe. A thin stripe is rarely associated with precancerous conditions or with cancer itself.*

she developed endometrial hyperplasia and clearly needed a hysterectomy if she wanted to continue with the estrogen. After some thought, she decided that hysterectomy was her choice. As it turned out, her uterus was quite small so that she was a good candidate for a laparoscope-assisted hysterectomy. She had the operation and recuperated so quickly that she was back in the gym after only two weeks.

How long should ERT continue?

There are certainly data from reliable scientific studies that say that ongoing ERT conveys many benefits and that the longer you take it, the longer you will enjoy the benefits. Women who find it distressing to think they will be taking ERT as long as they live should know that they can stop at any time. A widely held myth claims that it is dangerous to go on and off hormones, but in fact there is no danger whatsoever to stopping and starting.

What happens if I do stop ERT?

If you decide to stop, you do not have to taper off, since stopping ERT abruptly is not medically dangerous. However, you may be more comfortable if you stop gradually. In general, quitting "cold turkey" does not produce withdrawal symptoms, and most women do not suddenly get depressed or have other symptoms. A few who quit abruptly get significant hot flashes. These flashes usually go away

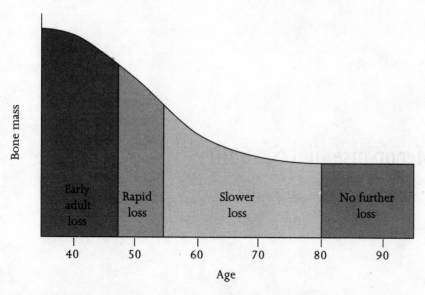

Figure 12. *Bone loss over time, showing periods of rapid and slow bone loss. Bone loss starts by a woman's mid-thirties. Without ERT it accelerates right after menopause. If ERT is taken and then stopped, the rate of loss increases.*

in a few months, but some women find them so uncomfortable that they go back on the ERT.

Of course, if you stop taking estrogen, you will lose its protective benefits. But if you are taking it to maintain strong bones, you will find yourself at age 60, for example, with more bone than you would have had if you had not been taking ERT since menopause. If you are taking it to protect against coronary artery disease, then the protection will end.

Is ERT addictive?

No, it is not like nicotine in cigarettes or other addictive substances. Usually women can stop without withdrawal symptoms, though a few have hot flashes.

9 Menopause and Sexuality

One of the myths of menopause holds that when a woman reaches menopause her sex life ends. As many women at midlife know, this is not true. But if menopause is a time of biological change, then for many women it is a time of sexual change also. Sexuality in middle age, as in other times of life, has physical, emotional, and even social components; so the changes that take place during the years surrounding menopause may be influenced by all these factors.

Physical factors may include changes in the structure and lubrication of the vagina that lead to discomfort or pain during intercourse, diseases (for example, heart disease or high blood pressure), or surgical repairs to correct incontinence, which could make sexual functioning difficult. Emotional factors include a woman's general outlook during menopause and her specific feelings about being menopausal. In the past, when female sexuality was presumed to be bound to reproductive capacity, women were thought to become disinterested in sex when they became menopausal because they were mourning their lost ability to produce babies. Although the close ties between reproductive capacity and sexual pleasure may be extremely meaningful to some women, they certainly are not significant to all women. For many, in fact, the certainty that pregnancy is no longer a risk heightens sexual pleasure.

Sexual functioning is also affected by self-esteem. A culture that holds that only young women are sexually desirable, or that sex is the exclusive province of the young, may make it difficult for an older woman to hold onto her self-esteem and to see herself as desirable. Women who feel that they are unattractive—too fat, too flabby, too saggy—may feel less inclined to sexual activity than women who have higher regard for themselves.

The most important element of sexual activity is a couple's response to their relationship and their ability to communicate within it. If someone comes to me and says her husband just isn't interested in sex any more or cannot perform, I ask her how she feels about that. Sometimes she is just as glad not to have a sex life. But if she has a sense of frustration and loss, then I try to help. As her physician, I want her to be comfortable and happy. I want her to realize that no single standard of sexual activity is acceptable whereas all others are not.

Often patients come to me for reassurance, which is not surprising in a society where sex is emphasized so strongly even though so much ambiguity exists. I cannot emphasize enough the importance of communication in a relationship. If you feel that your libido is diminished and you are worried about it, talk to your partner. If he really doesn't have any strong desire for intercourse either, you need not be upset any longer.

Difficulties do arise when one partner's desire is significantly different from the other's. Whether the woman wants sex and the man doesn't or the woman doesn't want sex and the man does, there is a problem. If both partners have active libidos and strong performance abilities and both are happy with that situation, then everything is fine. If neither of them has strong libido or performance ability and they are equally matched in desire, that's fine too.

It is also true that many forms of sexual functioning can be satisfying to both partners. As long as they are pleasing to both the man and the woman, oral intercourse and mutual masturbation are healthy forms of sexual activity.

What are the causes of sexual discomfort in postmenopausal women?

The most common problem reported to me is discomfort during intercourse. The primary reason is that without estrogen the vagina becomes dry, a condition known as atrophic vaginitis, and for many women (but not all) intercourse becomes painful, a condition technically known as dyspareunia. Unlike hot flashes or sleep disturbances, which improve with time, vaginal dryness gets worse the longer a woman is deprived of estrogen.

It makes sense to suppose that the vagina would be sensitive to loss of estrogen, since of all the bodily organs the vagina has perhaps the most estrogen receptors. When a woman's ovaries no longer produce estrogen, the walls of her vagina become thinner. The cells lining the vagina become flatter, less plump, and fewer in number. They do not produce as much lubricant as they did when stimulated by estrogen and they do not support the vagina as well. Nor are the vaginal walls as elastic and resilient as they were in the presence of estrogen.

An examining physician can see these changes with the aid of a speculum and make a quick assessment of a woman's estrogen status. Fatter women tend to be less afflicted with vaginal dryness than their thinner sisters, because fat produces a kind of estrogen called estrone.

Does the size of the vagina change after menopause?

The answer is a qualified yes. Women who remain sexually active tend to remain in better shape, vaginally speaking, than women who do not. The old "use it or lose it" metaphor is appropriate (though not exactly elegant) in this instance.

Does vaginal atrophy create problems other than uncomfortable intercourse?

Two problems that sometimes accompany vaginal atrophy are vaginal infections and urinary tract infections. As the walls of the vagina thin out and become dryer, these tissues are more easily injured and irritated and more vulnerable to infection. During your reproductive years the chemical climate of the vagina is slightly acidic, though the degree of acidity fluctuates during the menstrual cycle. This acidic environment discourages the growth of harmful bacteria but encourages the growth of your own vaginal flora, microorganisms that live in the vagina and fight infection. When the vagina becomes more alkaline, as it does when we age, it becomes more hospitable to hostile bacteria and less supportive of helpful ones.

Urinary tract infections occur with some frequency in older women for the same reasons. Just as the walls of the vagina thin out and are less well lubricated after menopause, the walls of the bladder, which also have many estrogen receptors, undergo changes and become more prone to infection. The friction and activity of sexual intercourse can exacerbate the process.

Does vaginal atrophy have causes other than estrogen depletion?

Women who have had radiation therapy in the region of their vagina, perhaps for cervical cancer, may have scar tissue in the vagina. In addition to the scar tissue's being less elastic than normal tissue, the vagina itself may have shrunk. Women who have had vaginal repair surgery for a prolapsed uterus, rectocele, or cystocele, may—rarely—end up with a vagina that is too narrow to function comfortably during sex.

Are vaginal changes reversible?

Virtually without exception, vaginal changes caused by inactivity, radiation therapy, or surgery are reversible. You can almost always get back into good vaginal shape, just as you can almost always get back into good physical shape generally.

I always tell patients who find intercourse painful after periods of inactivity or for other reasons to come in and talk to me. I have treated a number of women who had not had intercourse for ten years or so and then found a new partner. The first few times such women have intercourse they are going to be uncomfortable, especially if they don't use vaginal lubrication. I encourage those of them who are not on oral ERT to let me prescribe a vaginal estrogen cream, so that when they do become sexually active again, intercourse will not hurt. In addition to the physical distress, vaginal discomfort is a significant sexual turnoff for both partners.

Some of the women who come into the office are fifteen or twenty years postmenopausal, and their sex lives have gone from satisfactory to nonexistent—because they are uncomfortable. It is understandable that sex would not appeal to them if it is painful, but their husbands or partners are not happy with the situation. If these women are not willing to try oral ERT, I suggest vaginal estrogen, which can be applied in the form of a cream. And I have had husbands write me thank-you notes.

Another possibility is vaginal dilators, which a physician may prescribe to help restore the vagina to its normal size. Women who have scar tissue in their vagina or who have been sexually inactive for long periods often find them useful. The dilators are little cylinders in graded sizes, which you insert into the vagina with a lubricant such as K-Y jelly. They are made by different surgical supply companies in plastic, rubber, or glass. The smallest ones are narrow, perhaps the width of a couple of pencils. You leave them in for a few minutes each

Figure 13. *Vaginal dilators are rubber cylinders in graduated sizes that can be used to stretch the vagina.*

day, gradually increasing the size of the dilator that you insert. With the use of these dilators in combination with topical estrogen cream, most women can become functional again.

Some women whose vagina is too tight after surgery need more than dilator therapy. They have to return to surgery to have their vaginal repair relaxed; but this outcome is uncommon.

Do forms of sexual activity other than intercourse (for example, masturbation) help keep the vagina in good shape?

The fact that a woman doesn't have a male sexual partner doesn't mean that she must be sexually inactive. Many women who miss sexual activity when they become widowed or divorced turn to masturbation as a source of pleasure or stimulation. This substitute is perfectly all right and certainly contributes to keeping your vagina well lubricated.

Many women do not have sexual partners when they reach menopause. They may be single, widowed, or, more likely, divorced. At this time of life many women, switching their sexual orientation, turn to other women for sexual and psychological closeness. This too is a viable solution to sexual loneliness for many older women.

You should feel comfortable discussing these matters with your gynecologist, as should your gynecologist with you. One of the complaints sometimes leveled against male gynecologists, rightly or wrongly, is that many seem to assume that without a male partner a woman cannot be sexually active.

What therapies are available for postmenopausal vaginal discomfort?

Although hormonal and nonhormonal therapies are available for most symptoms surrounding menopause, the clear winner as far as vaginal dryness is concerned is estrogen in some form. There are lubricants for intercourse, which are satisfactory for the acute act; but for persistent vaginal dryness and the other complications that sometimes follow it (for example, vaginal infections or bladder infections), estrogen in some form is the only satisfactory solution.

The products available for lubrication specifically during intercourse include H-R or K-Y jelly or Lubrin, all of which are water soluble. One whimsically named product is Astroglide, made in California. When it first came out, it was available only in that state and people had to send away for it; now it is widely available. Certain high-quality massage oils can also give short-term pleasure and relief from dryness; these can be purchased over the counter. Although they will not hurt you, Vaseline and other petroleum-based lubricants are less satisfactory because they are sticky and tend to dry the vaginal tissues.

Are there nonhormonal lubricants that are intended to be used for vaginal dryness at other times?

For all-day lubrication both hormonal and non-hormonal products are available. The leading nonhormonal cream is called Replens. Although it can be used for intercourse, that is not what it is intended for. What it seems to do is to augment surface fluids in the vagina without stimulation by estrogen. You apply it three times a week on a regular basis, not just before intercourse. The company that manufactures it sends out literature that includes scientific studies suggesting that the product does cause an increase in vaginal lubrication without hormonal therapy.

If I am on oral ERT and still have lubrication problems, is it all right to use a commercial lubricant?

Certainly; you can use K-Y jelly or Astroglide or other products. Many of my patients find this solution satisfactory.

Will vaginal estrogen cream keep my vagina in good shape?

While oral estrogen is the best remedy for problems such as hot flashes, sleep-lessness, and bone loss, vaginal estrogen is very effective for vaginal dryness. My observations of patients suggest that women who are not using oral estrogen tend to get more vaginitis and more bladder infections if their vagina is dry and atrophic, and I sometimes recommend vaginal estrogen cream for these women also. The cream is not intended as a lubricant for intercourse, because the consistency is not ideal. It is meant to help the cells lining the vaginal walls produce the lubricant that you need to be comfortable during intercourse.

Do estrogen creams help with vaginal atrophy?

Women who don't want to or cannot take oral ERT can use vaginal estrogen creams, which stimulate the tissues of the vagina to produce their own lubrication. Very little estrogen is absorbed through the walls of the vagina, and usually the creams make a great deal of difference both in vaginal comfort and in reduction of infections. These creams, which come in the same brands as oral estrogen, are available by prescription only.

Who can use vaginal estrogen creams?

These creams are safe for virtually anyone. They are especially useful to younger women who have had premature menopause, either through chemotherapy or through surgery.

Brenda F. is 33 years old and has had breast cancer. Her oncologist has pursued the disease aggressively and prescribed chemotherapy to try to prevent recurrences. Chemotherapy often knocks out normal ovarian function, either temporarily or permanently, and consequently Brenda has undergone a kind of chemical menopause. Her oncologist does not approve of oral ERT, because many breast cancers, especially in younger women, respond to estrogen. Brenda is young and wants to be sexually active. Estrogen cream can be a big help to her, and her oncologist has no objection to it.

How do I use vaginal estrogen cream?

The cream is made by the same pharmaceutical companies that make oral estrogen, and it comes in those brand names (Premarin, Estrace, Ogen, and others). You apply it with an applicator, much like the applicators that accompany birth control creams, and insert it into the vagina two or three times a week at any time convenient for you. Bedtime is usually best, so that the cream doesn't leak out. If your own lubrication is not adequate even with the vaginal estrogen cream, you may also use K-Y jelly or Astroglide or the equivalent for intercourse itself.

Does vaginal estrogen cream get absorbed into the bloodstream?

Some of it does, but in general only a very small amount. The cream does remain in the vagina for a while (a day or a few days), and during this time the estrogen is absorbed through the vaginal walls.

Would vaginal estrogen cream have any consequences for my sexual partner?

No, it is not dangerous to your partner even if it remains in your vagina during intercourse. It will not have feminizing effects on him.

Are there any side effects of vaginal estrogen cream?

I have already suggested that vaginal estrogen cream, because some is absorbed through the walls of the vagina, is helpful to women who have frequent bladder infections. It may also aid women with urinary incontinence.

Some women are allergic to certain brands of estrogen creams. The tissues of the vulva and vagina are very sensitive to allergens, and occasional women experience itching and burning. The cause of the trouble may not be the estrogen itself, but the base in which it is dissolved. Since there are several brands, if one does not work, you can try another.

If you have not had intercourse for a long time, putting anything into your vagina may produce discomfort, even something normally nonallergenic such as K-Y jelly. For women in this situation I sometimes do a little arm twisting and suggest that they go on oral estrogen for a month to lubricate the vagina and replenish its cells enough so that they can then use topical estrogen cream.

How much does estrogen cream cost?

Like any form of estrogen, vaginal estrogen creams are expensive, in the neighborhood of twenty to thirty dollars a tube. The price differs from brand to brand.

Are there changes in female sexual responsiveness in middle age that are unrelated to vaginal discomfort?

Some women notice changes about the time of menopause that are not related to vaginal discomfort. They feel fine, sex is comfortable for them physically, but they notice that their sexual desire and their response to sexual stimulation have changed significantly. Perhaps they have less interest in sex, or when they do have sex they find it less enjoyable. They will say that they have no more flushes or other symptoms of menopause, but they have no interest in sex.

Remember that estrogen is a vasodilator. There is strong evidence that estrogen profoundly enhances blood flow to the pelvis as well as to other organs, including the brain. Progesterone, in contrast, may limit pelvic blood flow. Therefore many postmenopausal women who lack estrogen do notice a change in how they feel during sexual activity. This difference may have something to do with their lack of vascular engorgement in the pelvis.

Can ERT increase sexual desire?

When someone comes to me distressed because she has lost her sexual desire, I often suggest a month or two of ERT. Such a short regimen is not going to hurt her; the worst that can happen is that it won't help. If it doesn't, she can simply stop taking it. If the ERT does help, she can decide whether she wants to continue with it or not.

Does testosterone increase sexual desire in women?

The role of testosterone in mediating sexual drive in women is one of the controversial topics in gynecology today. Suppose someone comes to the office, concerned about her loss of desire, concerned about her partner and their sex life. She and her partner are getting along well; the cause of her lack of libido probably is not psychological or social. We try ERT, and although it improves her performance a little by making her more comfortable, she really would like to be more sexually interested. At this point I might suggest testosterone.

A lot of libido, however, is emotional, social, psychological, whatever you wish to call it. Testosterone will not solve lack of desire if you are angry at your partner or he is angry at you, or if you feel that you are getting old and unattractive, or if your partner is getting unattractive to you because he has put on fifty pounds and is out drinking beer with the boys all the time. If your previous basis for communication was limited to your children and they are out of the house now so you and your husband don't talk to each other, if he comes home and reads the paper or turns on the TV while you talk to your pals on the telephone, testosterone is not going to help. If, however, the roots of your lack of desire are physiological, or physiological and emotional jointly, then it may well make a difference.

Some researchers, both physicians and psychologists, feel that testosterone increases sexual desire in women and also promotes a sense of well-being. Studies show that it increases sexual desire, yet other papers in the scientific literature dispute that finding. My feeling is that the majority of practicing gynecologists would say yes, testosterone probably does increase libido. Among my patients who try it, about half say that it makes a big difference for them.

One of the arguments behind the belief that testosterone does not increase libido is that birth control pills lower a woman's testosterone production. A woman who is taking birth control pills has very little testosterone. But most women on the pill still have reasonably normal sex lives. Even though their endogenous testosterone production is low, their libido is intact. The whole issue is murky and complex.

As with the estrogen, I suggest that people try testosterone for a month or two. If it does not work for you, you can stop taking it.

Will taking testosterone make women masculine?

The first thing I usually hear when I suggest testosterone is something like, "Testosterone, that's the male hormone!" My standard counter is that yes, it is a male hormone, but women make it too—just as estrogen is a female hormone, but men make some also.

The dosages of testosterone that are generally given to improve libido are minuscule. They range from 1.25 to 2.5 mg of methyltestosterone, which really shouldn't masculinize anyone. Testosterone is sometimes prescribed for men, to improve libido or sexual performance, but in far greater doses; if a man were to take only 1.25 to 2.5 mg, he would not notice any change at all.

The masculinizing effects that too much testosterone could cause are facial hair growth and acne. Some women notice that their voice gets lower. Some women are very sensitive to testosterone and get hair growth rather quickly; for them, the dosage level is crucial. On the other hand, many older women get unwanted facial hair even when they are not taking exogenous testosterone. The reason is that our ovaries continue to make small amounts of testosterone even when they are no longer producing estrogen.

Can I take testosterone to enhance desire if I am interested in preserving fertility?

Testosterone is not an appropriate drug for women who are concerned about fertility. Although it may enhance desire, it may also have masculinizing effects on a fetus.

Is testosterone related to anabolic steroids?

Testosterone is a kind of cousin of the anabolic steroids, which athletes take (illegally) to increase muscle development and athletic performance. The side effects of the two are very different. Testosterone will not give you brain cancer; nor in the dosages we are talking about will it give you the kind of physique we see in muscle-building magazines. In fact, the male athletes who take anabolic steroids turn out to have very low testosterone levels because the steroids block their own production of testosterone. Many athletes who take steroids are sterile, a condition that is sometimes reversible and sometimes not.

Do masculinizing side effects go away when women stop taking testosterone?

Probably in one or two months of testosterone therapy, you will not notice an effect as profound as facial hair. But if you should grow facial hair, it will not disappear spontaneously when you stop the testosterone. New growth of facial hair will stop, however.

Will taking testosterone increase my risk of heart attack?

Although plenty of evidence shows that premenopausal women are less at risk for heart disease than men in the same age group, researchers do not yet know the precise role of testosterone in this statistical picture. In the dosages that we are talking about for libido enhancement, testosterone does not seem to have a significant effect on blood lipids or increase a menopausal woman's chances of having a heart attack.

In what ways can I take testosterone?

Like progesterone, pure testosterone does not get well absorbed orally, so several different methods have been devised to deliver it. One is a process called methylation, which is similar to the way progesterone is treated so that it can be absorbed. Methyltestosterone does get absorbed from the digestive system, but you cannot take it in high doses because it is toxic to your liver. Furthermore, the doses that would affect your liver would also give you other unwanted side effects such as facial hair. So the dosage of methyltestosterone that is usually prescribed is tiny.

Often testosterone is prescribed in conjunction with estrogen, so estrogen products are manufactured in combination with testosterone. Of the two basic varieties, one is a preparation called Estratest. It has a very small amount of testosterone added to the kind of estrogen used in Premarin. The dosage in Estratest is 1.25 mg of estrogen plus 2.5 mg of methyltestosterone. In another preparation called Estratest HS, the HS stands for half-strength. That is, the estrogen is 0.625 mg with 1.25 mg of methyltestosterone added. This is really the smallest amount that can have any noticeable effect on libido. Its side effects have been well studied, and the company that produces it will be happy to send you literature showing that this minuscule level of testosterone has no significant masculinizing effects and, more important, rarely affects the liver.

There is also a Premarin compound made with testosterone, but it has a larger component of methyltestosterone. The Estratest is 2.5 mg testosterone, or if you choose the HS version 1.25 mg of testosterone; the Premarin is 5 mg. It is an older product and less frequently used today.

If the Estratest does not work or if you do not want to take methyltestosterone by mouth because you are concerned about liver damage or because you have had hepatitis, injectable testosterone can be used. It is natural testosterone and thus does not affect the liver. Men who take testosterone because their own production has decreased get it in shot form; to maintain masculinization, to keep their beard, low voice, and other male characteristics, they have to take an amount of oral testosterone that would probably be toxic to the liver. The disadvantage is that the shots must be taken every four to six weeks.

An anecdote went around a recent meeting of the North American Menopause Society, a professional organization of physicians and researchers dealing with problems surrounding menopause. A physician forgot to warn some of his patients that he was going on vacation for two weeks. The women who were due for their shots were apparently calling the office to find out when he would return. According to him, or his patients, the testosterone made them feel so good that they missed it when they did not have it.

Another possibility is testosterone cream, which can be applied to the skin. Although a great deal of the testosterone is not absorbed, enough passes through the skin to help people with libido problems. No liver damage results, first because the cream is rubbed into the skin and thus bypasses the liver, and second because the hormone in these preparations is natural testosterone, not a methylated compound. Topical testosterone applied to the skin can also be used for lichen sclerosus et atrophicus, a vulvar disease. To use it, you dab a little on your skin once a day. You may find this process easier and more pleasant than an injection every four to six weeks. However, natural testosterone cream is not readily available commercially, so you and your physician may need to search around to find a pharmacist who can compound it.

Once I start taking testosterone, how long must I continue?

If you are taking testosterone to enhance libido and it seems to work for you, then you can take it for as long as you want; if it doesn't work for you, you can just stop. I have some patients who vary the routine to suit their needs. If they decide they want more libido, they take their testosterone; when they don't want more libido, they don't take it. So I have some women who take three Premarin and three Estratest tablets a week, that is, three tablets of estrogen alone and three tablets of estrogen-plus-testosterone. In short, they are mixing and matching.

Is there such a thing as male menopause?

Yes and no. Men certainly experience physical changes, including changes in hormone production, just as women do. Valid studies show that testosterone production decreases in men over the course of time, but the drop is much more gradual than the profound drop of estrogen production in women during their forties and fifties. Spermatogenesis, the production of sperm, decreases gradually in men. They don't make as many sperm, or as many viable sperm, as they get older; but they do continue to make some sperm into their seventies.

Certainly the physical changes of menopause have social ramifications for women. And to some extent the same is true of men. Both men and women face midlife social changes that may affect their attitudes or their self-image but, in my experience, those that women face are more profound and difficult. Yes, the man's mother is getting older, but usually his wife or sister is taking care of her. Yes, his children are reproducing and occasionally Grandpa takes care of them, but usually the chore is delegated to Grandma. Women face problems relative to rejoining the workforce, but men have been in the workforce for years and found their place in it.

Both men and women feel the pressure to look young and physically attractive, but again the pressure on women seems greater. Men are considered attractive at older ages than women, particularly if they have money or power. Even in the movie star set (a group of people selected in large part because they are more physically attractive than your average Jane or Joe) men have an easier time of it. There is no female counterpart on the screen, for example, of Harrison Ford.

So while we are all aware of the male midlife crisis, which might be the social equivalent of female menopause, in general men have fewer issues to deal with.

What about male sexuality in midlife?

Over time, testosterone production decreases in men. This fact may express itself in decreased sexual desire. Men may take more time to achieve an erection and the erection may not be as firm as it used to be. Or men may be slower to ejaculate.

These changes may be exacerbated by certain diseases that make it difficult for men to have intercourse as they age: high blood pressure, cardiac disease, angina, diabetes, and prostate problems. Men with any of these diseases can have problems with getting and maintaining erections, that is, the disease itself causes the difficulties. Another contributing factor, however, is the medication given for the disease. Many of the drugs that are used to block elevated blood pressure can also block sexual performance. In general they do not block desire, but they do block the ability to achieve an erection.

What prescription drugs can interfere with sexual performance?

A number of commonly used prescription drugs can inhibit sexual performance, both in men and in women. Among the most common are antihypertensives, that is, drugs that combat high blood pressure. Others are beta-blockers, used in cardiac disease and to treat angina and rhythmic disturbances of the heart, as well as high blood pressure.

Certain drugs prescribed for high blood pressure seem to block orgasmic response in women as well as men. Some women find that their response to sexual stimulation is lessened or just seems different. This reaction is uncommon but can be troubling.

If a woman comes to me concerned about the effect of antihypertensive drugs on her husband's sexual performance, I suggest that she talk to her husband's internist. Often men are unwilling to call their physician and say, "Look, I can't get an erection on this medication you gave me." Yet a telephone call is all that is needed. Dozens of drugs exist for lowering blood pressure. If one does not work, another one may be just as satisfactory in controlling blood pressure and not give the man an erectile problem.

If it is the disease itself and not the medication that causes the trouble, urologists are available who are skilled in the treatment of male dysfunction, and treatments are available ranging from the simple to the complex. Simplest are the oral medications that help produce an erection. Or chemicals can be injected into the base of the penis with a very small needle, which will cause an erection even if the man's blood supply to the penis is marginal. The man injects himself before intercourse, like a diabetic taking insulin. The nickname for the three drugs (papaverine, phentolamine, and prostaglandins) in the medication is PEP.

In addition to these drugs, there are mechanical options. Implantable pumps can be placed into the penis surgically. They use fluid as a means to pump up the penis.

Will testosterone increase libido in men?

Sometimes patients complain that their husband or partner has less libido than they do. The husband is not taking antihypertensives; he has no prostate problem; he can perform just fine — but he has little interest in sex.

This is a question for male urology experts. Certainly there are physicians who prescribe testosterone for men to see whether it enhances their sexual performance. But in the doses that men require, issues such as blood lipid levels need to be addressed by a physician.

What about sex after my partner has had a heart attack?

This important issue is addressed by almost all cardiac rehabilitation programs. Occasionally someone with end-stage coronary artery disease probably should not have intercourse, but in general once a person has recuperated from a heart attack, intercourse is quite all right. You should check with his cardiologist that your partner has recovered sufficiently and that there is no reason to be afraid of strenuous sexual activity.

As a gynecologist, I am frequently asked, "Will my husband have another heart attack if he gets sexually aroused?" I cannot answer that question; only the cardiologist who knows the degree of damage caused by the previous heart attack can assess that particular individual. Most of the time, after someone is fully rehabilitated from a heart attack, there is no reason he can't engage in full sexual activity.

If your husband or partner is not willing to raise the question with his cardiologist, you can certainly call the doctor yourself. Ask how much sexual activity is safe for your husband.

Is sex safe for women who have had heart attacks?

Again, check with your cardiologist. If you are getting on your treadmill and working out, if you are out walking, there is probably no reason not to have sex.

10 ● Fibroids, Incontinence, Itching, and Other Midlife Annoyances

Certain gynecological discomforts accompany middle age, no matter how healthy your habits, and can be classified as annoyances rather than as life-threatening illnesses. Among these problems are fibroids, incontinence, and vaginal itching. Although your mother may have been forced to put up with some of these difficulties, you may well be spared.

Fibroids

What are fibroids?

Called myomas in medical terminology, fibroids are technically defined as exuberant growths of the smooth muscle wall of the uterus. In this context "exuberant" merely means an excessive growth of basically normal tissue; the tissue grows too much but there is nothing pathologically wrong with it.

At least one in four women past the age of 30 has fibroids. It is important to emphasize that more than 99 percent of the time they are benign. They are not life-threatening and they won't harm you in any absolute sense. But they can make you bleed and give you pain. They can also cause infertility, which may be of concern to a small proportion of women who are approaching menopause. About 20 to 40 percent of women have fibroids by the time they are menopausal, with black women having a slightly higher frequency than white women.

How big are fibroids?

Fibroids come in sizes ranging from that of a pea to that of a small watermelon, to use common round objects as a basis of comparison. Physicians speak of them in terms of the size of a uterus during pregnancy: the size of a two-month pregnancy (comparable to a tennis ball) or a three-month pregnancy (comparable to a grapefruit). Often fibroids occur in groups, and women who have one fibroid are likely to have several.

Do fibroids grow slowly or quickly?

Fibroids can behave very erratically. Sometimes they appear suddenly, grow gradually to their maximum size, and remain that way forever. Other times they appear, jump to the size of a three-month pregnancy, remain that way for five years, then suddenly change again.

What causes fibroids?

No one knows precisely what triggers the growth of fibroids, though we do know that they are definitely estrogen dependent. Perhaps fluctuation in estrogen levels may play a role in their appearance. Since their growth is related to the presence of estrogen, fibroids tend to shrink or disappear when a woman goes through menopause and her estrogen levels fall.

At what age do women usually develop fibroids?

Fibroids can begin at any age. The youngest woman on whom I ever operated for fibroids was about 23 years old, but she was an exception. From the midtwenties on, the incidence of fibroids increases with age until menopause. Because they are estrogen dependent, fibroids do not ordinarily appear after menopause. Often they appear during the perimenopause, perhaps in response to fluctuating estrogen levels.

Are there risk factors for fibroids?

Fibroids are such a common phenomenon that it is difficult to determine whether there is a familial tendency toward them. There are no other known risk factors, so it is difficult to predict who will get them and who will not.

How can I tell whether I have fibroids?

You can have fibroids without realizing it, because they may not produce symptoms. The symptoms of fibroids are heavy bleeding during periods, pelvic pressure, the need to urinate frequently, backaches, and constipation. But you may have some or all of these symptoms without actually having fibroids since they can be indicative of other conditions.

How can fibroids be diagnosed by a physician?

Fibroids can be discovered by your physician during a bimanual (two-handed) pelvic examination. The physician places one hand in the vagina and the other on top of the belly and palpates, or feels, the fibroid. What the physician is actually feeling is not a lump in the uterus, but a changed contour of the uterus. Mentally the physician will compare the way the uterus feels with the way it would feel if you were pregnant, to get an estimation of size.

Fibroids can also be diagnosed through an ultrasound procedure, which is often used to confirm that what the physician is feeling is indeed the uterus with its fibroids and not a growth on an ovary. More sophisticated tests, such as MRIs and CT scans, can be used to diagnose fibroids, but these tests are more expensive and expose you to more radiation than ultrasound. Ultrasound is preferable and is usually an adequate diagnostic tool.

What symptoms do fibroids cause?

Depending on their size and where they are located, fibroids can cause symptoms varying from none whatsoever to very significant pelvic discomfort, including belly pain or a sense of pressure on the bladder or bowel. Many women who have fibroids feel that they have to go to the bathroom every ten minutes. If the fibroids become sufficiently large and are sitting on the ureters (the tubes that join the kidneys and the bladder), they can exert enough pressure to cause compression of the kidneys or force the urine backward, which can lead to serious problems. If they are pressing on the rectum, they will cause changes in bowel habits, for example constipation, or a feeling of fullness.

Fibroids can also cause bleeding, generally in the form of heavier periods; occasionally they cause bleeding between periods. Although many women with fibroids do not experience heavy bleeding, that is the main reason women with fibroids decide to have them removed.

Fibroids can cause backaches, especially during the luteal or second half of the menstrual cycle, when there is increasing edema or fluid retention in the pelvis. Occasionally fibroids cause severe pain, classically when they are "degenerating."

I have had patients with fibroids literally the size of small watermelons, who were annoyed at me for wanting them to have the fibroids removed. These women felt fine and had no bleeding or other distressing symptoms. I have had other patients with very small fibroids who were extremely uncomfortable.

Where in the uterus do fibroids grow?

Fibroids can be on the inner surface of the uterus, in the middle portion of the uterine wall, or on the outside. Some are a combination of all three. There are names for each location. The outer part of the uterus is called the serosa; fibroids in this area are called subserosal. Those in the uterine wall (mur is the Latin word for "wall") are called intramural fibroids. The mucosa is the inner lining of the uterine cavity, and these fibroids are called submucosal fibroids.

If your fibroid is growing off the back wall of your uterus and pressing toward your back, you will probably have a backache. If it is a posterior fibroid pressing on the rectum, you may well experience constipation.

The patients walking around with a baby-watermelon-size object inside, who were angry at me for proposing surgery, have subserosal fibroids. The fibroid is external to the uterine cavity; it is not troublesome; it is just there. Subserosal fibroids are the least symptomatic and they seldom cause bleeding problems because they are outside the main action site of the uterus. Women with erratic bleeding usually have submucosal fibroids, which can cause real problems even though they are only a half-inch in diameter.

Figure 14. Uterine fibroids can occur anywhere in the uterus. Although submucosal fibroids are usually small, their bleeding can cause significant annoyance.

Why do fibroids cause heavy periods or other bleeding?

No one knows exactly. But most people believe that in such a case the fibroid is breaking up the integrity of the uterine lining. Because of this disruption, the bleeding is heavy and erratic.

What is a degenerating fibroid?

Basically a fibroid can "degenerate," or collapse on itself, if it has outgrown its blood supply. Like muscle tissue, fibroid tissue needs oxygen. When it fails to get an adequate supply, the fibroid can cause severe ischemic pain. It is the same kind of pain you get when you have uterine cramps, but more severe. Once the fibroid degenerates, the tissue gradually disappears and the pain ceases. The process of degeneration usually goes on for several days, though not for several weeks or months.

Phyllis L., who came to me for her gynecological checkups for a number of years, started experiencing significant abdominal pain rather suddenly when she was in her late forties. She saw her internist, a very good internist, who thought her problem was appendicitis—but he wasn't sure because her symptoms did not fit those of classic appendicitis.

She went to one of the best surgeons in town, who also thought she had appendicitis, though he agreed that her symptoms were not the ordinary ones. Her abdominal pain got so bad that she went to the emergency room of the local hospital. Since I was her regular gynecologist, she asked if I could examine her, and I came to the emergency room before her surgery.

There was a lump on the right side of her uterus, without question, and her uterus was tender. The lump was not far from where her appendix would be located. I knew she had a fibroid in that area because I had examined her previously. At this point we did an ultrasound and visualized her fibroid, right where she was feeling the pain. We decided that her problem was a degenerating fibroid and we elected to treat her conservatively and give her pain medication. She stayed in bed for a couple of days and improved. When I reexamined her in my office some time later, the entire fibroid had disappeared. She has been fine ever since.

The phenomenon of degenerating fibroids is not uncommon in perimenopausal women, but occasionally a fibroid will degenerate during a pregnancy and again the situation is very uncomfortable. The only therapy during pregnancy is conservative: ride it out with bed rest and pain medication.

What is a prolapsed fibroid?

On rare occasions a fibroid may prolapse, or fall down, into the uterus. Most fibroids are merely little lumps, but sometimes they are on stalks that are called pedicles. If a fibroid on a pedicle prolapses, the uterus may try to expel it; but since the fibroid is attached to the uterine wall, the whole uterus tends to come along with the fibroid. The woman feels contractions like labor; her cervix actually dilates and thins out. The treatment can be either to remove the fibroid from its stalk or to perform a hysterectomy.

Can fibroids become cancerous?

While it is possible for fibroids to undergo "malignant degeneration," it is extremely rare. The possibility of a fibroid's becoming malignant is so remote that it is not one of the major reasons for hysterectomy. In terms of relative risk, having a fibroid removed because some day in the future it might become cancerous is like refusing to drive a car because some day in the future you might be killed in a crash.

Do fibroids always lead to hysterectomy?

Fibroids certainly are the most common indication for hysterectomy in the United States. Just because you have a fibroid, you are not an instant candidate for a hysterectomy, however.

If your doctor discovers that you have a fibroid and it is asymptomatic or not causing significant discomfort, he or she will probably ask you to come back in four to six months to see whether the situation is stable. If the fibroid is not growing or changing, then examinations will probably be scheduled at a wider interval.

Are there guidelines to how large fibroids should be allowed to grow before removing them?

A common criterion suggests that the size of a three-month pregnancy (equivalent to a grapefruit) is probably the largest your pelvis can accommodate without danger or discomfort. When a fibroid grows to the size of a four-month pregnancy (a cantaloupe), it may start pressing significantly on other organs. Usually at that point the woman is aware of its presence and may be quite uncomfortable.

Physicians begin to differ in opinion when the mass reaches the size of a grapefruit. My position is that anything larger than a cantaloupe, or four-month pregnancy, should come out. It is difficult to believe that any woman can be comfortable with a mass the size of a five-month pregnancy (or a honeydew melon) in her belly. She may have gotten used to the feeling and be able to put up with it, but it can't be comfortable. The more serious issue is that at this size the mass may well be compromising her ureters, the tubes from the bladder to the kidney.

Opinion on the size fibroid that must be removed surgically varies from gynecologist to gynecologist. Some physicians say you should have a hysterectomy if you have a fibroid the size of a two-month pregnancy; but since there is plenty of space in the pelvis for a mass the size of a tennis ball or even a small grapefruit, you probably don't have to have surgery for a fibroid this size unless you have significant discomfort. If your physician does tell you that you have a mass the size of a two-month pregnancy and that you should have a hysterectomy, it is advisable to get a second opinion. I would like to say that in the area where I practice no unnecessary hysterectomies are performed, but I cannot assert that with total confidence. If size seems to be your doctor's sole criterion for the prospective hysterectomy and you are in doubt, get a second opinion.

Another indication for hysterectomy is rapid growth of the fibroid. If a pelvic examination turns up a mass the size of a two-month pregnancy, and three months later that mass has grown to sixteen-week size, there may be cause for concern. What is growing in the uterus may not be a benign fibroid, but a malignant tumor. While sarcomas of the uterus are rare, they can occur. The only way to make sure that the mass is benign is to take it out and to examine every bit of it under a microscope.

The other criteria depend on the individual woman, her symptoms, and her response to them. If you are at the point where you can't tolerate the heavy bleeding any longer, or if you have gotten tired of having to urinate every twenty minutes and find that it interferes with your life, then you may elect to have a hysterectomy. If you have a backache that appears at midcycle and continues until your next period, you may well want a hysterectomy to relieve you of the pain. But these decisions are very individual, and only you can make them.

How about nonsurgical treatments for fibroids?

The key decision with fibroids is whether to intervene at all. It may be difficult for Americans, who are used to getting things done, to accept nonintervention, to accept having a fibroid and not trying to make it better, but often this is a wise choice. Biologically speaking, it is a kind of peaceful coexistence. If the fibroid doesn't bother you, if it isn't growing rapidly, and if it is smaller than a grapefruit, then leave it alone.

One of the easiest and least interventionist treatments for fibroids is menopause. Since fibroids flourish and thrive on estrogen, they tend to shrink during the perimenopausal period when the ovaries are producing very little estrogen. Fibroids often disappear altogether after menopause.

Another treatment, which mimics menopause, is the use of GnRH agonists (chemicals that act like GnRH). The GnRH stands for "gonadotropin-releasing hormone," and in the body this hormone is produced in the hypothalamus. During the normal menstrual cycle, gonadotropin-releasing hormone controls the pituitary gland so that it secretes the right amounts of follicle-stimulating hormone and luteinizing hormone at the right time; these hormones in turn contribute to the production of estrogen. Basically, GnRH agonists wipe out your estrogen production, and by depriving fibroids of estrogen you can control their growth. One of the most familiar of these drugs is Lupron, given as a monthly injection and often also used as a medication to control endometriosis. One of the first to use Lupron for fibroids was Dr. Andrew Friedman, who showed that within three months estrogen-deprived fibroids would shrink significantly, often to about half their former size. Unfortunately, when you stop taking the Lupron, your estrogen levels return and the fibroids are apt to grow back to their previous size.

Anita D., aged 44, came to me with fibroids that enlarged from the size of a grapefruit to the size of a substantial honeydew in less than a year. She decided to take Lupron to see whether it would control this rapid fibroid growth. After about three months the fibroids regressed, but the minute she stopped taking Lupron her fibroids began growing again. Within two months they had reached their former size. Her periods once again were miserable, with heavy flooding. Her fibroids were so large that when she walked into the office I could see the change in the size of her abdomen. Eventually she had to have a hysterectomy.

Can I take Lupron or another GnRH agonist for a long period?

Lupron has its drawbacks, so you cannot remain on it forever. The first drawback is cost, which as we have seen is something in the range of $300 to $400 a month. Second, Lupron is like menopause. Because it lowers estrogen levels, it causes all the consequences of menopause. In particular, doctors are concerned about osteoporosis: it has been shown that women who stay on Lupron for more than six months at a stretch begin to encounter bone problems. Women who take Lupron for a shorter time do not seem to have these difficulties. Presumably by taking Lupron you also lose the benefits of estrogen to your cardiovascular system, but it is osteoporosis that has been the concern of researchers.

Because of the adverse effects of Lupron on bone and on cholesterol, some physicians have decided on what is called add-back therapy. That is, they shut down ovarian function and estrogen production with Lupron, then add back a touch of estrogen as if they were giving ERT. While this approach preserves bone, it does not give optimal suppression of the fibroid.

For some people Lupron can be a real solution. Recall Cathy H., who found herself bleeding heavily in the supermarket one day during perimenopause. This incident occurred when she was 48 or 49 years old; with six months on Lupron, she has done well. Her endogenous estrogen levels declined enough so that her fibroids shrank, even though she still has them. She also still has some menstrual periods, but they are not very heavy and they are not very frequent. So the

Lupron seems to have taken her through a dangerous time when her estrogen levels were fluctuating rather wildly.

Will taking Lupron postpone menopause?

No. If you take Lupron for six months, it will not delay your menopause for six months.

Will birth control pills help fibroids?

Women with fibroids seem to have very individual responses to birth control pills. Some physicians believe that birth control pills increase fibroid growth; others say their use makes no difference whatsoever to fibroid growth. Some patients who have heavy bleeding seem to do very well on birth control pills, although the pill does not shrink the fibroid. Because birth control pills contain progestin as well as estrogen, the progesterone may help control the stimulation from the estrogen. The bottom line is that we don't know the exact relationship between birth control pills and fibroids. Therefore women with fibroids who take the pill, for whatever reason, need to be monitored.

If I have one fibroid, am I at increased risk for developing more?

Unfortunately, women who have one fibroid are likely to develop others later on. This may be an important consideration if you are thinking about surgery and trying to decide between removal of the fibroid and removal of the entire uterus including the fibroid.

What are the surgical options for fibroids?

Several surgical procedures are available for removing fibroids. The most familiar is the hysterectomy. Another procedure is the myomectomy, in which the fibroid is removed but the uterus remains more or less intact. Traditionally, myomectomies are performed with an abdominal incision. In the past ten years new procedures have been developed using a hysteroscope or a laparoscope. They are appropriate for removing some but not all fibroids. If the fibroids can be removed with the hysteroscope or the laparoscope, there is no prolonged recovery period because there is no major abdominal incision.

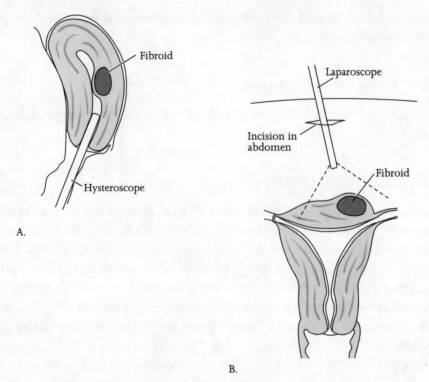

Figure 15. *The hysteroscope, inserted through the vagina, is used to remove fibroids from the inner wall of the uterus. The laparoscope, inserted through the abdomen, removes fibroids attached to the outer wall.*
A. Hysteroscopy
B. Laparoscopy

What are the advantages and disadvantages to these different procedures?

A myomectomy may be done surgically either with an abdominal incision or with a laparoscope, more commonly the former. The surgeries are more or less equivalent in terms of time in the operating room and blood loss. Recovery time after a myomectomy may be somewhat shorter, four weeks rather than six weeks, but it is still significant.

Myomectomies can be more difficult operations than hysterectomies and are often recommended for women who want to preserve their childbearing capability. Although it would seem easier to remove the fibroid than the entire uterus, a myomectomy can become difficult and sometimes involve more blood loss than a hysterectomy, because the fibroid grows into the wall of the uterus and has its own blood supply. In a hysterectomy the surgeon controls the bleeding, clamping off the large vessels to the uterus before beginning to cut. In a myomectomy there is no way to shut down the blood flow to the uterus, because the uterus is being preserved. To remove the fibroid, the surgeon must dig in to the wall of the uterus and peel off the fibroid, while the uterus is receiving its full blood supply. The bleeding can be reduced using operative tourniquets or packing towels around the blood vessels to temporarily press on them. These techniques are more or less successful, depending on where the fibroids are located in relation to the uterine blood vessels.

Because a myomectomy can involve significant blood loss, many physicians encourage the patient to have a blood supply available, preferably her own blood.

The other problem with a myomectomy is that the operation often causes adhesions afterward. Adhesions are formations of scar tissue that cause one organ to stick to another; with a myomectomy, the adhesions involve the uterus, which often adheres to the bowel. After the fibroid has been removed, the physician pulls the myometrium (the muscle wall of the uterus) back together and stitches it to stop the bleeding from the blood vessels that once supplied the fibroid. There are different surgical techniques and different coatings that the surgeon puts on the uterus after a myomectomy to minimize the risk, but myomectomy still has the reputation of being an operation that is likely to cause adhesions.

Although a myomectomy is the only surgical choice for a woman interested in preserving childbearing who must have her fibroids removed, the adhesions that may result from this operation can interfere with fertility. Furthermore, women who have had a myomectomy have a significant chance of needing a Caesarean section when they do become pregnant. Scar tissue and a general weakening of the wall of the uterus during the myomectomy may put a woman at risk of a ruptured uterus during labor. The only person who can tell whether a woman who has a myomectomy will need future Caesarean sections is the surgeon who performs the myomectomy. If you are interested in having children and must have a myomectomy, you should realize the possible complications and discuss them with your physician.

Marlene D. is 38 years old, recently remarried, and unsure whether or not she wants more children. She came in with a large fibroid, which was sitting right on her bladder so that she had pressure and needed to urinate frequently. I sent her to a urologist to be sure she did not have any other problems (which she did not), but through the cystoscope the urologist could see the fibroid pressing into her bladder like a little mountain. Because she wanted to preserve her fertility and had no other difficulties, a myomectomy was a good choice for her. Since the operation, her bladder problems have been much better.

Can fibroids be removed with laser surgery?

Yes, there are three tools that can be used for removing the fibroids during a myomectomy: the traditional metal scalpel, an electrified knife or probe called a Bovie cautery, and a laser. Laser surgery has no real advantage over traditional surgery. A laser is a knife—a knife made of a beam of light instead of metal, but a knife nonetheless. While there are procedures in which a laser is a superior tool, in a myomectomy it has no advantage over removing the fibroids with electrocauterization or a metal scalpel. But laser surgery gets good press and people are sometimes swayed to want procedures that are new.

Will ERT cause fibroids to grow?

No, probably not. Remember that the amount of estrogen you take in ERT is significantly less than what your own ovaries make endogenously during your premenopausal years. If you look at the estradiol levels in normal menstrual women, they range between 50 and 400 pg/ml during the menstrual cycle, which is quite a wide range. In menopausal women on ERT, the range is 50 to 80. So the menopausal woman who is happy walking around all month with an estradiol level of 50 has significantly less estrogen than the premenopausal woman who has a level of 50 for part of the month and a level of 400 for another part of the month.

Most women with fibroids can take ERT, though they should be watched by their physician to be sure the estrogen is not stimulating the fibroids to new growth. This follow-up is especially important during the first years of estrogen therapy because there is no way of knowing how an individual woman's particular fibroid will respond.

On occasion, however, women with fibroids can't take estrogen because their fibroids are stimulated by even a tiny amount of estrogen.

Vicki W. is an active and intelligent woman, the owner of a travel agency. She is absolutely miserable without estrogen, in terms of her personality and her mental outlook and her physical comfort. Even my office staff can notice the difference. When she is not taking estrogen, she has been known to call the office, get angry over the telephone, and yell at staff members; the minute she starts taking the ERT again, she calls back and apologizes.

For psychological reasons Vicki functions much better on estrogen. Unfortunately, she has fibroids. They are fairly small, ten- to twelve-week size at most, and on grounds of size there is no reason at all to take them out. But their location in the uterine wall makes them basically not removable without a hysterectomy.

Vicki is fully menopausal and therefore makes no estrogen on her own. I tried giving her estrogen without progesterone, but she developed hyperplasia; the lining of her uterus built up and built up, so eventually I had to give her progesterone, which makes her bleed.

So the question becomes, which is the worse evil? Should she feel wretched without the estrogen, having hot flashes all the time and feeling angry and upset? Or should she be bleeding heavily? There is no answer. My guess is that eventually she will opt for a hysterectomy. Her travel business takes her into many out-of-the-way spots. In fact, the last time she had a period she was vacationing on St. John in the Virgin Islands. The decision ultimately has to be hers; she alone must decide that her Jekyll and Hyde personality and the discomfort of heavy bleeding disrupt her life sufficiently that she wants to have a hysterectomy and continue her ERT.

Incontinence and Uterine Prolapse

Among the annoyances of having a middle-aged uterus and pelvis are problems of incontinence, the unwanted leaking of urine. Both the uterus itself and the ligaments that hold it in place are sensitive to estrogen. As estrogen production declines with age, both the uterus and the ligaments atrophy, causing what is known as pelvic relaxation, which means that your pelvic organs are no longer held firmly in place by their ligaments. Unlike most forms of relaxation, pelvic relaxation is not desirable. Women who have gone through term delivery of one or more children, almost always have some degree of pelvic relaxation.

The degrees of pelvic relaxation range from very mild to severe. With mild pelvic relaxation, your gynecologist doing a pelvic exam can feel the uterus coming down a little into the vagina. The uterus can slip so far down that it actually protrudes into the vagina toward the perineum, a condition known as uterine prolapse. A cystocele is a slippage or bulging into the vagina of the bladder, which normally sits above the front of the vagina; a rectocele occurs when part of the rectum bulges into the vagina through its weakened back wall.

One of the common symptoms that accompanies pelvic relaxation is stress incontinence, which is loss of urine when the pressure within the abdomen is increased by laughing, sneezing, coughing, or physical exercise such as running or jumping. Many women also experience stress incontinence during pregnancy.

Figure 16. *Weakening of the muscles of the pelvic floor can lead to bulges of the rectum (rectocele) or bladder (cystocele) into the vagina. The entire uterus can also fall (uterine prolapse). Some patients have all three conditions.*
A. Normal anatomy.
B. Rectocele.
C. Cystocele.
D. Uterine prolapse.

Once the baby has been delivered, the incontinence usually gets better; but it returns with future pregnancies and tends to get more severe with time.

Stress incontinence is a very common problem, and for many older women a serious one. There are women who are afraid to go on vacation because of it, or who must curtail certain activities—hiking, camping, sports. We all owe a vote of thanks to the actress June Allyson, star of a groundbreaking series of commercials that brought stress incontinence into the realm of public acceptability. For if people are willing to talk about an issue, some of the stigma disappears.

Is pelvic relaxation hereditary?

Uterine prolapse and pelvic relaxation seem to have more of a hereditary component than, say, fibroids. When a women tells me that her uterus is prolapsed, she often says that her mother had the same problem. I have one patient whose bladder was repaired when she was only 24 years old. Her mother apparently had the same problem, for she had seven children and seven bladder repairs.

What are the symptoms of pelvic relaxation or uterine prolapse?

Symptoms can vary according to the severity of the condition. In its milder forms, when the uterus and bladder have descended only slightly into the vagina, pelvic relaxation can cause back pressure and mild stress incontinence.

If uterine prolapse is severe, the uterus and perhaps the bladder will protrude from the vagina. In some cases of severe prolapse with cystocele, women experience the opposite of stress incontinence: they cannot urinate without manually holding up the bladder. Since the bladder has fallen into the vagina, the urethra is above it; the sac of bladder that remains below the urethra will not contract and empty unless it is pushed up above the urethra. Women with this condition are extremely vulnerable to urinary tract infections.

In addition, women with uterine prolapse and cystocele may feel pressure or fullness between their legs, a sensation described by some as "having my bottom fall out." Many women find the feeling extremely annoying; they cannot stand up comfortably because they experience so much pelvic pressure. Their mobility is decreased because they experience discomfort when they are walking or running, although they do feel better sitting or lying down. Other women with prolapse are less troubled by this sensation.

Can stress incontinence be cured without medication or surgery?

Simple first-line approaches will help many women. If you are overweight and have stress incontinence, you will do yourself a favor by losing the excess poundage. Heavy women have more stress incontinence because they have greater abdominal pressure, caused by the extra fat within the abdomen. If you lose the extra weight, the incontinence may disappear on its own. Second, if you are a smoker and you have chronic smoker's cough, you are doing yourself several disservices. The cough makes a smoker a bad surgical candidate; for even though a urologist may fix your bladder, the constant stress of coughing will undo the best surgery.

All women, fat or thin, smokers or nonsmokers, can benefit from the well-known Kegel exercises, which strengthen the muscles surrounding the urethra and vagina. The easiest way to describe the Kegels is to suggest that the next time you urinate, you stop and start the stream of urine. Of course you can do the exercises when you are not urinating, but the muscles you need to strengthen are the same ones that stop the flow. To do Kegels, contract these muscles and hold while you slowly count to five.

There is no such thing as doing too many Kegels. You can be too thin and you probably can be too rich, but you cannot do too many Kegels. If you drive, you might put a sign on your dashboard that says "Kegel." Then at every traffic light, at every toll booth, in every traffic jam, at every bit of construction on the turnpike, you will be reminded to do your exercises. You can't do much else when you are stuck in traffic, so you may as well make your boredom productive. My experience in clinical practice tells me that Kegels do help many women a great deal.

Does estrogen either in cream form or as oral therapy help with incontinence?

The success of ERT in treating incontinence is controversial in the scientific literature. One researcher, Linda Cardozo, a respected urogynecologist from England, has done controlled studies on women who take and do not take estrogen; her results did not show that ERT helped with incontinence. Nor could she demonstrate that degree of prolapse or severity of symptoms was improved by ERT.

My own experience tells me that ERT does indeed help some women. Women mention it in a kind of offhand way. They notice that they can jog or play tennis without becoming incontinent, though before starting ERT they had more difficulty with this problem. Or they talk about their hot flashes or their concentration, and then mention that, by the way, their urine problem is better.

If you do not want to take ERT orally, you can try topical vaginal estrogen creams, because for this purpose topical therapy is probably just as effective as oral systemic therapy. There are no contraindications for vaginal estrogen cream unless you happen to be allergic to the substance in which the estrogen is dissolved; almost no one is allergic to estrogen. Even most women who have breast cancer can use vaginal estrogen, because so little is absorbed. If your symptoms get better and you don't need an operation, fine. Unlike osteoporosis, in which you can stop bone loss but seldom rebuild bone that has already been lost, changes in urinary control are reversible. Estrogen will improve matters for the 70-year-old woman, just as it will for the 50-year-old woman.

Can pessaries help with incontinence?

Another approach to stress incontinence is mechanical. A device called a pessary can be inserted into the vagina to support the uterus and bladder. The most common type is a rubber or plastic ring designed to raise your pelvic organs, in the way stitches support it if you have a surgical bladder repair. The classic pessary looks rather like a giant diaphragm and is not much more difficult to put in. (Your gynecologist should be able to show you how.) Other types look like cubes or balloons.

A pessary is inserted temporarily, although it can be used over and over. Some women use it on an as-needed basis, for example when they are going running or participating in a sport; others leave it in longer. For people who are sexually active, it can obviously be a nuisance, but some women just remove the pessary when they have intercourse and put it in again later. In general, pessaries are used by women for whom intercourse is not an issue, especially older women who have uterine prolapse but are not appropriate candidates for surgery. Some younger women who are not ready for bladder repair surgery feel comfortable using one during exercise. Some women don't feel the presence of the pessary at all; other women have reactions ranging from annoyance to discomfort. The pessary may be hard to get in and out, and it may not cure the incontinence. Although there are different sizes and shapes, some women have such poor pelvic support that they can't keep any pessary in place.

Despite the disadvantages, I frequently suggest to my patients with incontinence or prolapse that they try a pessary. If they like it, they can avoid surgery. If

A.

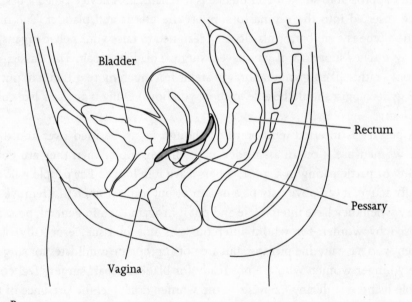

B.

Figure 17A. Pessaries are rubber devices that can help support the uterus, bladder, and rectum.
B. A pessary in place.

they don't like it, they at least have tried another nonsurgical option. Remember that a pessary is not a cure; it will not fix your prolapse. For some women it does not work. For others it works so well that surgery is not necessary. I would estimate that up to half my patients who try a pessary feel comfortable with it, at least on an as-needed basis.

Because pessaries support the prolapsed uterus or bladder whose pressure is contributing to urine leakage, they can help stress incontinence, especially for women who are weak or in poor health and could not tolerate surgery. They can also be useful for women who might elect surgery at some later date but would like to put it off to accommodate their schedule.

Edith L., a tough, smart, healthy 67-year-old former physical therapist, had a totally prolapsed bladder that made it difficult for her to be far from a bathroom for very long. Her health was not endangered, but she wanted her bladder to be fixed. An avid sailor, she also wanted to make a boat trip during the summer. A pessary enabled her to go on the trip and schedule her surgery at a more convenient time.

Is there incontinence other than stress incontinence?

Urge incontinence, clinically known as detrusor dyssynergia, is named for the detrusor or bladder muscle. Most people are aware of a symptom called spastic colon, also known as irritable bowel, a bowel that contracts too frequently and causes gas and diarrhea. Detrusor dyssynergia is irritable bladder. People who have this symptom feel the need to urinate when their bladder contains only 2 or 3 oz (60 to 90 ml) of urine instead of the usual 8 oz. A urologist or urogynecologist can measure the pressure in the bladder to find out how much urine the bladder contains when the patient feels the urge to urinate. Detrusor dyssynergia is not painful, but it can be embarrassing and inconvenient.

How is irritable bladder treated?

Detrusor dyssynergia is usually treated medically rather than surgically. One do-it-yourself approach is bladder training. If you are in a situation where you are near a toilet all day long, you might want to try it. You begin by urinating every hour on the hour, whether you feel the urge to do so or not. You keep this up for a few days and then start spacing the intervals to an hour and a half, then two hours, then longer. Although you may find it time-consuming and inconvenient to keep up this routine, you may also find it helpful, as some of my patients have reported.

Drugs are also a possibility for treating irritable bladder. The most commonly used is Ditropan, an anticholinergic drug that blocks the nerves in the bladder so they do not keep firing off messages that create the urge to urinate. Some physicians treat detrusor dyssynergia with imipramine and amitriptyline, antidepressants that go by trade names such as Tofranil and Elavil. Some of my patients are offended by the suggestion that they take an antidepressant, feeling that I am suggesting something is wrong with their mental health. But again, the antidepressant has an effect on those nerves in the bladder that keep sending the wrong messages. The antidepressant is prescribed in very low doses, lower than what is usually given to treat people with depression. Interestingly enough, small children who are nighttime bed wetters are also classically treated with imipramine.

These drugs will not help women who have stress incontinence or uterine prolapse. If they cough and sneeze or run and jump, they will still be incontinent. Many women have both types of incontinence, and it is important to find out from the patient just when the problem began, how much urine is lost, and so on.

Monica M. was troubled by the need to urinate frequently and was convinced that she needed surgery. She had never had children, so it was unlikely that she had stress incontinence, which is very uncommon in people who have not been pregnant. When she described her symptoms, it was evident that she had detrusor dyssynergia. She felt that she had to go to the bathroom all the time and that she had to get there in a hurry. She tried Ditropan and it worked well for her.

Can surgery correct incontinence?

Surgery is the most aggressive approach to stress incontinence and most of the time it corrects the problem. Before rushing into it, women should realize that no surgery is 100 percent effective and that all have the potential of coming undone. Just as a face lift sags with time and increased age, the structures supporting your bladder will do the same. Ten years from now you may need another operation.

Other factors influence the rate of success, for example the difficulty of the operation. Some repairs are relatively simple and some are more complicated. Some approaches, statistically more successful than others, are not performed frequently because they are complex and recuperation is arduous. The operation that is tightest and holds up the urinary tract structures most successfully has a high rate of complications.

When is surgery a viable option for incontinence and uterine prolapse?

When you have exhausted the other options and feel your quality of life is being compromised by incontinence or prolapse, it is time to consider surgery.

Still, I encourage my patients to wait until they have finished their child-bearing, because if you have a surgical repair, you may need a Caesarean section to save the repair, and a Caesarean section is a more difficult event than a vaginal delivery. Or if you have a vaginal delivery, you may need another repair operation.

A case in point is the woman mentioned earlier who had seven children and seven bladder repair operations. Unless her symptoms were so severe that she couldn't leave the house (and many women have such symptoms), the operations might have been delayed until later in her life.

Women who seek surgery because of discomfort from a cystocele should realize that any operation to correct the condition may result in some incontinence. If these women have trouble emptying their bladder because the cystocele forms a little reservoir below the urethra that never empties, they may find that they will be able to urinate much more easily; they may even become a little incontinent.

Alice B., an 80-year-old artist who keeps herself in good shape, had a huge cystocele that she had been controlling with a pessary. After a while the pessary just wasn't working and she found herself really hindered by her cystocele. Although nobody likes operating electively on someone who is 78 or 79 years old, this woman was a very vigorous person and her life was being seriously compromised. So we fixed her cystocele and she is a new person. She walks around all day in art museums; she stands at her easel and paints for hours; she carries around her large canvases and supplies and has become more active than ever.

Betty H. is about 70 years old and in terrific shape. Although she has a prolapsed uterus and a cystocele, she generally looks and feels wonderful. One of her hobbies is hiking. Eventually her cystocele began troubling her enough to keep her from doing what she wanted to do. Although her health was never in serious danger because of the prolapse, her activities were curtailed. After her prolapse was repaired, the quality of her life improved dramatically.

Although health is certainly an issue, quality of life is equally important in making the decision to have surgery.

What surgical procedures are available to correct uterine prolapse?

The most commonly performed surgery for this kind of problem is a vaginal hysterectomy with an anterior and a posterior repair. The first question patients ask when I describe the procedure is whether they have to have a hysterectomy; they want to know whether is it possible to leave the uterus in place. The answer is yes, it is possible. The surgeon can use a sling procedure to shorten the ligaments that support the uterus and hoist it back into the pelvis.

But if the uterus is falling into the vagina, why put it back in place, since gravity is going to tend to pull it down again? The ligaments that support the uterus have been badly stretched already, which is why the uterus prolapsed in the first place. So if the uterus is not removed, often the operation must be repeated.

If the woman who needs surgery for her uterine prolapse is premenopausal and is concerned about ovarian function, the ovaries can be, and usually are, left in place. After all, they are not part of the problem.

What are the surgical procedures for cystocele and rectocele?

Often uterine prolapse is accompanied by cystocele or rectocele or both. These are usually injuries associated with childbearing. A cystocele repair, also called an anterior repair, entails taking tucks in the fascia that supports the bladder to shorten and tighten it. Part of the procedure for repairing the cystocele is called a Kelly plication suture. It involves building up the tissue under the urethra, which raises it and thereby helps with incontinence. So there are essentially two components of repairing a cystocele: reducing the size of the cystocele and supporting the urethra.

Many women who have a cystocele also have a rectocele. The surgical repair of this condition involves reinforcing the tissue between the vagina and rectum, rebuilding that wall.

The Kelly plication suture, like many other operations, is named for the surgeon who invented it. John Kelly was chairman of the department of obstetrics and gynecology at the Johns Hopkins University School of Medicine for a number of years at the turn of the century and invented the Kelly clamp, commonly used by gynecologists in the operating room.

Dr. Kelly also made a significant contribution to literature. One year he asked a fourth-year student to repeat her training in gynecology because she did not seem to be terribly interested and hadn't done a very good job. Although she was almost finished with medical school, she announced that she didn't want to repeat the rotation and would rather just quit and go to Paris. Her name was Gertrude Stein.

What surgical procedures are used to treat incontinence without cystocele or rectocele?

Women who have only incontinence, whose bladder or rectum is not bulging into the vagina, are probably better served by a different operation. A number of surgical procedures exist for anatomic stress incontinence, all of which are variations on a theme. They involve attaching the bladder to some other abdominal structure and they differ on what structure to use as support.

One classic operation is the Stamey; another is the Pereira, both named for the surgeons who developed them. Stitches are inserted next to the urethra, and it is attached to some fixed part of the abdominal wall. In these procedures, the stitches go into the rectus fascia, the tight layer that covers the rectus (belly-wall muscles). In the past ten years this operation has become very popular and has more or less replaced the traditional Kelly plication suture because it works better, in general, if incontinence is the primary issue.

Another commonly performed surgery is the Marshall Marchetti Krantz procedure and its variations, of which the most common is the Burch. With the Marshall procedure, the stitches are placed into the covering of the pubic bone, the periosteum; in the Burch, the surgeon stitches into some of the other abdominal ligaments.

While most operations for uterine prolapse, rectocele, and cystocele are performed through the vagina, the procedures for incontinence alone are done wholly or partially abdominally. They have a high rate of success, about 90 percent, and success in these terms means complete continence. The 10 percent of patients whose operations are not "successful" do get some degree of relief. Very rarely does a patient experience no relief whatsoever.

Patients should know, however, that any of these procedures for incontinence may fail some years down the road. Although the operations remain successful forever for the majority who have them, a small proportion of women become incontinent again after a number of years.

Patricia G. has a severe eating disorder. A while ago I did a successful Marshall to treat her incontinence. At the time, she was successfully keeping her weight at about 140 pounds.

Pubic
bone

A.

Fascia of the
rectus muscle

B.

C.

Figure 18. *Commonly performed surgical procedures for stress incontinence. These involve tucking and tightening sagging tissues and sometimes attaching the bladder to another structure in the abdomen.*
A. Anterior repair.
B. Urethral sling, or Stamey suspension. In principle these operations are the same, but in the sling procedure a strip of material that passes under the urethra is attached to the fascia, whereas in the Stamey suspension stitches are inserted next to the bottom of the urethra and attached to the fascia.
C. Marshall Marchetti Krantz procedure.

Then she gained about 100 pounds, ballooning to 240. Her Marshall came undone with the extra abdominal pounds and she is again incontinent. Her urethra was stitched to the periosteum of her pubic bone, but the extra weight was too much for three or four stitches to support. Indeed, many gynecologists and urologists will not recommend a Marshall for someone who is seriously overweight.

What can be done if my surgical procedure fails?

The ultimate operation for people whose Stamey or Marshall has failed is the sling procedure. The surgeon takes a strip of tissue and slings it beneath the urethra, then attaches this structure up toward the pubic bone as a permanent support. Many surgeons use the rectus fascia, the very tense, very strong tissue that covers the muscles of the abdominal wall, to fashion the sling. Other surgeons use a nonreactive foreign substance such as Gore-Tex to make the sling. Today researchers are experimenting with injection of collagen around the urethra to make it tighter and build up more resistance within it, but the effects of silicone within the body twenty years into the future are not yet known.

What are the complications of these procedures?

Any surgery involves the risks of anesthesia and infection. In addition, patients should know in advance that they will have to have a catheter in their bladder for a while after the procedure. Some women experience little discomfort with the catheter; others dislike it intensely. If the patient needs a catheter, she will probably be given preventive antibiotics, since bladder infections can be a complication.

Because the surgery changes your anatomy, obstructing something that was not obstructed previously, you may have difficulty starting to urinate again. Formerly the bladder didn't have to work to empty itself; urine just flowed out, whether you wanted it to or not. Now that the surgeon has introduced an obstruction, the bladder has to work and strengthen itself to force urine out through the urethra.

Most people keep the catheters for three to five days after surgery, while the bladder muscles strengthen. The record among my own patients was three weeks. But nobody is catheterized forever after a Marshall or a Stamey.

One of the major complications of sling procedures, however, is that sometimes these operations hold up the urinary structures too well and people need to catheterize themselves or wear a catheter to start urinating again. On occasion the process can take months. Once in a while a patient will have to go back to the operating room to have the sling loosened a little. So unless someone has no control over her bladder at all, a sling operation is not the first option.

Who performs these operations?

Usually in the United States, a urologist will do the Stamey and the Pereira, whereas a gynecologist will perform the Marshall. In a Stamey, the physician uses a cystoscope, looking into the bladder five or six times during the procedure in order to place the stitches correctly. Most gynecologists are not trained to use cystoscopes, although some are. Urogynecologists usually perform sling operations.

Sometimes a gynecologist will do a Marshall to treat incontinence, as a kind of bonus along with a hysterectomy that is being performed to treat some other disease. It is becoming rare in the United States to have a Marshall performed independent of a hysterectomy. If you don't need a hysterectomy but need surgical treatment of incontinence, you will probably have a Stamey or one of its cousins.

If you are contemplating bladder surgery, you should discuss the procedure with your physician. If your gynecologist thinks you would benefit from a more urological approach, she or he will refer you to an appropriate urologist.

Vaginal Itching

Although there are several causes of vaginal itching, one major culprit is often yeast infection. Yeast cells along with other microorganisms live in the vagina all the time, normally held in check by its acid environment. When this balance is upset, yeast can become problematic.

How do I recognize a yeast infection?

The main symptom is itching. The infection is apt to be odorless, but it sometimes is accompanied by a vaginal discharge, classically described as white and curdy, something like cottage cheese. Some yeast infections have no discharge at all.

Who is vulnerable to yeast infections?

While women of any age may get yeast infections, older women not on ERT are more susceptible to infections of the vagina (vaginitis) and of the vulva (vulvitis). The lower estrogen levels that follow menopause result eventually in thinner vaginal and vulvar tissues, which are prone to invasion and irritation. Women who have diabetes are also at increased risk, as are women who are HIV-positive. I have diagnosed several women with diabetes because they came to me with recurrent yeast infections.

HIV also predisposes women toward yeast infections. Nowadays many people are paranoid about HIV and AIDS. I have had patients come in and say, "I just got my second yeast infection; I must have AIDS." I do HIV tests on women who have recurrent infections just because it is worthwhile to rule out the possibility, but I have never turned up any HIV-positives this way.

Many women who are plagued by yeast infections do not have either HIV or diabetes; they just get recurrent yeast infections.

Can I lower my risk for yeast infections?

You can do a few simple things to make yourself a less likely target. First of all, don't sit around in a wet bathing suit or in sweaty exercise clothes. The warm, moist atmosphere offered by these garments is an ideal growing environment for yeast cells.

Next, avoid unnecessary antibiotics. If you don't really need an antibiotic for bronchitis or some other condition, don't take one. While the antibiotics are busy killing off the bacteria that are giving you the bronchitis, they are also killing off your normal intestinal and vaginal flora (the bacteria that normally thrive there). These bacteria could be considered "good-guy bacteria"; they are basically lactobacilli that live in the intestines and vagina and secrete acid to protect the body from excessive growth of yeast. Often if a woman has been on multiple courses of antibiotics, her normal flora will be killed off and her body will be overburdened with yeast.

If you do have to take antibiotics, eat yogurt during the therapy. Buy natural yogurt, which contains live lactobacillus cultures (sometimes this type is more expensive than other yogurts). Or if antibiotic therapy has been lowering your natural vaginal flora and you find yourself susceptible to yeast infections, you can apply plain natural yogurt to the vagina and vulva. To many people this suggestion sounds gross, but it works and it is inexpensive. There are several ways to do this. You can dilute the yogurt and use it as a douche. Or if you have an old applicator for some vaginal medicine, you can fill it with yogurt and apply it that way. Or you can use a yogurt-coated tampon as an applicator. I suggest using the yogurt twice a day for four or five days to see whether you obtain relief.

What is the therapy for vulvitis or vaginitis caused by a yeast infection?

Often vulvitis or vaginitis has two components: the yeast infection itself, and an inflammatory component independent of the yeast and the scratching.

Various antifungal drugs, available over the counter or by prescription, attack the yeast cells. They come as creams or ointments and are applied directly to the infected area. The over-the-counter preparations cost in the range of $15 to $20; they are not inexpensive, but they are less expensive than prescription drugs and they may well work for you. A frequently used brand is Monistat, the commercial name of a drug called miconozole. Another common drug, clotrimazole, is sold commercially as Gyne-Lotrimin and Mycelex. As these preparations are used more and more commonly, certain strains of yeast are becoming resistant; but the significant majority of yeast infections will still yield to these over-the-counter medicines.

Topical antifungals are also available by prescription. They contain slightly different drugs, and fewer strains of yeast are resistant to them because they are less widely used. Commonly used prescription drugs are Terazol (terconazole) and Femstat (butoconazole). These are more expensive than the over-the-counter variety, but if your health insurance pays for prescription medications, they will cost you less out of pocket.

Recently many physicians have started to use systemic antifungals similar to the drugs prescribed for AIDS patients who have fungal infections. These drugs are effective, but because their long-term use has the potential of serious side effects they are still controversial.

There are also drugs such as oral nystatin, which is not a systemic drug. It is not absorbed into the bloodstream and it does not have side effects such as toxicity of the liver. When you take it, you decrease the load of yeast in your intestine. Sometimes I prescribe this drug for people who have increased vulnerability to yeast infections because of taking significant amounts of antibiotics. Because nystatin is not absorbed into the bloodstream, it does nothing for your vaginitis or vulvitis per se, but it does decrease your chance of reinfection with your own body yeast.

Since vaginitis or vulvitis may have an inflammatory component, doctors often recommend a topical anti-inflammatory agent if the antifungal therapy alone does not work. The fact that the itching fails to stop when you apply an antifungal cream doesn't mean that yeast didn't start the itching process in the first place. These agents are usually cortisone-like steroids.

Are there causes of vaginal and vulvar itching other than yeast infections?

Although vulvar cancer often makes its presence known through unrelieved itching, vaginal and vulvar itching is generally caused by something more benign.

Atrophic changes of the vagina and vulva can cause itching. Postmenopausal women who don't produce their own estrogen often are affected by such changes. Just as the skin of older people often gets irritated and itchy in winter when the air is dryer, these tissues too can become irritated.

Another condition that classically causes itching in the vulvar area, though it can appear anywhere on the body, is called lichen sclerosus et atrophicus, or LS&A for short. It is an inflammation, not an infection. Since it can be difficult to distinguish from vulvar cancer in physical appearance and in symptoms, your physician will probably recommend a biopsy. The tissue affected by LS&A looks whitish, rather than pink like normal vulvar tissue, the white color being caused either by scratching in response to itching or by the disease itself.

The condition is usually treated with topical anti-inflammatory drugs such as steroids. Sometimes LS&A is also treated with testosterone cream applied to the affected area. The amount of testosterone absorbed from the cream is not enough to produce masculinization.

Genital warts, caused by the condyloma virus, can also present with itching or burning. Sometimes, but not always, you can see warts on your skin. Your physician may want to examine you with a colposcope, because the warts have a classic appearance under magnification. A number of specific therapies are used to treat warts, including podophyllin, which comes from an herbal root, or TCA, tricarboxylic acid. Since warts are caused by a viral infection, antibiotics have no effect.

Another disease that can cause vulvar discomfort is something called vestibular vulvitis. More commonly seen in younger women than in older women, it is a frustrating disease to have and to treat because the physician cannot see much wrong except chronic inflammation. Typically women who have this disease go from doctor to doctor because no one can determine the cause of their discomfort. Even biopsies are not of much help.

Vestibular vulvitis can present with itching or with pain. Women sometimes complain of a burning type of pain, often in a horseshoe-shaped distribution around the bottom part of the opening of the vagina, then reaching back toward the rectum. Usually there is no pain in the rectal area itself. At the present time I have a young woman patient who has vestibular vulvitis periclitorally.

If you do have this problem, find a physician, either a gynecologist or a dermatologist, who is familiar with the disease. Ask your own doctor if he or she knows much about vestibular vulvitis, and if necessary ask for a referral to someone who does.

What is the cause of vestibular vulvitis?

No one knows for certain, but some researchers believe it may be related to previous chronic yeast infections or a chronic infection such as the human papilloma virus or the wart virus. Some women have vestibular vulvitis without any history of these other problems.

How long do these itchy conditions last?

Unfortunately, they can last months or even years, and some older women are significantly troubled by them. Even younger women are occasionally afflicted with vulvar itching. The first line of action is to try a little Monistat or another antifungal medication. If that doesn't relieve your symptoms in a week or two, you should see your doctor. A gynecologist can prescribe medicines that are not available over the counter. If your itching becomes chronic and does not respond to any medications, then your gynecologist will have to check on the possibility that you have vulvar cancer.

■ ■ Major and Minor Surgical Procedures

Abnormal vaginal bleeding may require surgical intervention for both diagnostic and therapeutic reasons. Surgical procedures range from minor operations, for example a D&C which can be performed on an out-patient basis, to major surgery such as a hysterectomy, which involves a stay in the hospital and a significant recovery period.

Dilatation and Curettage

What is a D&C?

The letters stand for dilatation and curettage. During the procedure, the cervix, the narrow opening to the main body of the uterus, is stretched or dilated, then the lining of the uterus is scraped out with a curette. The old slang among physicians for a D&C was "dusting and cleaning," and although the term is not quite accurate, it describes the purpose of a D&C, which is to clean out the glandular lining and get back to the underlying muscular layer of the uterus.

What are the reasons for a D&C?

In the context we are talking about, a D&C is performed for two principal reasons. The first and primary reason is diagnostic, to rule out or evaluate possible cancer of the uterus. The second is to help control bleeding.

A D&C is also the way most early-term abortions are performed. The physician may use suction curettage, but usually after the suction is performed the gynecologist will use a sharp curette to make sure that no tissue remains in the uterus. If a woman has a miscarriage and the placental tissue needs to be taken out, again a D&C is standard procedure.

Why do a D&C for diagnostic reasons when there are so many modern and sophisticated techniques for looking inside the body?

Modern technology has added some refinements that are helpful in diagnosing possible uterine cancer, and there many things that a physician can discover by an examination that uses ultrasound or x-ray studies. Ultrasound can sometimes show the presence of polyps or other growths. Ultrasound technology can reveal the thickness of the lining of the uterus, which is called the endometrial stripe because the endometrium shows up on the ultrasound picture as a dark stripe. If the endometrial stripe is narrow, something less than 6 to 7 mm wide, then only very rarely is there a chance of hyperplasia. Ultrasound is especially useful in evaluating women who are on ERT and have some unusual bleeding, perhaps because of uterine atrophy. If the endometrial stripe is wider, say 1.5 cm, the physician may say yes, this is a potential case of hyperplasia, let's do a biopsy and see what is going on inside the uterus.

CT scans and MRIs can also be helpful in looking at the inside of the body of the uterus and in diagnosing fibroids, for instance, but none of these fancy tests will show exactly what is happening to the individual cells that make up the lining of the uterus.

To rule out cancer, the physician must scrape out most of the lining of the uterus, perhaps not every single cell but enough to get a generous sample of all areas of the lining. The sample is then sent to a pathologist, who looks at it under a microscope and decides whether the cells are totally normal or whether, while not actually cancerous, they show changes that could become cancerous. These kinds of precancerous changes are called hyperplasia, which means "overgrowth," and the variety of hyperplasia that concerns physicians most is a condition called adenomatous hyperplasia. Adenoma means "gland," so adenomatous hyperplasia means excessive growth of glandular tissue. Left unchecked, adenomatous hyperplasia can proceed to cancer.

Why isn't a biopsy always an adequate test for precancerous changes of the uterine lining?

A biopsy is a mini-D&C. The physician dilates the cervix a bit and takes a pinch of tissue with a very small curette, an instrument about the width of a pipe cleaner with a sharp hook on one end. A D&C is a large-scale biopsy, and it takes tissue from all areas of the endometrium.

Most of the time a biopsy will suffice, because rarely is a cancer localized to one part or aspect of the uterus. Therefore in most cases a small sample will suggest what is happening throughout the uterine lining. However, in some high-risk women a D&C may be preferable, to check out every part of the endometrium.

What is a hysteroscopy?

Another refinement that modern technology has brought to the D&C is a tool called a hysteroscope. It is a long fiber-optic tube with a light at one end, and it is sometimes used in conjunction with video technology. What your doctor sees through the hysteroscope is projected onto a TV screen, so that you can see the inside of your own uterus on television.

With a hysteroscope the gynecologist can actually look into the uterus and see whether certain areas of the endometrium have abnormal-looking cells. If some areas look a little suspect, the gynecologist can scrape away that part of the endometrium. Hysteroscopes are especially useful to examine polyps, which are growths on the uterine lining. Hysteroscopes are also useful for examining fibroids, since your gynecologist can see what the growth looks like. While some gynecologists say that with the advent of hysteroscopy the D&C has become a thing of the past, most seem still to feel more comfortable scraping the lining to get a tissue sample and sending it to a pathologist to determine precisely what is going on.

What risks are associated with a D&C?

The major possible complications of a D&C, as of any invasive procedure, are bleeding and infection. During a D&C it is possible for the physician accidentally to put a hole through the wall of the uterus, which is called perforation. It is also possible to puncture the uterus with a hysteroscope, though it is less likely since that instrument is not particularly sharp. Perforations usually require no therapy unless they bleed, and even then a few sutures will usually do the job.

A few years ago a television documentary presented a special on hysteroscopy, with the message that hysteroscopies were good and D&Cs were not so good. For the next two weeks all my patients insisted on hysteroscopies and decided that they were definitely not going to have D&Cs. Television journalism aside, the prevailing opinion among gynecologists in this country seems to be that while hysteroscopy is a valuable adjunct, it should never replace the D&C as a bottom-line test for endometrial cancer.

How can a D&C be used to control bleeding?

One of the tricks of old-time gynecologists (and by "old-time" I mean people like me who were trained more than twenty years ago) was to use a D&C to help control heavy menstrual periods. Although there isn't any valid scientific reason why, the technique often seems to help. If polyps cause the heavy bleeding, then the D&C will get rid of the polyps and help get rid of the bleeding; but even those who have totally benign pathology will sometimes improve after a D&C.

I have worked with patients who had unpleasantly heavy menstrual periods; we have tried every trick known to modern science and when all else failed, a D&C has improved the situation. And of course it is a lot easier to recuperate from a D&C than it is to recuperate from a hysterectomy.

Yvonne P. is 47 years old. She is getting close to menopause and having a few hot flashes now and again. Her menstrual periods are very heavy, and although we have tried to control her bleeding nothing seems to help. She is a good candidate for a D&C, because classically the women who benefit from a D&C usually do well for a year, two years, or even three years, then their periods may start getting heavy again. Yvonne may be menopausal by the time her bleeding problem reasserts itself.

Some of my patients have had three D&Cs at about three-year intervals. Each time, they have improved for a long while, and in the nine-year interval they have reached menopause. By doing several D&Cs I have spared them a hysterectomy, which was my goal. Sometimes, unfortunately, I try a D&C and it doesn't make much difference. Then we have to go on to the next step, which may well be a hysterectomy.

Another advantage to a D&C is that for someone who is having unusual bleeding it will rule out endometrial pathology. Why is Yvonne, for example, having such heavy bleeding? Is it simply approaching menopause, or could she be harboring some hyperplasia? The advantage of the D&C is that the pathologist gets tissue to look at. Whenever I do a D&C, I send some tissue to a pathologist.

What is the recovery time from a D&C?

If you have a D&C, you will not be out of commission for weeks and weeks. Most women will feel some cramping the day of the procedure, comparable to the cramping of a heavy-duty menstrual period. A mild painkiller such as Tylenol or Advil will probably take care of it. Most women feel pretty well the next day. I tell my patients that for up to two weeks after the procedure they may experience some spotting and staining; it is not uncommon or indicative of anything dangerous.

As far as returning to normal activities including work, you can usually do so in a day or two. A great deal of the recuperation depends on what type of anesthesia you were given.

Can a D&C be performed under local anesthesia?

Yes, in most cases it can. The most commonly used anesthetic technique is a paracervical block, which means that something like Novocain is injected right into the cervix. It is the same as dental anesthesia, only in a different location. If this kind of anesthesia is used, the procedure can be done in a doctor's office.

A D&C with a paracervical block does cause some discomfort. The block anesthetizes the cervix, but it doesn't do anything to the inside of your uterus. A biopsy usually involves taking samples from different parts of the uterus to ensure getting representative sections, and different people have different sensitivities. How much discomfort a patient feels depends on the individual. I have had reactions ranging from "This is no big deal; why did you tell me it was going to be uncomfortable?" to "This is the worst thing that has ever happened to me in my life!" A middle-of-the-road group responds with "This is not fun, but who wants to go through general anesthesia?"

I tell a patient who is about to undergo any procedure under local anesthesia that if it gets too distressing she should say "Stop, I don't like this; I'd rather be asleep." Sometimes I have had to abandon a procedure because the patient is too miserable. Especially with postmenopausal women who are being evaluated for unusual bleeding, the cervix may be so tight that to get inside the uterus I have to stretch it hard, which can be uncomfortable and unpleasant.

If for some reason or other you undergo general anesthesia, remember that anesthesia has changed dramatically. Fifteen or twenty years ago, women would be admitted to the hospital the night before, have their D&C, and stay a day or two afterward. It was a big production. Nowadays, even with general anesthesia, the vast majority of D&Cs are done in out-patient settings, such as a surgicenter. You go into the surgicenter at about seven-thirty in the morning, your procedure is done an hour later, and you go home before lunch.

What kinds of anesthetics are used for a D&C?

Several modern drugs can be used for sedation or anesthesia in this sort of situation, where the patient does not have to be deeply anesthetized. The most common one is Versed, generic name midazolam, a short-acting sedative something like Valium. Another agent is Fentanyl, a short-acting narcotic, which behaves somewhat like morphine but wears off more quickly. The usual anesthetic agent is propofol (Diprivan is the trade name); it has replaced sodium pentathol, which used to make some people feel drugged for days. Diprivan looks rather like a piña colada, a whitish milky liquid, and acts like one, too: it works fast and wears off fast.

Endometrial Ablation

What is endometrial ablation?

It is a technique that uses a laser beam to remove the uterine lining with heat. The physician uses a hysteroscope to look at the inside of the uterus and under the guidance of the hysteroscope focuses the laser beam to "fry" the glandular cells that line the uterus. As in a D&C the goal is to get back to the underlying muscular layer. The procedure attempts to remove the entire layer; but even if the glandular tissue is not totally removed, the heavy bleeding is usually relieved.

Sometimes this procedure is presented as a new high-tech panacea, an approach without risks or complications, that can easily succeed where others fail. Endometrial ablation has its place in the range of available procedures, but it is not without risks or potential drawbacks.

Who is a suitable candidate for endometrial ablation?

Wanda C. is 47 years old and miserable with heavy periods. She has had a D&C, which did not relieve her problem. She has had a hysteroscopy, which did not reveal fibroids or polyps or anything pathological. She has tried progesterone and Ponstel but they didn't help either. She is definitely not interested in a hysterectomy. She has heard about endometrial ablation as a procedure that can destroy the glandular cells of the uterine lining, which after all are causing the bleeding, and stop her heavy periods.

Virginia E. is 42 years old. She is seriously overweight and has hypertension. Because of her obesity, she tends to bleed heavily. She, too, has tried progesterone and Ponstel, neither of which helped. Because of her obesity, she is not a good surgical risk for a hysterectomy.

Either of these women might be a reasonable candidate for endometrial ablation, Virginia because she is overweight and Wanda because she does not want a hysterectomy (which would be one way to cure her heavy bleeding). Women do not go into D&Cs lightly, nor should they approach endometrial ablation impetuously.

Is endometrial ablation difficult to perform?

Like any surgical procedure, endometrial ablation should be performed by a skilled practitioner, someone who has done it many times before.

There are potential problems with endometrial ablation. If the uterus is large, the laser must be used extensively. Through the hysteroscope the physician sees a piece about the size of a nickel at any one time, so he or she must move the scope and the laser around to see and remove all the endometrial tissue. This is not a problem if the woman has a small uterus, but it can be difficult if the uterus is large or if it has a lot of nooks and crannies. If, for example, a fibroid or two is outside the wall of the uterus pressing inward, the uterus will have an irregular shape.

Some physicians insist that a woman go on hormonal medication, say Lupron or danazol, for a month or two before the ablation. By suppressing FSH and estrogen production, which leads to stimulation of the lining of the uterus, the hormonal medication "flattens out" the lining and makes the procedure easier. The same physicians may also recommend continued hormone therapy for a month or two after the ablation, to let the endometrium scar and keep it from growing back.

What are the potential complications?

One potential complication of endometrial ablation results from the fact that the procedure is performed "underwater." That is, the physician instills water into the uterus itself to keep it from getting too hot, rather as the dentist uses water around an area being drilled. The medical journals have reported cases of women absorbing too much of this solution through the walls of the uterus, and at least one instance of a death related to such absorption. To be sure, this outcome is very rare.

Another possibility is bowel burn. If the laser penetrates the wall of the uterus, it can burn the intestine, which is very close to the uterus in the abdominal cavity. There have been numerous reports of bowel burn, and usually the patients end up with infection or peritonitis. The treatment is surgery to remove the piece of bowel containing the hole, and then antibiotic therapy. It is a serious complication and can even be fatal. To be perfectly honest, even as minor a procedure as a D&C can cause complications, though it is extraordinarily rare for death to ensue.

Some physicians will insist on performing a D&C before doing the ablation, just to make sure there is no abnormal pathology in the uterus. Your doctor does not want to focus the laser on cancerous tissue. Some physicians will insist on a D&C several months after the ablation, to make sure that the tissue has not regrown. So when you are talking about this procedure, you may be talking about a couple of D&Cs and some hormonal therapy as well.

The death rate from endometrial ablation is certainly much higher, and complications more common, than the public has been led to believe.

What else should I consider in deciding whether to have an endometrial ablation?

If you are having an endometrial ablation because, like Wanda, you are perimenopausal and have heavy bleeding resulting from hormonal problems, you should realize that in a few years you will probably be menopausal. If you decide to go on ERT after menopause, you will have to take progesterone, because no one can be totally sure that every gland in the uterus has been removed during the ablation. Suppose 5 percent of Wanda's endometrial tissue is left. That small amount will certainly not give her a substantial bleeding problem. But it can still become cancerous, so she will have to take progesterone and have a monthly cleanout bleed to protect her endometrium.

Are there safer ways to remove the endometrium?

A new technique is becoming available. It uses something called a roller ball— a sort of little electric ball that rolls around the lining of the uterus to scar the endometrium with electric current—rather than a laser, which scars it with intense heat. It is perhaps safer than laser ablation, because there is less risk of bowel burn.

Hysterectomy

Hysterectomy, the surgical removal of the uterus, has become the center of a controversy almost as heated as the turmoil surrounding ERT. The most commonly performed surgical procedure in the country two decades ago, hysterectomy was so routine that by 1975 one woman in three no longer had her uterus by age 60. The attitude underlying this extreme willingness to perform hysterectomies was that once a woman finished with her last planned pregnancy, her uterus became a useless organ; it bled, produced unwanted symptoms, and was potentially cancerous. Therefore it should be removed.

More recently, hysterectomy has come under the scrutiny of women's health advocates, who believe that the operation is performed much more frequently than is necessary. They note that the rate of hysterectomy is three times as high in the United States as it is in England and Western Europe, where health care standards are presumably similar. Studies have shown that the incidence of hysterectomy varies widely from one region of the United States to another. In the Northeast, for example, the rate is lower than in either the West or the South. Furthermore, the rate of hysterectomy can vary widely from community to community even within a small geographic region. Consequently, some observers believe that at least one-quarter of all hysterectomies done every year in the United States are unnecessary. These observers point out that the advice a woman receives about hysterectomy may depend on whether she has health insurance, on where she lives, and on the particular style of medical practice in her community. Finally, women's advocates have also attacked the medical profession for concealing from women the emotional and physical consequences of hysterectomy.

Perhaps because of the publicity generated by women's health advocates and perhaps because women in general are becoming more educated about their options, the annual number of hysterectomies has declined from its high in the late 1970s (725,000 in 1978) to about 578,000 in 1988. This 20 percent decrease has occurred despite an increase in the total number of women in their forties, the prime age for hysterectomy.

While all this controversy may complicate the decision on whether to have a hysterectomy, it certainly brings the issues into sharp focus. Each woman should realize her responsibility to understand the possible risks, benefits, and aftereffects of surgery; she should make her decision in conjunction with her caregiver on the basis of her own symptoms, her own lifestyle, and her own preferences.

WHEN IS HYSTERECTOMY APPROPRIATE?

How do I know I need a hysterectomy?

This question is one of the most common that women ask me. My standard answer is usually another question, "Do you think you need one?" In most cases hysterectomy is an elective procedure, not in the sense that a nose job or breast augmentation is elective, but in the sense that the reason for it is not life threatening. There is time to consider the options and make a thoughtful and informed decision.

Only on certain occasions must a woman absolutely have a hysterectomy. First and foremost is the presence of cancer. If a woman has cancer of the reproductive organs (uterus, cervix, ovaries, or fallopian tubes) she should in general anticipate having a hysterectomy. An exception might be a young woman in her twenties with certain kinds of ovarian cancer.

Another indication for hysterectomy is the presence of fibroids, benign tumors of the uterus, that have grown large enough to press on vital structures. Fibroids themselves do not inevitably necessitate a hysterectomy, for they can be small and cause little or no discomfort. However, large fibroids pressing against the ureters, the tubes that join the kidneys and the bladder, can cause compression of the kidneys or force the urine backward, which can lead to serious problems.

Another reason to have a hysterectomy is severe uterine prolapse. If the uterus has prolapsed to the point that it is actually out of the vagina, where it can become infected or ulcerated, a hysterectomy should be performed.

Finally, if a woman cannot keep up with her blood loss from severely heavy menstrual periods and is significantly anemic even though she is taking iron every day, she should think seriously about a hysterectomy if conservative therapies have not helped her.

The rest of the time the decision to have a hysterectomy is one that the woman herself should make in consultation with her caregiver. She has to feel that she is ready for a hysterectomy, that she wants it. The decision should not be made on the spur of the moment and it should not be made on a bad day. Suppose you have one or two days of very heavy bleeding every month; wait to decide about hysterectomy until a day when you are not bleeding.

Elective hysterectomy is determined by quality of life. The most common reason is the presence of fibroids that have not grown so large that they interfere with other important structures; the other principal reasons for elective hysterectomy are heavy bleeding and recurrent pelvic pain.

Are there ways to avoid hysterectomy?

In many cases there are, but they may require patience and toleration of symptoms. In our culture, which admires getting things done and requires decisive solutions to problems, many women are reluctant to wait and unwilling to tolerate discomfort if they do wait. But if you are approaching menopause and your fibroids are causing heavy bleeding, backache, pelvic pain, or frequent urination, you might wish to consider watchful waiting. Most fibroids shrink after menopause because they are estrogen dependent. If you can live with your symptoms and if your physician has determined that your fibroids are not growing rapidly or becoming dangerous to you in any other way, you can wait until after menopause to make a decision about hysterectomy.

If uterine prolapse is the reason you are thinking about hysterectomy, you might consider using a pessary. Although the pessary will not cure your prolapse, it may alleviate the symptoms by holding the uterus in place. Pessaries do not work for all women; nor do all women like them.

If heavy bleeding not caused by fibroids is your reason for contemplating hysterectomy, hormonal and nonhormonal therapies are worth trying before deciding on surgery. In many cases, the use of progesterone alone or of low-dose birth control pills can bring heavy or frequent bleeding under control. Supplementing dietary iron with iron pills can keep your hematocrit in a safe range.

What are the risks of having a hysterectomy?

With any surgery there is always a risk of infection. There is always a risk of blood loss. There is always a risk of problems with the anesthetic. And because the pelvic organs are packed closely together in a relatively small space and sometimes adhere to other abdominal organs, there is a danger of an inadvertent puncture of the bowel, bladder, or ureters. The risk increases for someone who has severe endometriosis or large fibroids. Obviously such a puncture, if found, can be repaired at the time of surgery.

Sometimes holes or fistulas develop after surgery when things do not heal properly, for example when a stitch gives way. The most common openings are between the vagina and another structure: a vesicovaginal fistula is a hole between the vagina and the bladder, a ureterovaginal fistula is between the vagina and a ureter.

Much as we would like to believe that everything always goes perfectly (in life as in surgery), things do go wrong. Severe problems are very uncommon. And they can usually be fixed. In general, however, it requires another surgery to repair the complications.

Does hysterectomy have any effect on PMS?

Frances H. is 40 years old and has significant PMS. She has finished having children and needs a hysterectomy because of large fibroids. Because she is only 40, she can look forward to ten more years of normal ovarian function. Should she have her ovaries removed?

One advantage to many women is that when the ovaries are removed, PMS symptoms frequently disappear. If a woman with severe PMS needs a hysterectomy for bleeding or some other reason, she should seriously consider having her ovaries removed. Some "PMS-ologists" have discovered that hysterectomy itself helps many but not all women with severe PMS, even though their ovaries remain in place. In light of our scientific knowledge today, this relief doesn't make sense, since PMS is a condition related to ovarian function and has little to do with the uterus. Perhaps the psychological dread of having a period is enough to trigger the PMS, or perhaps something subtle is happening hormonally that responds to the changed blood flow in the pelvis. No one knows, but physicians do report lowered PMS after hysterectomy.

Do postmenopausal ovaries have any significant function?

Although the ovaries no longer produce estrogen after menopause, they do make small amounts of androgens, which some researchers believe may contribute to libido. Some feminist groups suggest that even postmenopausally the ovaries are functioning in ways that are not known or understood; but basically the understanding of the scientific community is that the postmenopausal ovary does not do a great deal beyond producing androgens.

If I decide to have a hysterectomy, can I retain my ovaries?

This is another of the major questions pertaining to hysterectomy, one that I hear from patients at least once a week. If you are premenopausal and your ovaries are removed, you will undergo surgical menopause and can expect to experience hot flashes and other symptoms of menopause. Unless you are put on ERT postoperatively, the symptoms of menopause will be more severe than they would be if menopause were to occur naturally; for this reason women whose ovaries are removed usually elect to have ERT postoperatively. Occasionally women experience temporary hot flashes after surgery, even if the ovaries are left in place. This is not menopause and the symptoms are usually alleviated with temporary ERT.

Under certain conditions the ovaries absolutely should be removed. In other circumstances it would be better, but not essential, to remove the ovaries. And there are situations in which ovarian conservation is entirely a matter of personal preference.

Alice D. is an 18-year-old who has not yet had her family. She came to one of my partners with a large ovarian cyst that had to be removed. In a patient so young, the goal is to conserve as much functional ovary as possible. Therefore my partner did not want to remove the second ovary and wanted to save as much as she could of the ovary with the cyst. So she removed the cyst and sent a section of it to the lab for analysis while Alice remained in the operating room. When the pathologist examined the frozen section and found it benign, everyone was relieved. My partner finished the operation and closed the incision.

At the time of surgery the pathologist analyzing the frozen sections gives an instantaneous reading, which is not the final and decisive reading, since the frozen sections are only a few small bits of the diseased ovary. Later, in a more leisurely time frame, the pathologist looks methodically at every bit of tissue that has been removed. In the vast majority of cases the instantaneous reading is the same as the final decisive one.

Five days later, just as Alice was feeling better, the final pathology report came back. She had a borderline cancer, and the oncologists recommended that the rest of the ovary be removed. Unfortunately, Alice had to go back into surgery. The oncologists did not recommend removal of the other ovary.

Had Alice been 48 years old with the same grapefruit-sized mass on her ovary, the recommendation would have been to remove the uterus, tubes, cervix, and ovaries, a procedure known as TAH and BSO. A 48-year-old has only two or three more years of ovarian function. Since Alice has had one ovarian cyst, she stands an increased chance, perhaps 5 to 10 percent, of developing a cyst on her other ovary and needing major surgery again. If Alice had been only 40, the recommendation might have been to remove the diseased ovary, not just the cyst, but to leave the second ovary intact.

The recuperation time of the second surgery, as in Alice's case, when the remaining ovary is removed is not significantly different from the recuperation time when ovary and uterus are removed together. The second surgery is also a major operation. The potential complications of oophorectomy and TAH and BSO are similar. If the uterus is removed, the woman will not have to take progesterone with her postoperative ERT. Consequently, many gynecologists prefer to remove the uterus too, but the decision should depend on the personal preference of the patient.

Sandy R. is 32 years old and has finished her childbearing. She has significant pelvic pain. She has bilateral endometriomas (ovarian tumors of endometrial tissue outside her uterus) and has decided to have definitive surgery, to have her uterus removed. Even though she is only 32, she is better off having her ovaries removed also.

Basically Sandy has come in for pain; if her diseased ovaries remain intact, she still has the possibility of pain from her ovarian tumors.

Cindy T. is 45 years old. She is having a hysterectomy for heavy bleeding. Her ovaries are perfect; she has never had pelvic pain and has no reason to suspect she has endometriosis. Ten years ago she had a tubal ligation, and at the time her ovaries looked completely healthy. Now that she is 45, she has a small fibroid. Although she and her gynecologist have tried every known approach to control her bleeding, nothing has worked, so she has decided to have her uterus removed. Should she have her ovaries removed also?

Statistically Cindy, like other women, has a 1 percent chance of developing ovarian cancer and a 5 percent chance of developing something on her ovary, for example a benign cyst, that will require surgical exploration. Therefore she is likely to be among the 99 percent of women who do not get ovarian cancer; she is also likely to be among the 95 percent of women who will go through their later years with perfectly normal atrophic ovaries.

How long can Cindy expect to continue to have ovarian function if she decides not to have her ovaries removed? If her mother started having menopausal symptoms when she was 43 years old, or if Cindy herself has been having hot flashes, then her menopause might be imminent. She might want to hold off having a hysterectomy, hoping that with menopause the bleeding will abate. But if her mother went through menopause at age 58 and Cindy seems nowhere near menopause, then she will be losing quite a few years of potential ovarian function. There are some data to suggest that women who have a hysterectomy with their ovaries left in place may undergo somewhat earlier menopause secondary to the blood flow changes consequent to hysterectomy. In essence, the decision is Cindy's.

A postmenopausal woman who is having an abdominal hysterectomy should consider having her ovaries taken out because they are no longer making estrogen. But personal choice enters this decision also.

Do women who have their ovaries removed have problems adjusting to ERT?

In general, women do well with postoperative ERT. In my twenty years of practice I have had only two patients who had tremendous difficulty finding an estrogen that agreed with them. One woman now is taking injectable estrogen, because it seems to be the only thing that controls her symptoms without giving her severe headaches. The other cannot tolerate any estrogen at all. She was in her late forties when I removed her ovaries and she has proved to be allergic to every form of estrogen available, including all brands and routes of delivery—patches, tablets, and shots. But of the hundreds of women on whom I have operated, only these two have had difficulties. I always tell patients who are premenopausal that it may take some time and experimentation to find the ideal estrogen regimen, but eventually we will succeed.

Are there different kinds of hysterectomies?

Hysterectomies are performed either through an abdominal incision or transvaginally, through the vagina. In recent years a third type of surgery, a laparoscopically assisted vaginal hysterectomy (LAVH), has become available. In this operation, a combination of the transvaginal and abdominal hysterectomies, the uterus and cervix are taken out and sometimes also the ovaries and tubes. The surgeon uses a laparoscope inserted through small abdominal incisions to visualize the upper part of the abdominal cavity. The uterus is detached from its support structures through the laparoscope but taken out through the vagina, as are the ovaries and fallopian tubes (if they are removed too).

Are there conditions other than personal preference that determine which is the best procedure to use?

Once you and your physician have decided that a hysterectomy is necessary, you must choose one of these three approaches. Some people are candidates for any of the three available operations: abdominal, vaginal, or laparoscopically assisted vaginal; for other women one route is definitely preferable.

Part of the decision depends on your thoughts about ovarian conservation. You and your physician should also discuss the relative recovery times and the possibilities of complications such as bleeding and infection with each procedure.

Abdominal hysterectomy.

If you are going to have your ovaries removed, you should have either an abdominal hysterectomy or an LAVH. Although the ovaries can be removed vaginally, the process can be difficult, especially if their attachments are high in the pelvic cavity.

If there is a chance that endometriosis is involved (for example, if you are having significant pelvic pain), an abdominal hysterectomy or an LAVH is the best choice. If endometriosis is present, the physician will want to know about your ovaries. If the ovaries are involved and are attached by adhesions to other pelvic structures, they will not be easy to remove vaginally.

If you have a cyst on your ovary, a growth that could possibly be cancer, you are a candidate for abdominal exploration. Some physicians would argue that an LAVH would be equally appropriate, but most oncologists prefer that the cyst or suspicious growth be removed intact. They believe that by removing in pieces something that is possibly cancerous, they risk spilling malignant cells into the abdominal cavity. People who favor LAVHs argue that it is all right to take out the questionable growth in pieces because the surgeon washes the interior of the pelvic cavity after removing the abnormal tissues.

Vaginal hysterectomy

For other women, a straightforward vaginal hysterectomy is appropriate. Recuperation from this type is the easiest of all three procedures.

Diane T., mother of three children, has a problem with heavy bleeding. We believe the bleeding to be hormonally based, but after trying everything we have not solved her problem. Therefore we have decided to remove her uterus. She wants to retain her ovaries. Because she has had three pregnancies and deliveries, her uterus has descended somewhat into her vagina, so it should be easy to remove vaginally. Since she wants her ovaries to remain, there is no reason to use the laparoscope. This woman is a good candidate for a vaginal hysterectomy.

After the removal of her uterus by vaginal hysterectomy, examination of the uterine tissue by a pathologist revealed adenomyosis, that is, her uterine muscle was penetrated throughout by endometrial tissue. This finding explained why our conservative attempts to stop the bleeding had not succeeded.

If you and your doctor decide on a vaginal hysterectomy, you should be aware that the procedure may turn into an abdominal hysterectomy once the operation has begun. I always tell patients that until they are in the recovery room I cannot guarantee that I will successfully complete a vaginal hysterectomy. The reasons for the change in procedure may be bleeding problems during the operation or difficulty with the uterus descending into the vagina where it can be removed. When I am discussing with someone the possibility of having a vaginal hysterectomy, I sometimes give odds. I say, I am 90 percent sure that I can do this vaginally, but there is a 10 percent chance the operation will turn out to be abdominal. Or, I may say, there is only a 20 percent chance that I can do this vaginally, but I am happy to give it a try.

Laparoscopically assisted vaginal hysterectomy.

The third group of women can have an LAVH; these are people with no major abdominal problems, no large fibroids, no significant endometriosis, and no complicated pathology.

I have already mentioned Grace Q., aged 59, who chose hysterectomy because she did not want to give up ERT. Grace has serious arthritis, which she keeps under control by daily exercise. She has taken estrogen since menopause, but progesterone in any form gives her severe headaches. We tried ERT without progesterone, but she developed endometrial hyperplasia and needed a hysterectomy if she wanted to continue the estrogen. After considering her choices, she opted for the hysterectomy. A short recovery time was crucial because of her exercise regimen; since she had never had children, her uterus was quite small, which made her a good candidate for a laparoscopically assisted hysterectomy. She recuperated easily and was back working out at the gym after only two weeks.

Grace is a woman who can't afford to be out of commission very long; she needs her daily stint in the gym to keep her joints flexible. Abdominal surgery would have kept her from her exercise routine for several weeks and thereby increased her suffering from arthritis. The LAVH allowed her to resume her daily exercises and whirlpool promptly. She was an ideal candidate for that procedure.

What are the advantages and disadvantages of an LAVH?

The chief advantage is that the recovery time may well be shorter than with an abdominal hysterectomy. Many women do very well with an LAVH and are back in shape in no time at all.

One of my partners has a patient whom I had seen at the local gym for quite a while; although I didn't know her name, we always nodded and smiled when we saw each other. One day she came up to me and said, "Tell your partner that Jennifer is doing fine." I was startled when I realized that she had had an LAVH two weeks earlier and was in the gym doing a full workout. Of course, she was in spectacular shape to begin with and she might have done just as well with an abdominal hysterectomy, but I think having it done laparoscopically contributed to her quick recuperation.

On the other hand, some patients are slow to recuperate after the operation; they have, after all, undergone major surgery. They may not have had an abdominal incision, but the interior surgery is the same as that of an abdominal hysterectomy. The surgeon is cutting the same veins, arteries, and ligaments. These things are painful, yet because the patient has no scar on her abdomen she tends to get less sympathy.

Dr. Alan DeCherney, one of the foremost practitioners of laparoscopy in this country, has pointed out that this lack of sympathy is a real debit of laparoscopic surgery. One of his patients, from whom he had removed a benign ovarian cyst through the laparoscope, came back for her two-week postoperative checkup. He thought she would be happy about having had the procedure, but she told him that these had been the worst two weeks of her life. Even though she felt miserable, her friends and family had little sympathy for her; as far are they were concerned, she was feeling no pain whatsoever. If she had had a big scar on her abdomen to show for her trouble, she said, her friends and family would have been bringing her chicken soup and flowers instead of expecting to see her up and about.

Laparoscopic surgery certainly has its benefits, but it should not be considered painless surgery. For every Jennifer who is lifting weights at the gym two weeks postop, someone else feels dreadful. You must take these variations into account in anticipating your recuperative course.

I have mentioned the slight possibility that an LAVH, like a standard vaginal hysterectomy, will change into an abdominal hysterectomy while you are on the operating table, that some problem or complication will necessitate an abdominal incision. Therefore no one can be absolutely sure in advance that she will be back at work in two weeks.

Since an LAVH is a relatively new operation and not all physicians perform it, you should be sure to determine whether your doctor is familiar with the procedure. As with any operation, especially one that has a steep learning curve, you want to be sure that the doctor who will be operating on you has performed the surgery many times successfully, that is, without a significant rate of complications. You should find out whether your physician is credentialed to perform an LAVH. You should also determine whether you are a suitable candidate for the procedure, and if not, why not.

In group practice, often one doctor is better at a particular procedure and another specializes in something else. My own senior partner is one of the best abdominal surgeons I know, but he is not a vaginal surgeon. I do most of the vaginal surgery; he does our complicated infertility cases, which require special abdominal procedures. A third partner in our group is skillful at LAVH.

You may find it difficult or embarrassing to ask your doctor these questions, but it is worthwhile to do so. If you are an appropriate LAVH candidate but your own gynecologist does not routinely perform this surgery, ask for a referral to someone who has significant experience in the procedure. If you have a reputable physician and your relationship is solid, you should be able to get a satisfactory answer to your questions. If your physician is not experienced in performing LAVHs, he or she should be willing to tell you, "Yes, you are a reasonable candidate for an LAVH; no, I am not an experienced LAVH doctor."

Are laparoscopic hysterectomies less expensive?

If you do not have adequate health insurance, cost can be a major factor in health care decisions. Although it would seem that shorter hospital stays would make an LAVH cheaper than an abdominal hysterectomy, that is not the case. LAVHs are done with disposable surgical instruments (except for the laparoscope itself), and these instruments—the probes and stapling guns and suture devices used to tie off the blood vessels—cost about $2000. Because these instruments are difficult to sterilize and must be extremely sharp, they cannot be reused. Therefore the economic gain of a shorter hospital stay is more than offset by the cost of surgical instruments.

Is there such a thing as a laser hysterectomy?

Sometimes patients ask me about a laser hysterectomy. There really isn't such a thing. What most people are talking about is the LAVH, which uses a laparoscope, clips, and sutures, but not a laser. Lasers are used for other surgery, of course, but in many cases they do not have significant advantages over more traditional techniques.

GENERAL SURGICAL QUESTIONS

How can I prepare for a hysterectomy?

The better shape you are in, the better you will withstand the surgery and the more quickly you will recover. Being in good shape means getting aerobic exercise rather than doing sit-ups or push-ups to strengthen particular muscles. If you smoke, stop; or at the very least, cut down on the number of daily cigarettes. Smoking increases problems with anesthesia and causes additional discomfort after the surgery. If you have a smoker's cough, you will really feel it postoperatively.

Box 2. Questions to Ask Your Physician before Hysterectomy or Other Surgery

How long is the surgical procedure?

Is it advisable to store my own blood?

How long will I be in the hospital?

What complications can arise?

How will you deal with these complications if they do arise?

What type of pain will I have after surgery?

What will you use to alleviate the pain?

What type of anesthesia will be used? How long will I be under anesthesia?

Will I have stitches?

Will I have a catheter or an IV in me? For how long?

When will I be able to return to my normal routine—which includes work, exercise, sex, and driving a car?

When will I visit you postoperatively? How often will I see you after my first postoperative visit?

Source: Adapted from Karen Giblin, founder PRIME PLUS/Red Hot Mamas.

Get in good nutritional shape. Try to stay close to your ideal weight. If you are 40, 50, or 100 pounds overweight, lose as much as you can; significant overweight is a major risk for anesthesia and other surgical complications. Take iron to build up your hematocrit. The average American woman is well nourished and probably doesn't need too much in the way of supplemental vitamins, although taking extra vitamins can't hurt as long as you are reasonable. Get enough rest before the operation so that your immune system is not stressed by fatigue.

What should I discuss with my physician before surgery?

If you are taking medications, you should find out which are safe to take before surgery. Medicines that could be hazardous include common anti-inflammatories: aspirin, Motrin, Naprosyn, and similar drugs that many people use for arthritis, headaches, and other conditions. These drugs interfere with clotting and your doctor may ask you to stop taking them a few days in advance. You can ask for alternatives. Tylenol, for example, is perfectly safe.

Other drugs that you absolutely should not take if you are undergoing surgery are MAO inhibitors. People taking these uncommon drugs are restricted in their intake of cheese, wine, and nuts. If these foods are off limits to you and you are taking medication, be very sure that your physician knows about it. There are other drugs whose dosage your physician may wish to lower.

If you have allergies to any medications that your physician does not know about, you should mention them. Some people are allergic to iodine, which is sometimes used as a surgical scrub. If your physician knows, another antiseptic solution can be substituted.

If you have serious heart or lung disease, it is probably prudent to schedule a meeting with the anesthesiologist well before surgery so that everything can be understood and planned before the day of your operation.

What are autologous blood donations?

In this AIDS-conscious era, many women donate blood for themselves preoperatively. Since most of the time a hysterectomy is an elective procedure, you will have time to make what is called an autologous blood donation. As soon as you decide to have a hysterectomy, start taking iron. A few weeks before the operation, you may wish to donate a unit of blood at your hospital's blood bank, then build yourself up with more iron, and a few weeks later donate another unit, continuing this routine until you have given an adequate supply of your own blood (usually one or two units are enough). You can safely give blood about every two weeks; since the hospital and operating room will be booked for you three or four weeks in advance, you will have plenty of time.

Not every hospital has the facilities for autologous donations, but most do. If your physician doesn't discuss this issue with you, you should raise it yourself if you are concerned.

If you are unfamiliar with the blood supply laws in your state, ask your physician. In Connecticut, where I practice, the state's blood supply is extremely safe because all of the blood in the state blood bank is donated at Red Cross centers. Drug addicts who might sell their blood to make money have to go elsewhere. Furthermore, the word is out in the gay community not to donate. By law all blood in Connecticut since 1985 has been screened for syphilis, for HIV, and for hepatitis.

In other states in this country not all blood is donor blood. If you live in one of those states and cannot donate an autologous supply for some reason, you may want to contact the Red Cross about directed donation, that is, having your friends and relatives donate blood. Even this tactic is not without risk. Some blood bank directors believe that directed donations can be riskier than the general blood supply. Suppose you ask cousin George to donate blood for you. If, unbeknown to you, he is homosexual or perhaps has abused heroin at some point in his life, he may feel pressured to donate anyhow. It is naive to think that you can be sure about anyone else's sexual habits and experiences; I have seen many women who discovered after years of marriage that their husbands were bisexual.

What tests and evaluations are done before surgery?

Before you undergo anesthesia, your doctor will want you to have a cardiogram to be sure your heart is sound and a chest x-ray to be sure your lungs are clear. Usual preop blood evaluations include a blood count to see that you are not too anemic to withstand surgery. A clot of blood is sent off to the blood bank so that in case you need blood on an emergency basis (and you have not made an autologous donation), the blood bank will be able to give you blood that matches yours. Some doctors ask for a clotting study (called a PT and PTT) to see how long it takes your blood to coagulate.

Although the blood that is drawn for these tests may look like a large amount to you, it is not really very much at all. Three of the standard tubes contain 1 oz (30 ml) of blood.

What preparations are required the day before surgery?

People undergoing surgery should not eat after midnight the night before. If you're making your children's lunches the morning of the operation, don't even lick the peanut butter knife! If an anesthetized patient vomits, what is thrown up may be aspirated into the lungs and cause serious problems. Under elective circumstances no anesthesiologist will give anesthesia to anyone whose stomach contains food or liquid. Occasionally, however, the anesthesiologist will tell you that it is all right to take your normal medications with a sip of water.

Another thing you should do before surgery is take an enema. One of the major complaints after abdominal surgery is gas pain, and you can save yourself a lot of discomfort if you have an empty bowel. Usually I tell people to use a Fleet enema, which is all that is needed for most hysterectomies.

If your physician thinks you may have cancer of the pelvic organs, you will probably be asked to have a bowel prep, just in case the surgeon needs to do bowel surgery. Occasionally ovarian tumors can spread to the bowel, and in some instances the surgeon may have to take out part of the bowel. This does not mean that you are going to have a colostomy, but if your doctor is working near the bowel, it is advisable that the bowel be cleaned out.

Years ago it was standard procedure to come to the hospital the night before surgery. This practice allowed for the necessary tests and ensured that you didn't eat or drink anything after midnight. Today, because of hospital costs, most patients come in on what is called express admission. They have their blood tests, cardiograms, chest x-rays, and other preoperative evaluations as an outpatient in the week to ten days before surgery.

What kinds of anesthesia are available and what are the risks?

Most gynecological procedures can be done either under a general anesthetic or with an epidural or spinal anesthetic. General anesthesia puts the patient completely to sleep; she is hooked up to respirators that do her breathing for her, monitored by the anesthesiologist. When a spinal anesthetic is used, a small amount of Novocain or a similar drug is put into the space around the spinal cord. With an epidural anesthetic, a larger amount of the same type of medication is injected into the area outside the spinal space. A small soft tube or catheter remains in the back, so that the anesthesiologist can administer more medication as needed. Both a spinal and an epidural cause numbness from the chest down. In addition to the anesthetic itself, the anesthesiologist usually gives intravenous medications to make the patient oblivious to her surroundings. Although she continues to breathe on her own, she is not alert and not counting the minutes as they go by.

In most hysterectomies, the choice of anesthesia is up to the individual patient and what she feels most comfortable with. If you are deeply anxious about surgery and don't even want to see the inside of an operating room, you are probably better off with a general anesthetic. Occasional patients who have epidurals are aware of tugging and pulling; they are not in pain, but they do feel something happening. If this would distress you, general anesthesia is a better choice.

One advantage of a spinal anesthetic is that it wears off gradually. With a general anesthetic, you wake up and immediately feel the full brunt of the surgery. With a spinal, you are brought to the recovery room and the effects of the surgery assert themselves little by little.

There is little difference in risk between a general and an epidural anesthesia. With recently developed anesthetic agents, anesthesia is extraordinarily safe. While death from anesthesia does still occur, it is extremely rare. People who had surgery twenty years ago should know that the agents used today for general anesthesia are very different from the old-fashioned ones. So much surgery is done in out-patient clinics that it has been important to develop anesthetic agents that act quickly and wear off quickly. Formerly, when a patient stayed in the hospital for three days after a D&C, it did not matter that she was groggy. Nowadays, when she goes home right away, she needs an anesthetic that will wear off rapidly so that she can take care of herself at home. These quicker-acting agents have fewer side effects than the old ones did.

Furthermore, scare stories used to circulate about people who were paralyzed by spinal anesthetics. With current methods and techniques, there is no such danger. In the past, people often had severe headaches following spinal anesthesia, caused by a leak of cerebrospinal fluid from the puncture where the needle introduced the anesthetic. Today's needles are so small that postoperative headaches are a rare complication, and anesthesiologists have medications that can help alleviate the few spinal headaches that do occur.

THE OPERATION

Which organs are removed during a hysterectomy?

Technically the word "hysterectomy" means removal of the hystera, the Greek word for "uterus," but today the operation almost always includes the cervix; the fallopian tubes and the ovaries may also be removed.

The technical names for these operations describe the organs that are involved. If the entire uterus (that is, the fundus, or body, of the uterus) and the cervix are removed, the operation is called a total abdominal hysterectomy, abbreviated in the gynecology literature as TAH.

About forty years ago one of the commonly performed procedures was something called a supracervical hysterectomy, which meant that the uterus was taken out but the cervix was left in place. Another name for this operation was subtotal or partial hysterectomy. Common sense lay behind this approach, since most of the maladies that necessitate a hysterectomy are remedied by taking out only the fundus of the uterus. Without the uterine corpus, symptoms such as bleeding, fibroids, and pain usually can be cured. Still, the cervix in and of itself has no function, and now physicians tend to take it out routinely as part of a hysterectomy, because it can become cancerous. An occasional physician will perform a supracervical hysterectomy if a patient specifically asks for it. Last year I did one, my first in about thirteen years, in answer to a patient's strong request. The issue has become somewhat controversial for two reasons: some women believe that the presence of the cervix contributes to sexual satisfaction; and a few investigators believe that it helps support the vagina when the uterus has been removed.

A supracervical hysterectomy may be appropriate in an emergency situation, perhaps when someone is bleeding postpartum. Sometimes the patient is critically ill, and a hysterectomy is easier if the cervix remains in place. Removing it may increase the risk of infection or further blood loss.

When women speak of a "total" hysterectomy, they usually mean the uterus, the cervix, both ovaries, and the fallopian tubes. In strict medical terminology, however, a total abdominal hysterectomy means removal of the entire uterus including the cervix. The abbreviation for removing everything—uterus, cervix, ovaries, and tubes—is TAH and BSO, total abdominal hysterectomy and bilateral salpingo-oophorectomy. The term "salpingo" comes from the Greek word for "tube," while oophorectomy, sometimes called ovariectomy, refers to removal of the ovaries. In terms of the risk of complications and recovery time, the procedures are basically the same whether or not the ovaries and tubes are removed.

Often when a gynecologist is performing a hysterectomy, he or she will talk about taking out the appendix at the same time, which adds perhaps five or ten minutes to the operation. Sometimes patients request it, and although appendicitis is more common in young people, it can strike at any age. While the appendix does not serve any biological function, some people have an emotional attachment to it; others as a matter of policy want nothing removed that absolutely doesn't have to be removed. It is very important that your physician respect your wishes and do what is emotionally comfortable for you.

What exactly does the surgery entail?

The most common form of hysterectomy is abdominal. After the patient has been anesthetized, the surgical team washes the vagina with an antiseptic solution. The reason for this prepping is that later in the operation an incision will be made in the vagina, and decreasing the germ count lowers the risk of infection. The physician then inserts a catheter into the bladder to keep it empty and minimize the space the bladder occupies in the pelvis.

The abdomen is then cleaned and the top part of the pubic hair shaved off. Whereas formerly the whole pubic area was shaved, now only enough shaving is done to keep hair from getting into the incision. The rest of the abdomen is draped with towels to create a clean field around the incision.

The surgeon then makes the incision. Two kinds of incisions can be made for an abdominal hysterectomy. One is up and down, going from just beneath the belly button down toward the pubic bone. An up-and-down incision is useful if the surgeon needs a large area within the pelvis to work, for example to remove a large fibroid or if there is strong suspicion of cancer. Otherwise many surgeons favor a Pfannenstiel incision, a low transverse incision popularly known as a bikini cut. A Pfannenstiel is more attractive cosmetically than an up-and-down incision and tends to heal a bit faster.

Beneath the skin is a layer of fat. Some people have a little; some people have a lot. The surgeon cuts through the fat and encounters the fascia, the layer that really holds other structures together. Fascia is like tendon tissue, shiny and white and tough. Usually the surgeon incises the fascia sideways and takes it off the muscles beneath it.

The rectus muscles beneath the fascia are two straplike muscles that run up and down parallel to each other, from the ribs to the pubic bone. In the midline there is a little space between the two rectus muscles; sometimes in a late pregnancy, the uterus bulges out in the separation between the rectus muscles. In a nonpregnant woman, the rectus muscles are quite tight and lie close together.

The surgeon separates the rectus muscles and pushes them to the two sides. Occasionally, to get more room, the surgeon will have to cut the rectus muscles a little, but at the end of the operation the muscles will be sewn together and will heal. Patients do not have to worry about having their strength diminished or their abdominal wall permanently weakened.

The next layer is the peritoneum, which lines the body cavity. Since the intestines and other structures lie right beneath it, the surgeon carefully makes a little nick in it, then extends the incision with direct visualization. Usually this incision is vertical. The surgical team moves the bowel and the muscles out of the way with sterile packs, all of which are numbered and labeled, so that they will not get stuck or lost in the belly. The team puts in retractors to hold the abdominal wall and the bladder out of the way for better visualization.

After the physician manually palpates the organs in the pelvis—the liver, the intestines, the lymph nodes, the kidneys, and so on—checking for abnormalities, the hysterectomy proper begins.

If there is a lot of scar tissue or adhesion, the surgeon removes it to restore normal anatomy. Working from the top down, he or she locates and cuts the round ligaments that support the uterus at the top. If the ovaries are being removed, they are isolated from their blood supply (the ovarian artery and vein) and from their attachments in the pelvis and removed. If the ovaries and fallopian tubes are to remain, they are isolated from the uterus. Since the bladder sits right on top of the uterus and cervix and is attached to them, the surgeon must separate these organs, a procedure known as taking down the bladder flap.

Next the uterus and the cervix are divided from the broad ligament, the uterine blood supply, and the cardinal ligaments that attach them to the side wall of the pelvis. The surgeon has now reached the level of the top of the vagina. Unless the patient has cancer, no vaginal tissue will be removed, so the surgeon makes an incision at the cervicovaginal junction and divides the cervix from the vagina.

Since the uterus is now separated from the vagina, from the side walls of the pelvis, and from the ovaries, it can be removed through the abdominal cavity. The surgeon puts several stitches at the top of the vagina to stop bleeding and to reattach the vagina to the ligaments that formerly supported the uterus. The vagina is now attached to the cardinal ligaments and the round ligaments.

Once that is done, the bladder flap is tacked back over the top of the vagina. This procedure creates a significant change in the anatomy of the bladder, which is now sitting more or less where the uterus was located. Accordingly, women who have had a hysterectomy will be aware for a week or so after surgery that urinating feels different.

When the uterus and vagina have been resuspended, the surgeon may do an appendectomy, detaching the appendix from the fat surrounding it and from the bowel and snipping it off. The surgeon then removes the packs and the retractors and closes the various layers, starting with the peritoneum and working outward, closing and stitching the muscle layers, the fascia, the fat, and finally the skin. There are several different ways of closing the skin. If you prefer one way to another, talk to your surgeon ahead of time. If you don't like clips or you want a specific kind of suture, let your surgeon know.

A vaginal hysterectomy is an abdominal hysterectomy in reverse. The patient is in stirrups and usually two assistants are holding retractors to keep the side walls of the vagina out of the way while the operation proceeds. The operation begins at the cervix, with an incision all the way around its circumference. After pushing the vaginal tissue away from the uterus, the surgeon makes a small incision in the posterior cul de sac, which opens into the abdominal cavity. The patient's position, with her head a bit downward, keeps the intestines out of the way. Much of a vaginal hysterectomy is done by feel. After pushing the bladder off the uterus from below, the surgeon makes an incision anterior to the uterus. Through these incisions the surgeon feels along the uterus, working upward to its top, clamping and cutting and stitching, until the uterus is detached from its pelvic ligaments. Since all of this is done as much by feel as by direct visualization, the pelvic structures have to come down easily. If the patient proves to have endometriosis or adhesions, it is at this point that a vaginal hysterectomy may become abdominal.

Interestingly enough, one of my patients who has fared the best after a hysterectomy was a woman on whom we intended to do a vaginal hysterectomy. Her uterus did not descend, so we had to make a change partway through. Logically her swift recovery makes sense. We did vaginally what is easy to do through the vagina. Then we did abdominally what is easy to do via that route. She was home from the hospital in three days, eating, and feeling comfortable. At her postop check three weeks later, she said that she had never felt ill for even one day.

The procedure for an LAVH is a combination of the two previously described. The surgeon begins at the top, making two small abdominal incisions through which the laparoscope is inserted. The cutting of the ligaments near the top of the uterus and division of the uterine artery and vein are done via the laparoscope, through which the surgeon can visualize the interior of the pelvis to see whether or not there are adhesions. The bladder flap and uterine vessels are taken from above. From below, the surgeon takes the cardinal ligaments and withdraws the uterus through the vagina.

Once the uterus has been removed in a vaginal hysterectomy, the surgeon sews up the peritoneum and reattaches the ligaments to the top of the vagina. When all the reattachments have been made, the surgery is complete. There is no skin, no fascia, nothing else to close. For this reason the healing process often takes less time with a vaginal hysterectomy.

How long does a hysterectomy take?

The length of surgery depends on whether other procedures, for example a bladder repair, are being done at the same time. The average hysterectomy takes anywhere from an hour and a half to three hours, depending on how much surgery is undertaken. Ask your physician for an estimate. But remember to tell the relatives or friends who are waiting for you to add an hour or two to that time. You may spend a little while waiting outside the operating room; once inside, it takes a half-hour or longer for the IV to start and the monitoring devices to be hooked up.

Anesthesiologists as a group are chatty people, and they may spend time talking with you to help you relax. Some hospitals have more rigid schedules than others; your physician can give you an estimate of how long relatives may have to wait beyond the scheduled operating time.

What can be done for postoperative pain?

Twenty years ago the standard treatment for postop pain was Demerol or morphine, given by injection every three or four hours—sometimes with an antihistamine such as Vistaril added to give better pain relief, sometimes just straight Demerol. When the pain decreased, oral pain medications were substituted.

Nowadays there are better ways to administer these drugs. Among the most significant improvements is something called patient-controlled analgesia (PCA), which means that you are hooked up to a little pump and given a controller. You can push this "joy buzzer" every 6 to 10 minutes and a dose of painkiller drips right into the IV. If you push the button more frequently, say every minute, the pump will dispense the drug only every 6 to 10 minutes. Interestingly enough, it turns out that people require less analgesia if they can control its frequency.

Before the pump came into use, the posthysterectomy patient would get her shot of morphine or Demerol, go to sleep for about two hours, wake up in pain and get another shot, go back to sleep, wake up in pain again, and so on. But with the PCA, she can keep dosing herself and control the pain. Because the doses are small, she remains more alert. Most women need to keep the PCA going for a day or two after surgery, though some use it for longer or shorter periods.

Another modern technique for pain control involves giving a spinal containing narcotic medication before the surgery. This kind of medication is called intrathecal narcotics and gives pain relief for up to twenty-four hours after surgery. You can have intrathecal narcotics even if you are going to have a general anesthetic. Some physicians even keep the epidural in place after surgery so that more medication can be introduced. The advantage of putting the narcotic into the spinal or epidural space instead of the brain is that it doesn't cause grogginess. The patient is alert but the pain is deadened.

RECOVERY AND RECUPERATION

What pain medications are available to take at home?

The two major categories are narcotics and anti-inflammatories. Narcotics include codeine, Demerol, Percodan, or Vicodin. A narcotic nasal spray called Stadol is absorbed through the nasal mucosa and gives satisfactory postop pain relief. Anti-inflammatories include Motrin, Naprosyn, Toradol, and a host of other widely available drugs. For postoperative pain the drug of choice depends on what kind of hysterectomy you have had and how much pain you are experiencing. If you have had an abdominal hysterectomy, you will probably need a narcotic for a few days beyond surgery. Some physicians send patients home with both narcotics and anti-inflammatories.

Is there a danger of becoming addicted to pain medications?

Although people worry about addiction, it is not a real danger. Studies have shown that you have to use painkilling narcotics every four hours for a month to become addicted. After the first week or two, most people don't need much in the way of pain medication.

Narcotics do cause constipation by decreasing the activity of the bowel. Since many people have difficulty getting their bowel function back to normal after surgery, overuse of narcotics can increase the problem. There is a delicate balance between being comfortable and not drugging the bowel. The major advantage of anti-inflammatories is that they don't usually cause constipation.

You can mix and match your pain medications. If you are reasonably comfortable during the day with a couple of Tylenol or a couple of Motrin, stick with those medications. At night, when pain tends to increase and you are trying to get some sleep, take a Demerol or Vicodin or use your Stadol.

What is the recovery period after hysterectomy?

If you have had an abdominal hysterectomy, you should anticipate a six-week recovery period. That time frame is based on the healing of the stitches that hold the fascia. Recuperation time is an individual matter dependent in part on your age, in part on your physical shape, and in part on factors that perhaps cannot be anticipated. If you are a debilitated 50-year-old, you will probably take considerably longer to recover than a 65-year-old who is in terrific shape.

Even if you are having a vaginal hysterectomy, you should anticipate six weeks' recovery time. Part of the reason is that a vaginal hysterectomy can easily turn into an abdominal hysterectomy, and your postop schedule should reflect this possibility. A second reason is that I don't think women should make unreasonable demands on themselves. I want them to be kind to themselves and enjoy the luxury of an available six weeks. If you feel terrific and want to go back to work earlier, all right. But if you don't, you won't have to be angry with yourself or disappointed with the pace of your recovery; such moods are far from therapeutic.

Most of my patients are eager to know in advance when they can go back to work. A hysterectomy is major abdominal surgery and though you may not be in actual pain two weeks after surgery, you are sure to be tired and need a rest period in the afternoon, no matter how tough-minded you may be. If your job is fairly sedentary and does not involve any lifting, it is probably all right to go back to work two weeks after surgery as long as you limit yourself to half-days. If your job involves sitting in front of a computer managing your accounts or writing your novel, work from nine to noon but plan to take a nap in the afternoon. If you work in a nursing home and have to lift patients, you should wait six weeks before resuming your regular job activities. Whether you have had an LAVH, an abdominal hysterectomy, or a vaginal hysterectomy, the six weeks' prohibition before lifting still applies.

After six weeks you may think you are back to normal in terms of energy and comfort, but about three months after surgery, you may wake up one day and really feel totally recovered. About a dozen years ago, before gallbladders were removed by laparoscopy, I had mine taken out. I was back at work in three weeks and was running in four weeks. If you had told me that I didn't feel 100 percent recovered, I would have disagreed. But, retrospectively, about three months after surgery I was out running one day and it hit me that I felt better. I hadn't felt bad in the interim, but suddenly I felt truly recovered. This seems to happen to most people after a hysterectomy.

In general, during this interim period you can do whatever you normally do, but you might want to do it less intensely than you did before surgery. Yes, you can go skiing, but you might not want to do the giant slalom. Yes, you can go bowling, but you might not want to bowl the three games you normally do.

Therefore you should organize your life around this projected recovery time. If you are a schoolteacher and don't want to miss school, have your hysterectomy at the end of June. I have one patient who skis avidly all winter and goes boating all summer. I performed her hysterectomy between the two seasons. Some women prefer to have their children in school during the recovery period; other mothers find the school year busier than summer as far as child care is concerned, because heavily scheduled activities involve more driving.

What symptoms should I watch for after a hysterectomy?

Be alert for bleeding. Most people have some staining or discharge from the vagina as the stitches at the top of the vagina dissolve, but the discharge is usually less than the bleeding of a normal menstrual period. Occasionally a stitch gives way and the vaginal area can bleed; this kind of bleeding may happen weeks after surgery and may be as heavy or heavier than the flow of a menstrual period. Report it to your physician.

You should not be having fevers higher than 100 degrees. If you do, call your doctor. As far as pain is concerned, you should be feeling better, not worse, as each day goes by. You will probably go home from the hospital with pain medications; if you find that you need them more rather than less, call your doctor. Pain and fever could be signs of infection.

You may also feel some hot flashes related to changes in your estrogen levels, whether or not your ovaries have been removed. If you did have an oophorectomy and your ovaries were working full tilt before they were removed, you may need a fairly large dose of estrogen. If you were going through menopause already at the time of your hysterectomy and oophorectomy, you may need less estrogen. But if you notice menopausal symptoms—hot flashes, sleep problems, and so on—call your physician about these also, as they probably indicate that your estrogen dosage needs adjustment.

If your physician has put you on ERT after your hysterectomy and you notice unpleasant side effects of the estrogen (for example, queasiness or headaches), let him or her know. You can have your dosage changed or switch to another route of administration. For these reasons you should keep an open dialogue going with your physician during the early weeks of recovery.

What restrictions are there on diet or physical activities?

You can eat and drink whatever you wish, but until your bowels are working well you should avoid onions or broccoli or whatever makes you feel bloated. Gassiness isn't dangerous, but it is uncomfortable after surgery. If you are no longer taking narcotics for pain control, alcohol in moderation is all right, but if you are taking narcotics, you should be very careful about drinking. Pain medications and alcohol can interact strangely and can even be dangerous, so do not take your two Demerol tablets with a glass of wine.

Avoid strenuous activities or anything that will put your abdominal muscles in jeopardy. Don't do your sit-ups; don't do your laundry; don't pick up your vacuum cleaner or your 32-pound grandchild. I had a patient who saw her granddaughter every day. The child, who was as attached to her grandmother as to her mother (an operating room nurse), even came into the waiting room outside the operating room and sat on the stretcher, unable to let her grandmother out of her sight. My principal postop instruction to the patient was that she could not pick up the child, though she could hold her on her lap.

Although doctors used to tell women not to go up and down stairs, the current feeling is that stairs are all right if you do them slowly and infrequently. Take one step at a time. Don't go up and down twenty-seven times a day; two or three times a day is enough for the first week or two. Don't carry anything. Plan your day so that you don't find yourself wanting to run upstairs for your book and then your glasses and then something else. You can sleep upstairs, but you may want to take your afternoon nap downstairs in the living room.

I don't want my patients to drive for the first week or two after surgery. The rationale for this restriction is that it is fine to drive under normal conditions, but if a child darts in front of your car and you have to slam on the brakes, I can guarantee that it will hurt.

In addition, I tell my patients not to have intercourse until I have had a chance to see that everything is healing well. Some doctors say their patients should wait a month; others say six weeks. This is not to say that you can't have sexual stimulation or orgasmic responses, it just means that you should not have anything in your vagina until you are well healed.

I tell my patients that it is all right to shower and even to get the incision wet, though some surgeons would disagree. Taking a tub bath is different, because it is difficult to get into and out of the bathtub. Sitting in the water is not a problem and won't lead to infection; the difficulty is the climbing over the edge of the tub.

What are the emotional aftereffects of hysterectomy?

This issue is a delicate one and of course differs from woman to woman. In my own experience as a physician, very few patients have regretted the decision to have a hysterectomy as long as the decision was theirs to begin with. Most women are very accepting of the idea of the operation once they have decided to have it.

When my patients who have had a hysterectomy come back for a routine annual checkup, I ask each how she is doing and (as a joke) whether she wants a uterine transplant. The answer is usually along the lines of "Are you crazy?" Another answer I hear frequently is, "I should have had this done a long time ago." My standard comeback is, yes, but a long time ago you weren't ready for it. Although the quality of your life is much better now without the heavy bleeding or the backache or whatever, emotionally you were not ready for the hysterectomy until you decided to have it.

The emotional issues can be particularly strong when the ovaries as well as the uterus are removed. Questions of femaleness, of sexuality, and of sexual response should be addressed before the operation. They are so complex that for some women who have finished their childbearing, even having a tubal ligation brings a lot of concern. (Many men do not want to have vasectomies for similar reasons.)

For other women a hysterectomy is nothing more than an operation, a physical procedure akin to having an appendix removed. They must decide whether they want to go through the operation and whether they have time for the recovery period, but the decision doesn't carry a lot of emotional weight.

Since the operation is in most cases an elective procedure, the decision is more difficult than some to make. If gallstones in your common duct are causing you significant pain, it is easy to say to the surgeon, yes, take them out. If they are just sitting there in your gallbladder and not bothering you, the decision is more difficult. Do you want to go through all that pain and discomfort when you don't feel bad in the first place?

If you have decided to have a hysterectomy and you mention it to friends, you will soon discover vast numbers of women eager to discuss their experiences with you. Many will tell you that their operation was no problem and assure you that you will feel great afterward. But others will tell you horror stories. They will pull out the tale of Great-Aunt Julie's hysterectomy, how awful it was, and how it ruined her life. Very much the same kind of thing happens when you are pregnant, and in both cases it is wise to listen with a grain of salt and keep in mind the source.

If something really gets under your skin, call your doctor. If you feel foolish calling your physician with your worries, call your doctor's nurse, who will probably know the answer to your question. Most nurses have been through a lot of patients' hysterectomies and can tell you what goes on.

Is there such a thing as posthysterectomy depression, caused by the physical effects of the procedure itself?

Some experts believe that there may be a biochemical cause for the depression some women feel after hysterectomy. They reason that pelvic surgery causes a drop in beta-endorphins, those natural "feel good" chemicals released by the brain, and that this decrease could cause the depression.

Will having a hysterectomy interfere with my sex life?

Many women experience some pain during intercourse the first few times after a major operation. This response is temporary.

Other women find permanent changes. If as part of your usual orgasmic response you have uterine contractions, obviously you will not have them after a hysterectomy. After a hysterectomy you will have no cervix, but unless you are among the women whose pleasure involves pressure against the cervix, the hysterectomy should not affect your sexual response. Most of my patients tell me that their husband or partner is not markedly aware of the cervix being gone. If you retain your ovaries, you probably will notice little change as far as libido is concerned. If you had your hysterectomy because you were troubled by endometriosis or fibroids, you may be much more comfortable during intercourse because this painful tissue is not being jabbed.

The other issue is the ovaries, which affect vaginal moisture and, possibly, libido. Estrogen keeps the vagina moist, and if your ovaries are taken out, you will have to deal with the problem of vaginal lubrication. If you do not go on ERT postoperatively, your choices are standard lubricants such as K-Y jelly or vaginal estrogen. The ovaries are also implicated in libido or sexual desire. In addition to estrogen, they produce small amounts of testosterone, even post-menopausally. Some researchers believe that androgen production by the ovaries is responsible for libido, while others believe that testosterone only heightens aggression.

If you find that you suffer from loss of libido, estrogen preparations that also contain small amounts of testosterone may be helpful. One of the most commonly used is Estratest, which contains testosterone—not enough to give you a beard, facial hair, or acne, but enough, supposedly, to increase libido if lack of androgens is responsible for your disinterest in sex. Some postmenopausal women who still have their ovaries find it helpful. A small percentage of women who take testosterone notice an increase in aggressive feelings.

In addition to these physical issues surrounding hysterectomy and sexual response are the psychological issues, which can be complex. Consider the analogous situation of a man who has a vasectomy and thereafter finds himself impotent. Is his impotence related to his vasectomy? Not anatomically, but if his self-image requires that he be able to impregnate women to be truly masculine, his vasectomy may well interfere with his sexual functioning. If, before vasectomy, he fears he will have a problem functioning sexually, then he probably will.

The same thing can be said of a hysterectomy. If a woman thinks she will have a problem with sexuality after she has a hysterectomy, then she probably will. If her self-image as a sexual being is tied into having a uterus, even though she may be past her childbearing years, hysterectomy may well be a problem for her. Therefore a woman for whom hysterectomy is an elective procedure should make her decision very carefully; she might want to consider going to a counselor before her operation.

12 Cancer of the Reproductive Organs

America is a cancerphobic society; the disease is the one that for whatever reason we fear more than any other. But one reason I became a gynecologist is that I have a reasonable chance to cure a lot of people. Most gynecological cancers can be detected early and have high cure rates. That alone is sufficient reason for you to continue your gynecological checkups even after menopause.

The most common gynecological cancers are, in order of frequency of occurrence, breast cancer, uterine cancer, cervical cancer, and ovarian cancer. There are also cancers of the vulva, which are very rare, and tumors of the vagina, which are even more rare.

What can I do to protect myself from cancer in general?

Cancer is caused both by external factors (chemicals, viruses, radiation) and by internal ones (hormones, immune conditions, and inherited genetic factors), which over a period of time work alone or in concert to produce cancer. Some of these factors are within your control and some are not. At the risk of boring repetition, the practices that constitute a healthy lifestyle also have cancer-protecting attributes.

The American Cancer Society estimates that in 1994 about 165,000 lives were lost to cancer because of tobacco use, all of them preventable. Another 17,000 people will die cancer deaths related to excessive alcohol use, frequently exacerbated by smoking. Don't smoke; don't use chewing tobacco or snuff (probably not a huge temptation for readers of this book, though once when I was in training I almost ordered unnecessary tests on a middle-aged woman patient who spat out a great glob of tobacco juice); don't drink much alcohol; don't eat a diet heavy in fat; don't spend unnecessary time out in the sun; and do protect your skin with sunscreen.

Smoking, as everyone knows, is a prime contributor to lung cancer, oral cancers, and cancer of the bladder, as well as to heart disease. In fact, it seems that smoking contributes indirectly to cancer in many organs of the body—one more reason to stop. Obesity increases risk of breast and uterine cancer. Heavy alcohol consumption is an important factor in liver cancer and cancers of the oral cavity. On the positive side, a lifetime of exercise seems to be a factor that reduces cancer risk. A study of women who had attended the same college found that those who had not actively taken part in athletics developed 86 percent more breast cancer and 153 percent more uterine and cervical cancer than the women who had participated in college sports.

Another way to protect yourself against cancer is to have regular checkups. In Chapter 13 is a discussion of which physical exams and tests you should be having in addition to your gynecological checkups.

Can I lower my risk of cancer through diet or nutrition?

Many factors contribute to your risk of cancer, and while you cannot assume that you will never get cancer if you follow the dietary guidelines suggested by the American Cancer Society, you can certainly know that you have done what you can, nutritionally speaking, to keep your risk low. Current research suggests that diet does play an important role in establishing your relative risk for cancer.

Keep your weight in the desirable range. People who are 40 percent or more overweight have an increased risk of colon, breast, prostate, gallbladder, ovarian, and uterine cancers.

Eat a diet that includes many different foods. The American Cancer Society recommends the kind of diet already endorsed by the American Nutrition Society. The ideal diet includes a variety of fruits and vegetables and high-fiber foods such as whole-grain cereals, breads, and pasta. Studies have shown that eating a lot of vegetables and fresh fruits decreases your risk of cancer of the lung, bladder, rectum, stomach, and esophagus.

Cut down on total fat intake, as a diet high in fat seems to be a factor in the development of breast and colon cancers. High-fiber foods are a healthy substitute for fatty foods. Limit consumption of alcohol if you drink at all. Cancer of the larynx, throat, esophagus, and liver occur more frequently among heavy drinkers, especially those who also smoke cigarettes or chew tobacco.

Don't eat much salt-cured, smoke-cured, or nitrite-cured food, which means cutting down on ham, bacon, and processed meats such as bologna. They seem to contribute to the development of cancer of the stomach and esophagus, diseases that are more prevalent in parts of the world where these foods are a dietary staple.

Do birth control pills raise my risk for cancer?

I always find it ironic that when teenagers come in asking for birth control, many of them are reluctant to take the pill because they believe it is going to give them cancer. On the contrary. No data show that birth control pills increase the risk for any kind of cancer, but reliable studies suggest that birth control pills reduce the risk of endometrial cancer and ovarian cancer.

Breast Cancer

Anyone who reads the newspapers or watches television these days has been made aware that one of every nine women in this country will develop breast cancer. This statistic, while alarming, is not quite as devastating as it may seem at first glance; it does not mean that if you take a group of 25- or 50-year-old women, one in nine of them will get breast cancer. The numbers are developed over a woman's whole expected life; that is, of women who live to be 81, one in nine may expect statistically to have developed breast cancer at some point in her life.

Breast cancer is the most common gynecological cancer, and its incidence increases with age. Furthermore, its frequency in the general population has risen at about 2 percent a year since 1980. Recently the rate seems to have leveled off at about 108 per 100,000. One reason for the apparent higher incidence seems to be the expanded use of mammography, which has led to greater detection of the disease in early stages. It is also true that the incidence of breast cancer

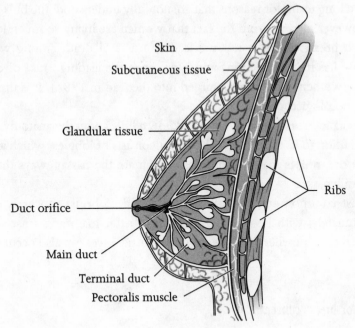

Skin

Subcutaneous tissue

Glandular tissue

Ribs

Duct orifice

Main duct

Terminal duct

Pectoralis muscle

A.

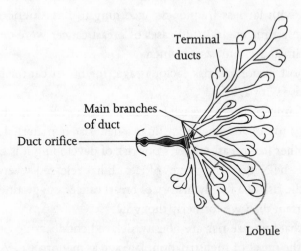

Terminal
ducts

Main branches
of duct

Duct orifice

Lobule

B.

*Figure 19A. The structure of the breast. B. The structure of the breast showing one lobe
with its ducts and lobules.*

has increased long term, for reasons that are not fully understood; the bulk of the increase, however, derives from the fact that women are living so much longer.

Although breast cancer is not the leading cause of death among women (heart disease has that distinction) and is not even the leading cause of cancer death among women (lung cancer surged into the lead in 1987), it is the most prevalent gynecological cancer.

To understand breast cancer, you must know a little about the anatomy of the breast. In addition to its fatty tissue, the breast consists of lobules, which are the areas where the milk is made, and ducts, which are the passageways through which the milk passes.

The most common and most worrisome kind of breast cancer is ductal cancer. Fortunately, with better technology and better mammograms, we are finding ductal cancer earlier than we did in the past. Cancer can also occur in the lobules.

Who is at risk for breast cancer?

The highest risk factor is femaleness, the risk of being a woman. Men do develop breast cancer, but with far less frequency. According to the American Cancer Society, in 1994 an estimated 182,000 cases of breast cancer were detected in women and an estimated 1,000 cases in men.

The second most important risk factor is age, for breast cancer incidence continues to increase with age.

A third risk is family history, especially on the maternal side. It has been standard epidemiology to suggest that if your mother, sister, maternal aunt, or maternal grandmother had breast cancer, your risk of developing it is increased. Recently, however, the National Institutes of Health has released several studies that deemphasize the risk of a family history of breast cancer, suggesting that this factor is less important than we formerly thought.

Other factors that increase risk are obesity, delayed childbearing or no children, early age at the onset of menstruation, late age at menopause. Women of higher education and socioeconomic status are more at risk for breast cancer than women who are less well educated and less well-to-do. Studies of breast cancer in countries where the traditional diet is lower in fat than in the United States suggest that low fat intake lowers risk of the disease. Some research has suggested that high alcohol intake correlates with increased risk of breast cancer, but the studies are not definitive.

Most of these risk factors are not under your control. You probably will not decide on the age at which you bear your first child in order to minimize your risk for breast cancer. Nor can you control your family history, your gender, or your age. Therefore the American Cancer Society suggests that your best course of action is screening and early detection.

How important a risk factor is family history of cancer?

A couple of studies funded by the National Institutes of Health suggest that family history plays less of a role than we formerly suspected.

What seems to be of greatest concern is premenopausal breast cancer. If your mother got breast cancer when she was 70, that fact has a minimal impact on your statistical chances of getting the disease. If she had breast cancer when she was 30, that is a different story.

The relatives who are most important to your statistical chances are your mother and sister and your maternal aunt. If your grandmother had cancer, or your cousin six times removed, then your family history is statistically less meaningful than if your mother had the disease.

The actual genetics of this is unclear. Any woman who has a family history of the disease should be aware that she is at higher risk and should be watched more closely.

Am I at high risk if women on the paternal side of my family have had breast cancer?

Statistics show that women with a history of cancer on their father's side are not at such high risk as those with a history on their mother's side. Nevertheless, someone who has difficult breasts to examine—for example, breasts with chronic lumpiness—or who has had several biopsies, even though they were not premalignant, should be followed closely.

Part of the reason is your state of mind. If you have a family history of cancer on the paternal side and you worry about increased risk, your doctor should respect your desire to be followed vigilantly.

A.

B.

C.

D.

E.

If I have a strong family history of breast cancer, should I consider having my breasts removed so that I don't get breast cancer later on?

Occasionally patients come to me worried about their family history and their own risk for breast cancer. They are considering a mastectomy, even though they have not developed any indications of breast cancer. I have talked to my surgeon colleagues and they say that prophylactic mastectomies are very rare, except in cases where a woman has had cancer in one breast and shows signs of atypical hyperplasia in the other. Breast cancer is a worrisome subject, but I would certainly urge anyone to get a second opinion before having a prophylactic mastectomy.

What are the recommended guidelines for breast examination?

The three approaches to breast examination are self-examination, examination by a physician, and mammography. It is vital to realize is that no single method alone is sufficient; you should conscientiously pursue all three.

First is monthly self-examination. A woman knows her breasts and their topography, so to speak, better than anyone else. Although she may not know what a malignant lump feels like, she can detect subtle changes. The best time to do a monthly breast exam is right after your period, if you are still having periods, since a regular routine is easier to remember. If you are menopausal or a perimenopausal woman on ERT, just pick a convenient time.

Second is an annual breast exam by a physician, either your gynecologist or your internist. At the first exam, your physician will make a baseline study, per-

Figure 20. *Five simple steps to monthly self-examination.*
A. *Check the breasts while bathing; lumps may be easier to feel when your skin is wet.*
B. *Place your right hand behind your head and use the sensitive finger pads of your left hand to feel the right breast as you check for thickening, lumps, or other changes. Then use your right hand to examine your left breast in the same manner.*
C. *With your hands at your sides, examine your breasts in a mirror, looking for any change in size or contour, or any dimpling of the skin. Raise your hands over your head and again look for changes.*
D. *Gently squeeze each nipple, checking for discharge.*
E. *Lie flat and put a pillow under your right shoulder. Place your right hand under your head and use your left hand to feel the right breast and armpit for lumps. Then place your left hand under your head and use your right hand to examine your left breast and armpit.*

haps jotting down notes or making diagrams, to establish a working knowledge of what your breasts are like. At future exams you doctor can note any changes. If such changes need to be followed more closely, your physician may recommend breast exams at six-month intervals instead of once a year.

Third is mammography, which is important in finding lesions or lumps that may be too small or too subtle to feel. Mammograms do not pick up all lumps, however, and sometimes you can feel a lump that does not show up on the x-ray; in fact 7 to 10 percent of breast cancers that you can feel do not show up on mammograms. This fact does not mean that mammograms are useless. It means that you have to couple them with self-examination and examination by your doctor to get maximum protection. To minimize the discomfort of a mammogram, you can cut down on caffeine for a few days before the exam. Not only will this increase your comfort, it will make the x-ray easier to read.

Do I need a mammogram if there is no history of breast cancer in my family?

Absolutely. My patients ask me this frequently and the answer is a resounding yes. Most women who develop breast cancer do not have a known family member who has had the disease.

How often should I have a mammogram?

The standard recommendations from the American Cancer Society are a baseline mammogram between ages 35 and 40, a mammogram every other year between the ages of 40 and 50, and annual mammograms thereafter.

Mammography for women in their forties is currently controversial. The National Cancer Institute has stated that mammography during that decade does not increase life expectancy in women who are later diagnosed with cancer. However, all the major health organizations such as the American College of Obstetricians and Gynecologists and the American Cancer Society still believe that early detection is valuable and that it is worthwhile to have mammograms between the ages of 40 and 50. There is no argument that mammograms at least every other year for women in their fifties are of real value.

If a woman is at particular risk for breast cancer, her doctor will instruct her to get more frequent mammograms. Sometimes abnormalities are discovered on mammograms that are not significant enough for a biopsy, but that should be followed on serial mammograms more frequently than once a year.

Are there tests other than mammograms that can be used to detect breast cancer?

Probably no one likes having a mammogram, and many women find them uncomfortable. While no technique yet developed by modern science detects breast cancer as accurately as a mammogram, some techniques can be used as adjuncts to supplement what a mammogram shows.

If you have a lump that you can feel and want to know whether it is full of solid matter or filled with fluid, ultrasound can help. Sound waves outline the area that has a texture different from the surrounding tissue. Ultrasound does not detect the kind of small calcium deposits that often appear on a mammogram, sometimes triggering a diagnosis of breast cancer.

Women occasionally ask about MRI, or magnetic resonance imaging, to evaluate the breast. Several articles have appeared in the media saying that MRI imaging is marvelous and that it is less painful than a mammogram; but in terms of evaluating the tissues, of pointing out areas in the breast that may be suspect, or of suggesting whether suspicious tissues are actually cancerous, MRI is still an experimental technique. It is also a very expensive test, costing more than a thousand dollars for a single study.

Thermograms measure heat production by tissues and were popular for a while, on the premise that cancer produces heat. However, the sensitivity of these tests did not prove helpful in the long run in screening for breast cancer.

For the present, mammograms remain the most important test for breast diagnosis, and no replacements are on the immediate horizon.

Do silicone breast implants increase the risk of cancer?

No studies have shown that they increase risk.

Should women with silicone breast implants have the implants removed to prevent possible problems later on?

As the possible drawbacks of silicone breast implants have been broadcast by the media, many women who have gotten them either for cosmetic reasons or for breast reconstruction have started to worry about potential problems. Among the difficulties that women have experienced are pain and lumpiness. Sometimes biopsies have revealed scar tissue around the capsule that surrounds the implant itself. Other women have reported problems of a systemic nature, symptoms that resemble rheumatoid arthritis for example (though no scientific studies have demonstrated a relationship between arthritic symptoms and breast implants).

If you are not experiencing problems, there is no reason to have the implants removed just because you might have problems sometime in the future. If you have lumpiness or breast pain, or symptoms of a vague or systemic nature that you think might be caused by your implants, report them to your primary care physician, who can consider them thoroughly with you and evaluate whether or not they are related to the implants.

With so much publicity about breast implants, it is easy to acquire tunnel vision and attribute all kinds of symptoms to the implants. The danger is that you might have some other potentially serious condition that you are overlooking because of ascribing your symptoms to the implants.

What are fibrocystic breasts?

When you do your breast self-exam, you may find that your breasts feel lumpy or bumpy. You probably have also noticed that this condition changes throughout your menstrual cycle. About 60 to 70 percent of women in this country have lumpy breasts at one time or another. The lumps are caused by a high incidence of the fibrous tissue that is part of normal breast tissue; fibrous breasts are also prone to cysts, which are fluid-filled sacs.

This condition is sometimes called fibrocystic breast disease, but in fact it is not a disease. Formerly it was known as cystic mastitis, which implied an inflammation of the breasts, but that is not the case.

Are women with fibrocystic breasts at increased risk for cancer?

In general, you are not at increased risk for developing breast cancer if you have fibrocystic breasts. However, some women have fibrocystic breasts whose cells divide and reproduce faster than the cells of normal breast tissue. If these rapidly growing cells develop atypical changes, then these women are at a risk for cancer that is four times greater than the norm. The condition of overly rapid growth is called hyperplasia and the condition of odd-looking cells is termed atypia. If you fall into this group of women who have hyperplasia with atypia, you should increase your attention to breast self-examinations and be sure you carry them out early in your menstrual cycle when your breasts are easiest to examine. If you find any subtle changes, call your doctor.

Fibrocystic breasts are harder to examine because they are lumpy to begin with. It is difficult in self-examination to tell a benign lump from something that might be potentially dangerous. It is also a little trickier for the radiologist to read a mammogram, because the breasts are a bit denser.

How does breast cancer develop?

Like other cancers, breast cancer develops through a series of gradual changes, which progress from normal breast tissue to full-fledged cancer. The first step is fibrocystic changes that are nonproliferative. You have more changes in the fibrous tissue and an increased tendency to form cysts, but the cells themselves are not growing abnormally.

The second step is proliferative fibrocystic disease, or hyperplasia. The cells divide faster than normal cells but look like normal cells.

The next stage is called atypical hyperplasia. The cells are growing and dividing abnormally fast and some of the fast-growing cells have unusual characteristics (atypia). The presence of hyperplasia with atypia is an early warning that the breast is at increased risk for developing cancer.

Next is carcinoma in situ. If you were to look through a microscope at the individual cells, you would see cancerous changes occurring; but these cells are not invading adjacent cells. It is just that there are changes within each individual cell.

Finally, invasive carcinoma occurs. The cancerous changes are invading adjacent cells and may or may not be invading blood vessels or lymph nodes.

The sequence is the same for ductal cancer or for lobular cancer, but the prognosis is different. In ductal cancer, the cancerous cells occur within the ducts that serve to transport the milk. In lobular cancer, the cancerous cells occur in the lobes where the milk is produced. Therapeutic approaches vary for different types of breast cancer.

If I find a lump in my breast or have a mammogram that shows unusual areas of tissue, what should I do?

You should first call your primary care physician, who can examine you and confirm that what you have found needs to be investigated. Your primary care physician will most likely refer you to a surgeon, who will set about determining what the lump is. Is it benign, perhaps a cyst? Or is it cancerous? Although gynecologists certainly examine a lot of breasts and order a lot of mammograms, very few of them are trained to do breast surgery. In this country almost all breast surgery is done by general surgeons.

The kinds of lumps that can be felt are called, in medical terminology, discrete and vague. Discrete lumps are very different from the surrounding tissue. Vague lumps are less distinguishable from their surroundings and usually not so hard.

If someone has a vague lump in her breast and is a heavy caffeine drinker, her physician may take her off the caffeine, give her vitamin E and vitamin B6, and see whether the lump goes away. If your doctor makes these suggestions, it is absolutely imperative that you take them to heart and that you follow the lumpy area closely yourself and call your doctor immediately should there be any change. You should also return for a breast exam in the next month or two, at some point early in the menstrual cycle.

Most lumpy areas or vague lumps can be followed safely through one or two menstrual cycles, but if after two menstrual cycles (with vitamin B6, vitamin E, and no caffeine) the lump has not gone away, it usually needs to be biopsied to be sure it is not a cancer. Although cancers can manifest themselves in very obvious ways, they can also be nebulous and indistinct. Therefore any lump, vague or discrete, has to be dealt with.

If the lump is discrete it might be a cyst, which is a fluid-filled sac. One approach is to aspirate the lump with a needle. If the lump does not disappear, as a cyst does when it is aspirated, the specialist will recommend a mammogram (if one has not already been done) and perhaps an ultrasound study. An ultrasound will determine whether the lesion is solid or cystic but multiloculated; that is, whether it is a single cyst that has just one sac or has walls within it. Multiloculated cysts may not disappear when aspirated. If the lump is solid, the next step in the diagnosis is a biopsy.

What does a breast biopsy involve?

If a lump persists and needs to be removed for diagnostic purposes, usually a surgeon will remove it surgically. This procedure, called an excisional biopsy, is followed when the lump can be located by palpation. It can be done in a surgicenter as an out-patient procedure, either with some kind of sedative and a local anesthetic or with local anesthetic alone.

The anesthetics are injected into the breast; the surgeon makes an incision and removes the lump. It is taken out in its entirety, along with a rim of the normal tissue around it, to be sure that the whole lump is removed. The tissue then is sent to a pathologist for examination under a microscope.

Another kind of biopsy is a needle-localized biopsy. This technique is used on lesions that are too small to be felt (or cannot be felt for other reasons) but are seen on mammograms. When this happens, the surgeon uses the mammogram as a guide to find the lesion. This technique also is performed as a out-patient procedure, again with a local anesthetic with or without sedation.

Before the actual surgery takes place, the patient goes to the x-ray department of the surgicenter or hospital. Her breast is cleansed, a local anesthetic is injected, and with the aid of the x-ray machine a guide needle is inserted into the breast, to point toward the lesion. After this needle is in place, the radiologist takes another mammogram to confirm that the needle has localized the lesion.

The needle is taped in place and patient goes to the operating room, where the surgeon uses the guide needle to locate the lesion. Sometimes after the incision has been made the surgeon can feel the lesion and can be sure then that all the suspect tissue has been removed. In other cases (for example, when the tissue in the suspect area looks different from the surrounding tissue) the surgeon will send the excised tissue back to the x-ray department to confirm that what was removed includes the entire suspect area. When the complete lesion has been removed, it is sent to the pathologist.

A new type of biopsy called an stereotactic needle biopsy is now being used in some institutions. It is similar to the needle-localization biopsy, because it uses a mammogram as a guide, but a needle is used to remove some of the tissue, which again is sent to a pathologist for examination. Although this technique is still in the experimental stages and cannot be universally used, in some cases it eliminates the need for surgically excising the lesion.

Do women whose biopsies are diagnosed as benign need any special followup?

The appropriate followup depends on what the biopsy actually showed. The woman whose biopsy was benign but displayed hyperplasia with atypia belongs to a group with somewhat increased risk and needs to be followed carefully. She should have a mammogram in six months; usually an annual mammogram is recommended thereafter.

If the lesion was a cyst and no other cysts appear, or if it was a solid lesion like a fibroadenoma or a fibrocystic tissue with no atypical hyperplasia, then the guidelines of the American Cancer Society suggest that routine mammograms are probably adequate, especially if there is no family history of cancer. However, many physicians like to see such women six months after the biopsy to check on the healing process and to note the appearance of the breast in the area where the biopsy was done. There can be significant scarring after a biopsy, and it is important to know whether that has occurred. The scarring will be a permanent feature of the breast and will figure in the physician's baseline assessment for future examinations.

What is the treatment for breast cancer?

If the cancer is in the ducts, the treatment involves removing the lump and sometimes the breast. In the past, the only treatment for ductal cancer considered safe in this country was a mastectomy. The standard operation involved removing all the breast tissue of the affected breast and taking samples of the lymph nodes in the adjacent armpit.

In 1989 a large-scale scientific study showed that a lumpectomy was as effective as a mastectomy. If a woman had one and only one cancerous area in the breast, if the area was less than 2.5 to 3.0 centimeters in size (a little more than an inch) and the tumor cells were not terribly aggressive (that is, they did not look particularly malignant under the microscope), then the lump could be removed safely without taking the entire breast. For many women this is a desirable choice, since cosmetically a lumpectomy is much less disfiguring.

What is the difference between a mastectomy and a lumpectomy?

A mastectomy, which is the common term for a "modified radical mastectomy," involves removing the breast tissue and sampling some of the lymph nodes in the armpit or axilla. A lumpectomy, also known as a partial mastectomy, involves removing the cancerous lump along with a rim of normal tissue, plus axillary dissection. Axillary dissection refers to a separate operation in which the tissue in the armpit is removed along with anywhere from 6 to 25 lymph nodes. After lumpectomy a course of radiation therapy usually lasts six weeks.

Who is a candidate for a lumpectomy?

Despite what you read or hear in the media, not everyone is a suitable candidate for a lumpectomy, which will usually be accompanied by axillary dissection and radiation therapy. The two most important factors in determining who can have a lumpectomy are the number of cancerous areas, and (if there is only one area) the size of the lump. If more than one spot of cancer exists in the breast, a condition that physicians call multifocality, radiation is not adequate therapy to prevent recurrence. If the lump is larger than 3 cm, or about an inch and a quarter, it is difficult to remove the lump cosmetically along with a rim of normal tissue. Even if a woman has a large breast, so that a lump bigger than 3 cm could be removed, a lump this size increases the possibility that there are other cancer cells within the breast.

What kinds of breast reconstruction are available after a mastectomy?

Many women who have mastectomies want breast reconstruction. The time schedules for performing this procedure vary. One approach is immediate reconstruction, whereby the surgeon carries out the mastectomy and the plastic surgeon performs the reconstruction at the time of the initial surgery. Another approach is to wait six months to a year before doing the reconstruction.

Immediate reconstruction is a joint approach involving the cancer surgeon and the team of plastic surgeons who do the reconstruction. The decision is based on where the reconstructive tissue is going to come from. If someone with a tumor smaller than 3 cm has difficulty deciding whether she wants a mastectomy or a lumpectomy, she might speak to a plastic surgeon to learn the pros and cons of immediate reconstruction.

The pros are primarily emotional, doing away with the emotional stress that often accompanies the wait of six months or a year for reconstruction. Many women choose to wait, however, because with immediate reconstruction comes a 25 percent increase in complications, which can include infection and inadequate healing of the skin over the implant.

What materials are used for reconstruction now that silicone is no longer employed?

Depending on individual body type, tissue can be removed from other parts of the body, such as the abdominal wall. Saline (saltwater) implants are also used. And though silicone is banned officially for elective reconstructive surgery for cosmetic purposes, it is still technically available for cancer patients. Several of the companies that manufactured silicone in the past are no longer making implants, so availability is very limited.

Where does chemotherapy fit into this scheme?

Chemotherapy used to be reserved for patients whose cancer had spread to their lymph nodes. Today evidence from studies in this country and around the world shows that if a tumor looks very aggressive under the microscope, even though there is no spread of cancer to the lymph nodes, a woman is at increased risk of recurrence or of developing cancer somewhere else in her body. Therefore the current recommendation is that chemotherapy is appropriate for women with aggressive tumors, even if they have no lymph node involvement.

What drugs are used for chemotherapy?

In chemotherapy the needs of each patient must be considered individually. One kind of chemotherapy involves manipulating hormone levels. Some cancer cells have receptors called estrogen and progesterone receptors, meaning that estrogen and progesterone molecules attach themselves to the cancer cells and stimulate the growth of the cancer. Each cancer that is biopsied is examined for these receptors. If the estrogen receptors are positive, the patient may benefit from an antiestrogen drug such as tamoxifen, whose trade name is Novadex. Other kinds of chemotherapy attack rapidly dividing cells regardless of their receptor status.

What is the tamoxifen prevention trial?

Since 1981 tamoxifen has been studied to see how effective it is when used as chemotherapy after surgery. For women who have had breast cancer, tamoxifen has proved to be quite effective in preventing the development of new cancer in the opposite breast. In 1992 the U.S. government decided to see whether women at high risk for breast cancer might benefit by being put on tamoxifen even before they had any signs or symptoms of cancer. Women are eligible for the study only if they are considered to be at high risk. If, for example, you have a mother and a sister who both developed breast cancer at age 40 and you don't have any children, you would be considered a potential candidate for this study. Each woman must realize that there are possible side effects of tamoxifen and that it has not yet been proved beneficial to women who have not already had cancer.

If you are interested in participating, consult your primary care physician to understand the implications of the study and the side effects of the drug.

What are the possible complications of tamoxifen?

There are two major risks from a gynecological point of view. One is the significant increase in cancer of the uterus; the other is the incidence of phlebitis, a potentially serious inflammation of the veins. There is also a possible benefit. In addition to its effectiveness in preventing recurrences of breast cancer, the drug reduces cholesterol levels and it is hoped that it will reduce the risk of heart disease, the leading cause of death in older women.

Women should realize that taking tamoxifen is not a simple matter like taking a vitamin or an aspirin. Tamoxifen is a very complicated drug, both a form of estrogen and an antiestrogen at the same time. Its effects on veins and on the uterine lining come about because of its estrogenic qualities.

For women who have had breast cancer, the drug's proven benefit in preventing new cancers outweighs its risks. For women who have not had breast cancer, the preventive value of this drug is not yet known because the study is so new. Women who are taking tamoxifen should have regular checkups so as to treat any uterine cancer as early as possible.

Can someone who has had breast cancer have ERT?

A number of oncologists believe that so little is known about the physiology of breast cancer and its relation to hormones that any woman who has had breast cancer should not be on hormonal therapy. The issue is highly controversial. Many women with a severely compromised quality of life, because of significant hot flashes or atrophic changes in the vagina, feel that their symptoms are so overwhelming that ERT might make sense for them. The risk-benefit relationship must be carefully weighed by the woman and her health care provider.

Can someone who has had a biopsy that showed atypical hyperplasia have ERT?

If a woman is at high risk for breast cancer, either because of her family history or because she had a biopsy that showed atypical hyperplasia, she should be aware of the risks imposed by hormonal therapy. In this case, however, the decision of whether or not to take ERT has to be individualized; there is no one right answer for everybody.

Uterine or Endometrial Cancer

Endometrial cancer is cancer of the lining of the uterus, the endometrium. It is a relatively rare disease, about six times less common than breast cancer, and it is also a cancer that grows slowly and is likely to be diagnosed early. Unlike many forms of cancer (pancreatic, ovarian, or stomach cancer), uterine cancer makes its presence known because most of the time it causes bleeding early in the process. With this early warning, uterine cancer is ordinarily quite easy to cure.

When the disease is confined to the body of the uterus, cure rates are about 95 percent. A scientific study a few years back compared women with and without endometrial cancer who had similar risk factors for heart disease, diabetes, high blood pressure, and so on. Surprisingly, the group without endometrial cancer did worse statistically than the group with cancer. This finding certainly does not mean that endometrial cancer is good for you, merely that cancer did not prove to be the lethal issue for most of the women in the group.

What are the warning symptoms of uterine cancer?

Irregular bleeding is the first warning. It is not the kind of bleeding you get when the length of time between your periods shortens from twenty-eight days to twenty-one days. Nor is it the heavy bleeding that women experience perimenopausally (though heavy bleeding does occasionally accompany uterine cancer). The bleeding that most women get with uterine cancer is sporadic spotting, the kind that comes for a few days or a week and then goes away and comes back again.

Who is at increased risk for uterine cancer?

Uterine cancer is a disease that has classic associated risks. Unlike breast cancer, where risk seems to increase with age, endometrial cancer apparently peaks around age 50. While younger women can get the disease, they very rarely do so.

Among the classic risk factors, obesity is far and away the most significant. Whenever I see a massively obese woman, I see a hysterectomy in the making. I also feel a certain sympathy for the gynecologist who will have to penetrate all that fatty tissue to get to the uterus. The reason fat women get cancer of the endometrium is that fat tissue makes estrogen, so these women are basically on unopposed estrogen replacement therapy. Their fat is making plenty of estrogen even when their ovaries are not.

Some of the other risk factors, diabetes and high blood pressure, may be associated with obesity but may also be independent of body weight. That is, if you are obese you are at increased risk for high blood pressure and diabetes; but if you have one of these conditions even if you are not obese, you are still at increased risk for uterine cancer. If you are a slender diabetic, your risk of uterine cancer is higher than that of the average population. If you are an overweight diabetic, and many diabetics do have a problem with weight control, you are at significantly increased risk.

Another important risk is that of not having children. A woman who has had eight pregnancies is at much lower risk for cancer of the lining of the uterus than someone who has had one child. Delayed childbearing also seems to increase risk, but only minimally.

Women who are on ERT but do not take progesterone are at some increased risk for uterine cancer. Depending on which scientific paper you read, that risk is estimated at anywhere from two times to as much as eight times that of the normal population. That may sound like a greatly increased risk, but if you are talking about a disease that affects one in a thousand people, as opposed to eight in a thousand people, you are still talking about a very rare disease.

Taking progesterone and having periodic cleanout bleeds reduce risk to just about that of the normal population, although progesterone will not prevent uterine cancer in every single case. Some women will get the disease regardless of their hormone status.

Taking tamoxifen as a prevention therapy for breast cancer increases the risk of endometrial cancer, in that tamoxifen has estrogenic properties.

You might notice that this pattern of risk resembles the pattern for breast cancer. Factors common to both are increased risk with age, late age at first live birth or never having children, early age at onset of menstruation, and late age at menopause. The genetic factor is much lower in endometrial cancer, however.

The reason for the similarity in risk for the two diseases seems to have something to do with estrogen. Women have high estrogen levels during pregnancy, but it is a type of estrogen different from that which nonpregnant women produce. Also, progesterone is present in extremely high levels during pregnancy. It seems to be this profile of different hormones that offers a protective effect against breast cancer and endometrial cancer.

Because of the similarity in risk pattern, women who have had endometrial cancer are at high risk for breast cancer. They should be sure to keep up their regular mammograms (but of course so should everyone).

Taking birth control pills, as we have seen, reduces the risk for endometrial cancer, just as it does for ovarian cancer.

Are there precursor stages to endometrial cancer?

Before a full-blown cancer of the endometrium develops, the tissues go through precursor stages just as they do with other cancers. Cancer is classified according to its location and its severity, that is, how far it has spread. These stages involve various kinds of hyperplasia.

Adenomatous hyperplasia refers to excessive growth of the glandular cells that make up the lining of the uterus. The term "adenomatous hyperplasia" indicates that a given sample of uterine tissue contains more than the normal number of glandular cells. Adenomatous hyperplasia with atypia means that there are more than the normal number of glandular cells *and* those cells look different, not ordinary. It is adenomatous hyperplasia with atypia that may lead to endometrial cancer.

Many physicians believe that simple adenomatous hyperplasia is not a serious threat, that only when the pathologist starts seeing atypical cells is there reason to worry.

If endometrial cancer is discovered in the precursor stages, is surgery necessary?

Adenomatous hyperplasia, even with atypia, can be treated medically, without surgery. Many gynecologists treat it with progesterone. Since adenomatous hyperplasia seems to be a condition of excess estrogen, the addition of progesterone will bring the hormones into balance and actually reverse some of the hyperplasia changes.

Ursula R. is 48 years old and perimenopausal. Fair and slim, she has a family history of coronary artery disease. She has adenomatous hyperplasia with atypia. Ursula has tried progesterone in every known form and whatever kind she takes, she feels awful. She gets headaches and she feels out of control emotionally, although when she is not taking progesterone she is a very stable, intelligent, responsible person.

Because she is fair and slender, she is at high risk for osteoporosis and should probably take ERT to protect her bones. Because she has a family history of CAD, she should go on ERT to reduce her risk of coronary artery disease. If she could tolerate the progesterone, I would give her progestins and repeat biopsies and D&Cs to see whether the progesterone could get rid of her atypia. Since she cannot tolerate the progesterone, her only choice is to have a hysterectomy.

The usual approach to adenomatous hyperplasia is to give progesterone and then do a biopsy in another three months or so, to see whether the extra growth is gone. Because this kind of cancer is not ordinarily fast growing, we have the luxury of time to try medical approaches before resorting to surgery.

What are the stages of uterine cancer?

As with most gynecological tumors, there are four stages. Stage I disease is confined to the body of the uterus or, as it is called, the uterine corpus. Disease of this sort is the easiest to treat. Stage II disease involves the uterus and the cervix as well. Although the cervix can be considered part of the uterus, there is an important difference. Lymph nodes are close to the cervix, and if these are involved it is possible for the cancer to spread from this location. In stage III disease the cancer is no longer confined to the uterus and cervix but has started spreading to other pelvic organs, to the ovaries, to the tissue around the uterus, to lymph nodes outside the uterus. Stage IV disease has distant metastases; fortunately we see very little of it. The vast majority of women who present with endometrial cancer are stage I, which means that they can be cured.

Edith C. came to my office last year after a single episode of bleeding. She is 73 years old, postmenopausal of course, not using ERT, and healthy as can be. Edith is not fat; she is not diabetic; and she plays eighteen holes of golf several times a week. In short, she is in great shape. We did a D&C and discovered that she had stage II disease; so I performed a hysterectomy. Fortunately, she came in with her first episode of bleeding; she did not delay; she did everything right, and there is a very good chance that she will be cured. She did have the bad luck to have her disease progress to stage II before she had any unusual bleeding. Now, a year later, her golf handicap is unchanged and she is as active as ever.

Life expectancies range from a 95 percent cure rate (which means that 95 percent of people with the disease will be alive in five years) with stage I cancer to a 10 percent rate with stage IV disease.

What is the therapy for endometrial cancer?

The classic therapy for stage I disease is a hysterectomy. Unless there is some very good reason for not doing so, the ovaries are also taken out. The reason is that estrogen stimulates the cancerous cells, and if any are left somewhere in the body, the estrogen will cause them to grow. Sometimes the surgeon will take out a few lymph nodes. In any case the uterus is always sent to the pathologist after removal. The pathologist's report determines whether follow-up therapy is needed.

What does the pathologist look for?

He or she will look at the tissue of the uterus under the microscope and grade the tumor according to several criteria. First will be an evaluation of how close to normal the cells within the uterus look. The least malignant tumors are called well differentiated; the cells in them look quite a bit like normal tissue, but there is more tissue present than under normal conditions. Poorly differentiated tumors, on the other hand, contain cells that do not so closely resemble normal tissue.

The pathologist will also investigate the degree of penetration, how far the tumor has invaded the muscular area. Another term for penetration is myometrial invasion, which means penetration by the cancerous cells of the myometrium or muscular wall of the uterus. Most of the time when the tumor is well differentiated, it has not penetrated very far through the wall of the uterus. Pathologists grade the penetration in percent: taking the entire width of the uterus as 100 percent, the pathology report will state that the tumor has permeated or invaded 5 percent of the distance, or 20 percent of the distance. A tumor that has penetrated only 5 percent of the distance through the uterine wall is very well confined.

Although a D&C will tell something about the differentiation of the cells and the rate of cell division, the only way that penetration can truly be evaluated is from the hysterectomy specimen itself. This grading or staging after surgery will often determine whether you need further therapy.

If your doctor tells you that you have some abnormal cells in your endometrium, you needn't panic. You don't have to fear that because you have abnormal cells you will quickly die of cancer. Just as you have the luxury of time with abnormal Pap smears, you have a relaxed time frame to make decisions about adenomatous hyperplasia. You can treat it; you can try progesterone; you can have repeat biopsies. Unless your D&C has shown that you have invasive cancer, don't feel that you have to have a hysterectomy immediately.

Liz H., a very chubby 56-year-old, had a D&C in November that showed that she had stage I endometrial carcinoma. The treatment for it was a hysterectomy, but the proposed timing was unfortunate. She wanted to put off the operation for a month because the six-week postop recuperation period would take her into the middle of the Christmas season, and she wanted very much to be with her family during the holidays. I didn't see anything wrong with the slight delay, but I got some opposition from the oncologist. At any rate, we waited a month and performed her operation before Christmas. She had a very small focus of disease in her uterus. Now it is three years later and she is fine. Her cancer at the time of the surgery has not spread. The disease has not recurred, and her chances of remaining cancer-free are greater than 90 percent. However, I worry about her because her weight is 250 pounds and she is at high risk still for diabetes and high blood pressure.

What kinds of follow-up therapy might be recommended after a hysterectomy?

One common follow-up, even for innocent-looking stage I disease, is radiation. Perhaps 8 to 10 percent of women with very mild-appearing disease get a recurrence at the top of the vagina after their hysterectomy. Gynecologists and radiotherapists have found that if you give some radiation to the top of the vagina, a very localized area, you can significantly reduce the chances of a recurrence.

Years ago physicians would put a bit of radium into the vagina and leave it there for a day. Now we use potent but very focused x-ray beams, given in three separate five-minute treatments. This gamma med, as the procedure is called, does not have side effects. There is no burning of the skin and the patient does not lose her pubic hair. The top of the vagina is not scarred in a way that might make it difficult to have intercourse. The gamma med reduces the risk of recurrence from 8 or 10 percent down to 1 or 2 percent.

If the disease has progressed further, additional radiation therapy is usually recommended. Or different kinds of chemotherapy are given, some of which are very helpful. Hormonal therapies based on progesterone prevent hot flashes in situations where the gynecologist is not comfortable giving estrogen.

Among my patients are a number of nuns, all of whom because of their celibate lifestyle are at increased risk for endometrial carcinoma and breast cancer. (In contrast, their celibacy protects them from cervical cancer and sexually transmitted diseases.) One of the sisters is a little plump and has mild diabetes and hypertension, both of which are risk factors for endometrial carcinoma.

Ten years ago she did have endometrial carcinoma and I performed a hysterectomy. Since then she has been taking progesterone for prevention of hot flashes. Recently she developed breast cancer, which seemed independent of her progesterone therapy, and indeed it was progesterone-receptor negative. Nevertheless, her oncologist did not want her on any hormonal therapy. Without the progesterone she was having really unpleasant flushes.

We have been trying different medications to control the flashing and have settled on Bellergal. She feels better, but not as well as when she was taking the progesterone.

Can women who have had endometrial cancer take ERT?

If the uterus and ovaries are surgically removed, menopause will come on immediately and often with significant symptoms. The question of estrogen replacement to relieve symptoms is controversial and centers on whether, after the hysterectomy, cancerous cells are left anywhere in the body. If there are none, then virtually every physician would feel comfortable giving ERT to relieve hot flashes and other symptoms.

In cases where it is impossible to be sure that every single cancerous cell has been removed, different doctors take different approaches. Some say that if the woman is free of cancer five years after the operation, ERT is safe. Of course, by then many women no longer have hot flashes. Other doctors say that since most women with endometrial cancer are overweight and their fat produces estrogen anyhow, they will probably not have intense menopausal symptoms and will not need ERT for relief. Certainly they won't have to worry about osteoporosis, because their fat protects their bones.

What about slim women? Although they are at lower risk, some of them do get endometrial cancer. Should they take ERT after their hysterectomies? Here the issue gets most controversial and there is no clear-cut right answer. The best procedure is for you to talk to your physician. If your symptoms are severe and your doctor does not want to give you ERT, you might consider a second opinion.

Are hysterectomies for uterine cancer ever done vaginally?

Hysterectomies for cancer are almost always done abdominally, in part because an abdominal hysterectomy gives the best view of what is inside the pelvis. In rare conditions, for example if a woman is grossly overweight and her body fat is a real impediment to the abdominal procedure, or if she has had many children and her uterus is prolapsed, the surgeon may opt to do the procedure vaginally.

How do the treatments for endometrial cancer affect sexuality?

While women who have had gamma med basically experience no side effects, women who have had total pelvic irradiation can have some scarring in the vagina. For these women, it is important to continue to have intercourse to prevent further contraction of the vagina. If vaginal dryness is a problem, lubricants are available.

Many gynecologists would also feel comfortable recommending estrogen cream because of the small systemic absorption. Some would rule it out, because they believe that if even a small amount of estrogen is absorbed through the vaginal walls, it risks stimulating further cancer. Again, this is an area where women must discuss the issue with their gynecologist.

Can women who have had a hysterectomy for endometrial cancer take testosterone to increase libido?

This issue is only mildly controversial. Many researchers feel that testosterone increases libido and find no reason why a woman who has had a hysterectomy for endometrial cancer cannot try testosterone therapy. If her doctor does not want to prescribe estrogen to oppose the testosterone, then the two of them will have to work through a period of adjustment to find just the right dosage: enough testosterone to increase sex drive, but not so much that it causes masculinizing symptoms.

There are physicians, however, who believe that since some of the testosterone will be metabolized into estrogen, women who have had endometrial cancer should not take testosterone or perhaps any other steroid.

Does ERT increase my risk of uterine cancer?

Today it is known that unopposed estrogen (that is, estrogen given without progesterone) can increase the risk of cancer of the endometrium because it causes the endometrium to grow. During her premenopausal years, a woman sheds the lining of her uterus every month during her menstrual cycle. But after menopause, unless progesterone is given and withdrawn to mimic the menstrual cycle, the endometrium just continues to grow, sometimes resulting in hyperplasia.

Cervical Cancer

Cervical cancer is a disease that peaks in women in their thirties and forties, so if you are reading this book because you are a perimenopausal or menopausal woman, you have passed your peak risk period for getting this disease. It is also a rare form of cancer and generally a slow-growing one.

What is cancer of the cervix?

The cervix is the opening of the uterus into the vagina and could be considered part of the uterus. But while there are cancers both of the cervix and of the uterus, they are very different diseases. They are discrete because of the different cellular makeup of the cervix and the endometrium, or lining of the uterus.

The lining of the uterus is composed of glandular tissue, whereas the outer part of the cervix is covered with what is called squamous tissue. Glandular tissue is made up of large, chunky, column-type cells; squamous tissue is made up of flat cells, the kind that also constitute skin. The tissue that covers the inner part of the cervix resembles the tissue that lines the uterus; it is glandular tissue.

The less common of the two kinds of cervical cancer is called adenocarcinoma of the cervix; this disease resembles cancer of the uterus and it affects the columnar, glandular cells that cover the inner part of the cervix. The other kind is squamous cell carcinoma, which affects the flatter squamous cells that are mostly on the outer part of the cervix.

To understand cervical cancer you have to understand how the cells of the cervix change during a woman's lifetime, starting out as one kind of cell and transforming themselves into another. This process, called cell differentiation, takes place right after puberty, in the teenage years. During this time the cells change from columnar, cube-shaped cells to flatter squamous cells. The technical term is "squamous metaplasia."

During squamous metaplasia the cells already in the process of transformation may receive an insult of some kind that will cause them to undergo further changes. These further changes will not show up until a woman is in her twenties, thirties, or forties. It is easy to think of cervical cancer as a disease of

Superficial

Upper two-thirds:
normal flat
layered cells

Deep

Lower one-third:
abnormal cells
with large nucleus

A.

Basement
membrane

Superficial

Upper half:
normal cells

Deep

Lower half:
abnormal cells

B.

Actively
dividing
cell

Superficial

One or two layers
of normal cells.

Abnormal cells with
large nuclei.

Deep

C.

Many
actively
dividing
cells.

Figure 21. *Stages of cervical dysplasia.
The cervix is composed of several layers
of cells, which normally become flatter
toward the surface. In cervical dysplasia,
also called cervical intraepithelial neoplasia (CIN), these cells lose their typical
layered appearance and seem to divide
more actively and erratically.
A. CIN 1: Mild dysplasia.
B. CIN 2: Moderate dysplasia.
C. CIN 3: Severe dysplasia.*

younger women, because the further someone gets from the time when the cells are changing, the less likely she is to get cervical cancer.

It is important to know that cervical cancer is a disease that can be apprehended and cured before it becomes full-blown. Seldom does someone's cervix go from totally normal to cancer in a very brief period. Hence the value of Pap smears.

How is cervical cancer diagnosed?

The vast majority of cervical disease in this country is diagnosed through Pap smears even before it becomes cancerous. Since women routinely began to be given Pap tests, the incidence of cervical cancer has dropped drastically.

What are the stages of cervical cancer?

Like cancer of the uterus (endometrial cancer), cervical cancer is classified according to the amount of tissue involved. The changes to the cells of the cervix happen superficially at first. As time goes on, the changes go more deeply into the cell layers. As long as the cancerous-type changes are confined to cell layers above what is called the basement membrane, the condition is fully curable by local therapy. This stage is not yet cancer; the changes involve only a part of the superficial tissue, and the condition is referred to as dysplasia.

In the early stages, cell changes are not really invasive cancerous cells, since cancer implies the ability to spread; this stage is called carcinoma in situ. The changes occur slowly, so you and your physician have a long period to deal with them. Indeed, it is highly unusual for somebody to proceed from mild to moderate to severe dysplasia to cancer in a matter of months. Such changes usually take years. All the same, I certainly do not recommend that people give up having Pap smears every year. If you do have an annual Pap test, your chances of getting invasive cancer are almost zero.

Microinvasion is a stage of minimal penetration of the basement membrane. Such cancers, although technically invasive, are still relatively easy to cure. Microinvasion as a stage falls between carcinoma in situ and stage I.

Stage I cervical cancer is confined to the cervix and the uterus. Stage II cancer has spread locally, to the top of the vagina. Stage III cervical cancer has spread a little farther, sometimes to the lower part of the vagina, toward the side walls of the pelvis, sometimes to the ureters, which enter the bladder right next to the cervix. Stage IV cervical cancer has spread still farther, perhaps extending backward or forward and involving the bladder or the rectum.

If I have an abnormal Pap smear, must I have treatment quickly?

A few years back, Scandinavian researchers did a massive study on a group of more than ten thousand women. Several thousand had documented carcinoma in situ of the cervix, that is, carcinoma that did not penetrate the basement membrane. The researchers did nothing for these women; they simply watched them over a ten-year period to see what happened. One-third reverted to normal pathology; they got well with no intervention. One-third stayed the same. The final third progressed toward cancer. But the time frame was ten years, not twenty minutes.

Although I am not advocating that we fail to treat carcinoma in situ just because the Scandinavian study said that some of these women get better spontaneously, I want to emphasize that if you have an abnormal Pap smear—and many women will at some time in their life—do not panic. Proceed slowly. Repeat the Pap test; have biopsies. But don't get involved with radical therapy because of one or two abnormal Pap smears unless a biopsy shows that you have invasive cancer. You have time to talk to your doctor and to get another opinion if you want.

What causes cervical cancer?

Researchers are trying to discover what kind of agents produce the insult that initiates, however slowly, these cancerous changes. Are these agents chemicals or viruses or bacteria? Scientists do not know for sure, but they do know that the substances that trigger the changes are associated somehow with intercourse.

Right now the leading candidate is something called the human papilloma virus, or HPV, the virus that gives you genital warts. Often people who have cervical cancer have had episodes of genital warts (researchers have actually been able to grow strains of the wart virus from tissue samples of women who have cervical cancer).

If you have had genital warts, don't assume that you will automatically get cervical cancer. More than fifty strains of condyloma or papilloma virus produce genital warts; only about three can give you cancer. In fact, the condyloma virus is very common. Many, many women carry HPV around with them, just as many people carry some other virus that doesn't always make them sick, like herpes in their mouth. Some experts believe that 100 percent of women who are sexually active in the United States have been exposed to the virus. Most women mount their immunological defenses against it and have warts at worst, but often no symptoms at all.

Other theories about the cause of cervical cancer exist, and the final answers are not yet in. As I explain to my teenage patients, we know that it has something to do with sex, but we don't know what.

Who is at high risk for cervical cancer?

Whatever the agent that brings about precancerous changes to cells of the cervix, we know that people who are exposed to multiple sexual partners are at increased risk of cervical cancer. We also know that women who have early intercourse are at increased risk of cervical cancer, unless they protect themselves with condoms.

Because changes are taking place in your cervical cells when you are in your late teen years, you are more at risk if you have intercourse at that time. If you wait until you're 22 years old to have intercourse, most of these changes will have already taken place, so you are at lower risk than someone who has intercourse before she is 20. To the question "Can sex give you cancer?" the answer is yes, absolutely. It matters how many different partners you have had and how early you began having intercourse.

Early childbearing also seems to have an effect. If you have children when you are young, obviously you have been having sex early also, but some factor in childbirth itself apparently increases risk. Women who have had many children are at higher risk than women who have had few children.

Thus someone who first had intercourse at age 24, who then married and had only one partner for the rest of her life, is a low-risk candidate—unless her husband has had multiple partners. If that is the case, then he increases his wife's risk for cervical cancer.

Another risk factor is HIV. Anyone who is HIV-positive, who is infected with the virus that causes AIDS, is at higher risk for cervical dysplasia or cervical cancer itself.

Does genital herpes increase the risk of cervical cancer?

Probably not. People used to think that herpes was a risk factor, that getting herpes set you up for cervical cancer, but this is no longer considered to be the case. The data that led to the earlier conclusion were based on the fact that women who had had herpes seemed to have a higher incidence of cervical cancer. What is true is that women with herpes are more likely to have multiple sex partners, early intercourse, and more children. Thus the risks for cervical cancer are similar to the risks for genital herpes. Women who have genital herpes are likely, then, to fall into a high-risk category for cervical cancer.

What is a Pap smear?

Named for Dr. George Papanicolaou, a Pap smear is a sampling of the superficial cells of the cervix. The physician swabs the cervix, scrapes off some cells, and puts them onto a slide so that a pathologist can look at them and tell what kind of cells are being sloughed off. Are they normal-looking cells? Do they look like cancer cells? Or do they look like something in between, something on their way to becoming cancer?

I emphasize to my patients that a Pap smear is a guide. It is not a definitive test. It may suggest that everything is fine, that no cells are present that look at all cancerous or precancerous. But it may suggest that some cells should be further investigated. The test will not invariably show what is going on in terms of cell changes in the cervix, but it will show that there *are* changes and allow the physician to cure the condition well before it becomes cancer. Most of the changes that we see on Pap smears are benign or precancerous; almost all of them can be cured with small interventions.

What happens if I have an abnormal Pap smear?

Suppose you have a Pap smear done and it shows a cervical abnormality. If the abnormality does not seem severe, your doctor may recommend repeating the Pap smear in another few weeks, because often the body can heal itself if left to its own immunological devices.

If you return in three months and the smear is still abnormal, what kind of evaluation is next? Most gynecologists will suggest something called colposcopy—looking at the cervix with a colposcope, which is a sort of giant microscope. The procedure can be done in the doctor's office without anesthesia. Through the colposcope the abnormal tissue really does look different from the tissue surrounding it. It has different blood-vessel patterns, and the cells vary in shape, size, and perhaps density. During the procedure the physician will snip off little bits of the most irregular-looking tissue and send them to a pathologist, who will look at them under a regular microscope and tell your gynecologist what is going on.

Often the pathologist will discover that the problem is merely an inflammation, not in any way linked to cancer. Other times the pathologist will say that the problem is caused by infection with the condyloma virus, hence the abnormal Pap smear, but there are no cellular changes that could be worrisome.

Cervical biopsies are slightly uncomfortable, but from personal experience I can tell you that they aren't nearly as uncomfortable as endometrial biopsies; I was able to go right back to work in the clinic after I had my cervical biopsy, many years ago.

What does it mean if my gynecologist says I have dysplasia or neoplasia?

Several names, pretty much synonymous, are used in the medical terminology to refer to changes in cell growth and appearance. The oldest is "dysplasia," which literally means "abnormal growth." Cervical changes were classified by degree as showing mild dysplasia, moderate dysplasia, or severe dysplasia.

Another term used by physicians is "cervical intraepithelial neoplasia" (CIN). The "intraepithelial" means that the cellular changes are in the epithelium or outer layer of the cervix; these changes are not deep, they are not invasive cancer. The "neoplasia" connotes unusual cell changes but in this context does not imply invasive cancer. While CIN is definitely not cancer, it is often classified in grades, as cancer is: CIN 1 corresponds to mild dysplasia, CIN 2 is moderate dysplasia, and CIN 3 is severe dysplasia.

Some physicians refer to severe dysplasia as carcinoma in situ. I don't like to use that terminology, because the word "carcinoma" makes people nervous. Carcinoma in situ and severe dysplasia are essentially the same thing. What the "in situ" means is that the carcinoma is above the basement membranes; it is not invasive. If you take care of it, you should be cured and unless you have HIV infection, you should never have to worry about the disease again.

Is cervical dysplasia a forerunner of AIDS?

It is true that cervical cancer is often associated with AIDS; that is, women who are HIV-positive are at increased risk for cervical cancer. But the opposite is not necessarily true. Just because a person has cervical dysplasia, she is not at higher risk for AIDS.

Cervical dysplasia is much more common than AIDS; if you do have cervical dysplasia and you are worried about AIDS, have an HIV test. However, the vast majority of women with cervical dysplasia do not have AIDS.

If I have cervical dysplasia, will I need to have a hysterectomy?

The therapy for cervical disease depends on its severity. None of the several approaches to cervical dysplasia involve radical surgery. If a patient has severe dysplasia, desires sterilization, has painful menstrual periods, and really wants a hysterectomy, then she could have one. In general, few women end up with a hysterectomy for dysplasia.

What is cervical cryosurgery?

Cryosurgery is a surgical therapy that involves freezing. The physician takes an instrument that looks like a magic wand and places it against the abnormal area on the cervix. Nitrous oxide gas is passed through the tip of the wand, which gets very cold and actually freezes the cells. Soon the abnormal area looks like a little iceball on the cervix. The frozen area is allowed to thaw and then is refrozen. This freezing and thawing kills the superficial cells, which are sloughed off, and the body generates new, healthy, nondysplastic cells.

Another approach, which also kills the superficial cells so that the body sloughs them off, is laser surgery. This technique utilizes heat rather than cold and actually vaporizes the diseased cells.

Both laser surgery and cryosurgery can be done in an outpatient surgery center or in a physician's office.

What is a cone biopsy?

Some physicians recommend taking out a chunk of the diseased tissue. This procedure, called a cone biopsy, is a little more complicated than cryosurgery or laser surgery, and it is a bit more aggressive in that more tissue is removed. A cone biopsy can be done in one of two ways, with a cutting tool—a scalpel or a laser—or with an electrical wire. The choice depends on your gynecologist's preference and on what your cervix looks like.

Either procedure can be done in an office setting, though most are performed in a surgicenter with a little sedation. Usually the sedation involves a local anesthetic such as Novocain for your cervix and something like intravenous Valium to calm your nerves, although some women elect to have general anesthesia.

With either a scalpel (a "cold-knife conization") or a laser, the surgeon removes a small, cone-shaped wedge of cervical tissue and inserts a few stitches around the area where the tissue was excised.

The newest technique is called a LEEP, which stands for "loop electrical excision procedure." A very hot tungsten wire with electric current passing through it is employed to remove a cone-shaped wedge of tissue. The advantage of the wire procedure is that it cuts through the tissue easily and cauterizes the blood vessels at the same time, thereby controlling the bleeding. There is very little of the charring of the edges of the incision that occurs when a laser is used for the cutting. For these reasons many physicians have switched to the LEEP procedure.

What are the risks and possible complications of cone biopsy?

In terms of cure rates or complications after surgery, the procedures for cone biopsy are all comparable. As with any surgery, you should make sure your operation is performed by someone who has done it many times, but the risks of cone biopsy are negligible. The risk of infection or bleeding is always present in surgery; but with cone biopsies, the risk is small and most people do well.

Many women do experience significant cervical or vaginal discharge for a few days or a few weeks after cone biopsy. The amount of discharge and the time it lasts differ from woman to woman, rather than from one type of procedure to another. The most significant discharge seems to occur after cryosurgery.

Does a cone biopsy interfere with fertility or childbearing?

A cone biopsy does not affect your fertility. Nor does it give you an incompetent cervix, that is, a cervix that will not sustain a pregnancy. It is rare for women to experience problems with childbearing after a cone biopsy.

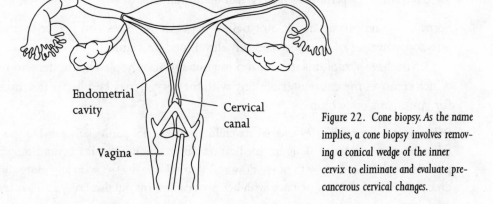

Endometrial
cavity

Cervical
canal

Vagina

Figure 22. Cone biopsy. As the name
implies, a cone biopsy involves removing a conical wedge of the inner
cervix to eliminate and evaluate precancerous cervical changes.

What kind of recovery period should I anticipate if I have a cone biopsy or LEEP procedure?

Since the procedure is minor enough to be done in a surgicenter or a doctor's office, the recovery period is short. The vaginal discharge may last for a few weeks.

The only restriction on your activity is that you should abstain from intercourse while your cervix is healing, a period of two to three weeks. Usually your physician will check you at that point to be sure that you are healing well. A Pap smear is not useful as a diagnostic tool until the cervix is fully healed.

When should I have another Pap smear after a cone biopsy?

Most physicians recommend waiting for about three months, but sometimes the cervix is not completely healed even then and the Pap smear is not readable by the pathologist.

The first accurate postoperative Pap smear usually shows that the abnormal cells are gone. After that, most physicians recommend a repeat Pap test more frequently than once a year, perhaps every six months for a year or two; thereafter, if nothing abnormal turns up, it is common to space the Pap smears further apart again.

Is a hysterectomy ever performed for cervical abnormalities?

Some old-time physicians do not believe in cone biopsies and prescribe hysterectomy instead of the more recently developed procedure.

If you have symptoms in addition to your cervical dysplasia, a hysterectomy, which removes the entire uterus along with the cervix, may be a better treatment for you than a cone biopsy.

Daisy M. is in her midforties and has six children. She is not particularly reliable about following instructions or taking her medication. She comes to the office complaining of periods that last ten days, with heavy flow and clotting. She doesn't want any more children and she is really incapacitated with her periods. It turns out that Daisy also has cervical dysplasia.

Daisy is a suitable candidate for a hysterectomy. Instead of removing part of her cervix and letting her cope with her heavy periods and with birth control, we can offer her a hysterectomy. It will give her the sterilization she would like and solve her bleeding problems as well.

Finally, a hysterectomy may be indicated if cervical changes have progressed beyond carcinoma in situ. Conservative therapy mandates a patient who will follow up and be reliable about coming in for examinations. If you don't wish to take on this responsibility, then conservative therapy is not for you.

Is it appropriate to ask for a tubal ligation also, if I am having a cone biopsy?

Some women come into the office needing a cone biopsy and ask for a tubal ligation at the same time. They would prefer not to have their uterus removed, which is a personal preference that should be respected, but they would like sterilization. Fifteen years ago I seldom did a cone/tubal, because these are two very different procedures that achieve the same result as a hysterectomy, a single procedure. Today I do perform them. The two procedures are simple enough that doing both at the same time is not a problem. In general, recuperation from a cone/tubal is rapid. A hysterectomy is major surgery and requires a much longer recuperation period.

What are the therapies for more advanced stages of cervical cancer?

Most women with cervical cancer are diagnosed early through Pap smears, usually in the precancerous stages. The early detection is possible because these women bleed. When they do, they go to their gynecologist and their disease is discovered. The bleeding patterns with cervical cancer are different from those of endometrial cancer. Women with cervical cancer often notice bleeding after intercourse; seldom do they complain of heavy periods.

With stage I cervical cancer there are two options for treatment. One is radiation therapy, which is quite effective. The other is radical pelvic surgery, which involves removing the uterus and taking out the lymph nodes next to it.

One advantage to surgery as a treatment for cervical cancer is that most women who get the disease are fairly young. They have functioning ovaries. Cervical cancer, unlike endometrial cancer, is not related to estrogen, so there is no reason to remove the ovaries. Radiation therapy, in contrast, will eliminate ovarian function, which is not desirable in younger women. Not only can the surgical approach preserve ovarian function, but it can usually preserve sexual function by keeping the top of the vagina intact without scarring.

Many physicians recommend some radiation therapy adjuctively because of the risk of involvement in lymph nodes that have not been taken out. And there are some new protocols that involve chemotherapy.

What are survival rates for stage I cervical cancer?

They exceed 90 percent, which means that 90 percent of women treated for stage I cervical cancer will be alive five years later. In fact, if you have lived five years beyond your treatment, you are likely to live a great deal longer; cervical cancer, unlike some other forms of cancer, generally recurs quickly if it recurs at all. For women who are HIV-positive, survival rates are less reassuring.

If I have a hysterectomy for cervical cancer, can I keep my ovaries?

One of the main reasons for performing a hysterectomy as opposed to radiation therapy for cervical cancer is that the ovaries can be preserved. Intensive radiation to the pelvis destroys ovarian function, which brings on premature menopause. Since cervical carcinoma is not estrogen sensitive, someone who has had a hysterectomy for cervical cancer can keep her ovaries, and should be encouraged to continue having intercourse.

What kind of physician should treat someone with cervical abnormalities?

Any board-certified gynecologist should be able to take care of cervical dysplasia and perform a cone biopsy or whatever therapy is appropriate. You do not need a cancer specialist for this kind of treatment.

If the cancer has spread beyond the cervix and become invasive, it is a good idea to consult a specialist—either a gynecological oncologist or someone who works in conjunction with one. Obviously radiation therapy should be directed by a specialist in this field. If you are going to have surgery for invasive cancer, you should choose someone who is a specialist in cancer surgery and has considerable experience. The kind of radical hysterectomy appropriate for invasive cervical cancer is different and technically more difficult than a simple hysterectomy for fibroids or for stage I endometrial cancer. Your surgeon need not be someone who has been board certified in gynecological oncology, but he or she should be skilled in radical pelvic surgery.

Ovarian Cancer

Ever since Gilda Radner died of ovarian cancer in 1989, this disease has received significant publicity. Among gynecological cancers it is hardly the most common, far less so than breast cancer or uterine cancer. Ovarian cancer accounts for only 4 percent of the cancers among women. About one woman in a hundred will develop ovarian cancer, while about one woman in nine, if she lives into her mideighties, will develop breast cancer.

It is not the incidence of ovarian cancer but its mortality rate that makes it such a threatening disease. Generally ovarian cancer is discovered late. Most uterine and cervical cancers present with stage I disease, but many ovarian cancers present with stage III. Women who have cancer of the uterus or cancer of the cervix tend to bleed at unusual times. Women with cancer of the breast can often feel a lump or see a change in their breast. With ovarian cancer, women usually don't bleed from their vagina and usually don't feel a mass in their abdomen.

What are the warning signs?

The symptoms that send women to their physician are usually the signs of extended disease. The most common symptom is a sense of fullness or bloating in the abdomen, which comes not from the size of the abdominal mass but from fluid collecting in the abdomen, a condition called ascites. What makes the diagnosis difficult is that most women regularly feel fullness or bloating at some time of the month. So if you are more than 40 years old and have vague digestive symptoms (stomach discomfort, gas, distension) that persist and can't be explained by another cause, you might talk to your gynecologist about the need for an evaluation for ovarian cancer.

Who is at increased risk for ovarian cancer?

Basically, any woman is at risk for ovarian cancer. Older women are at increased risk because incidence of the disease peaks between the ages of 70 and 75, in contrast to cervical cancer, which peaks in one's thirties, and endometrial cancer, whose highest incidence is in one's forties. Accordingly, women should continue to see their gynecologists to be checked for ovarian cancer. Many women feel that when they reach menopause they don't have to keep on seeing their gynecologist; after all, they aren't having difficulties with their periods. Nor are they at much risk for cervical cancer, which tends to be a disease of younger women. But if they haven't had their ovaries removed, those ovaries need to be checked, either by a gynecologist or by an internist who knows how to do a pelvic exam.

Those with a family history of the disease, as Gilda Radner's example points out, have increased risk. "Family history" means not so much one relative as several relatives who have had the disease. Though having a mother or sister who has had ovarian cancer does increase your risk somewhat and signify that you should be closely followed, having a strong history, with several relatives who have had ovarian cancer, does put you at very substantially increased risk. The families in which ovarian cancer is a problem tend to have many members who have had the disease, not just one or two.

Amy L. is a patient of mine in her thirties. Her mother had ovarian cancer and her mother's sister died from it. Her mother's sister's daughter, Amy's cousin, was diagnosed with the disease recently. In this kind of family it is clear how to proceed. Amy had her second child when she was about 32. She waited until the infant was getting along well enough that Amy could go to the hospital and have her ovaries taken out. All the physicians treating Amy and Amy herself felt that this was unquestionably the right move.

Women who have had breast cancer are at increased risk. Women who have never had children are more likely to develop ovarian cancer than women with children. Smokers are at slightly increased risk for ovarian cancer, although the increase in risk is not so great as it is with lung cancer or bladder cancer. Countries that are industrialized report higher rates of ovarian cancer than countries that are not.

Are there ways to lower my risk for ovarian cancer?

You can't lower your risk for ovarian cancer, as you can for cervical cancer, by postponing your first intercourse or limiting the number of your sexual partners, but there are factors that reduce risk.

Women who have never been pregnant are more likely to get ovarian cancer than women who have had several children. Theoretical reasons have been suggested for these statistics. Some researchers believe that the ovarian changes that eventually lead to cancer come about because of ovulation, and while a woman is pregnant she does not ovulate. Thus by reducing the number of her ovulations, she reduces the number of times when ovarian changes might take place.

For the same reasons, birth control pills apparently protect significantly against ovarian cancer: women on the pill are about 50 percent less likely to get the disease than comparable women who are not. The protective effect seems to last for a considerable time after the woman has stopped taking the pill. Consequently, if someone tells me that she is terribly afraid of getting ovarian cancer, I suggest that she start taking birth control pills.

Are there ways to check on the history of ovarian cancer in my family?

The Gilda Radner Familial Ovarian Cancer Registry at the Roswell Park Cancer Institute in Buffalo, New York, is a data bank of familial histories. The registry maintains a hotline (800-682-7426) that you can call between 8:30 A.M. and 4:00 P.M. eastern time. The head of the registry is Dr. Steven Piver, whose job it is to disseminate any information that you might need. When I called him about Amy, he concurred in the decision, believing strongly that Amy was at such high risk that she should have her ovaries removed even though she was only 35 years of age.

Do people get ovarian cancer who do not have a strong family history of the disease?

Familial cases make up only a small percentage of the women who have ovarian cancer. There is a good side and a bad side to this fact. The good side is that if you have just one relative who has ovarian cancer, perhaps your mother, it does not mean that you are at greatly increased risk. Your mother, or cousin, or sister— whoever—might be one of those nonfamilial, sporadic cases. If you have several relatives who have died of ovarian cancer, then you probably are at increased risk. The bad side is that you are not home free just because you do not have a relative who has had ovarian cancer.

Do fertility drugs increase my risk for ovarian cancer?

A brouhaha recently erupted over whether fertility drugs such as Clomid and Pergonal increase the risk of ovarian cancer. Large-scale medical studies suggest that it is not the Clomid or the Pergonal that increases risk for ovarian cancer, but the fact that women who have never been pregnant are at higher risk. Not surprisingly, many women who take these drugs are women who have never been pregnant; some do not succeed in becoming pregnant, unfortunately, and therefore fall into the higher-risk group.

A second connection between fertility drugs and ovarian cancer is that women who are taking fertility drugs in order to increase their chances of getting pregnant are not taking birth control pills, which would protect them from ovarian cancer.

Are there ways to detect ovarian cancer early?

Most ovarian cancer that is picked up early is found during routine pelvic exams. The American College of Obstetricians and Gynecologists recommends an annual exam to screen for ovarian cancer.

Some people believe that ultrasound technology can detect ovarian cancer, but its uses are limited. First of all, ultrasound is not cost effective. A pelvic exam with ultrasound costs somewhere between two hundred and three hundred dollars. If the ovarian tumor is so small that a gynecologist cannot feel it, it may not be picked up by the ultrasound. This is very different from mammography, where x-ray technology is extremely helpful in detecting breast cancer.

Ultrasound is useful, however, in determining the nature of an ovarian growth. If your physician notes during an exam that you have an ovarian mass, ultrasound can help determine whether it is benign or malignant. Fluid-filled cysts are much less likely to be cancerous than those that have some solid components.

Certain blood tests have been given a lot of attention in the press lately, but these tests are not reliable enough to be used for routine screening. One is called a CA-125, and a newer one is known as a C19-9. These marker tests look for high levels of certain carbohydrates (CA-125 and C19-9) in the blood, since elevated blood levels of these carbohydrates are correlated with ovarian cancer.

The correlation is not like the association, for example, between spina bifida and alpha fetal protein. In the case of a fetus with an incompletely closed neural tube (the channel that holds the spinal column), the mother's blood shows an elevated blood level of alpha fetal protein because the fetus is making this protein. It leaks out through the opening in the defective neural tube and gets absorbed into the mother's blood, where it can be measured. It is logical, then, that a woman pregnant with a fetus that has spina bifida will have elevated levels of alpha fetal protein in her blood.

With CA-125, however, the association between the marker and ovarian cancer is not unique; the test gives many false positives and many false negatives. Women who have endometriosis often have elevated CA-125, as do some women who have fibroids. Occasionally women with chronic thyroid disease have elevated CA-125 readings. And many women who do have cancer of the ovary have perfectly normal CA-125 blood levels.

Because of the unreliability of CA-125 tests, they are not useful for screening the general population, but they can be helpful in particular situations. Suppose someone has had cancer of the ovary and her ovaries were removed. After the surgery her CA-125 level went down. Her doctor can use the test as a way to check for recurrence of the disease.

Or suppose someone has a familial history of ovarian cancer that is not clear-cut.

Louise T. is in her early thirties. Her mother had ovarian cancer as a young woman. It is possible that Great-Aunt Natasha had it also, but since she lived in Russia and the stories about her are hearsay (no one in America ever met her), we can't be sure whether Natasha died of ovarian cancer or something else. Louise is anxious. She hasn't had her children yet and doesn't want to have her ovaries removed.

How can Louise's doctor monitor her closely? One way is to increase the number of pelvic exams to two per year. Another way is to alternate a pelvic exam with an ultrasound every six months. A third way is to follow Louise's CA-125 level and observe possible changes.

Are all ovarian tumors cancerous?

Definitely not. If your doctor says you have a mass on your ovary, chances are that it is *not* malignant. The overwhelming number of ovarian masses are benign, even in women who are as old as 60.

Are there different kinds of ovarian cancer?

In order to understand the different kinds of ovarian tumors, some of which are not cancerous, you must know something about the structure of the ovary. It is made up of three kinds of tissue: the epithelium, the capsule surrounding the ovary; the tissue of which the eggs themselves are composed; and the inner stromal tissue that supports the eggs.

The most common tumors are epithelial tumors, on the outside rim of the ovaries. The most common epithelial tumors are called serous cyst adenocarcinomas, which means that they contain fluid or serum. Some cancerous tumors of the epithelium contain a jellylike substance; these are called mucinous cyst adenocarcinomas. Both mucinous cyst adenocarcinomas and serous cyst adenocarcinomas can have solid material within them also.

Tumors of the inner structure of the ovary are called stromal tumors. These tumors can make hormones and may cause hormone-related problems. For example, granulosa cell tumors produce estrogen. Women with such tumors may have symptoms such as bleeding, because they are producing very high levels of estrogen. Women who have tumors of the stromal tissue, which produce testosterone, may come into the office complaining of masculinization—excessive facial hair, acne, and aggressive behavior. These tumors are rare but occasionally seen in older women.

Tumors of the egg tissue itself are called germ cell tumors or egg tumors. The most common are cystic teratomas, also called dermoid cysts. They are very rarely cancerous and are most common in younger women. They can have almost any body tissue inside them—hair, teeth, cartilage, neural tissue. After all, the egg is a totipotent cell, able to make any kind of cell found in the body; so it makes sense that disordered egg cells can also make body tissues. Because the diseased egg cells are not fertilized, they are not "turned on" in the normal way; indeed, scientists don't know what does turn them on and make them start dividing. One of the ways these tumors used to be diagnosed was by taking an x-

1. Stroma

2. Layer of eggs; egg (follicle) maturation occurs

3. Cortex (epithelium); outer lining of ovary

Figure 23. *The normal ovary contains three types of cells. The central supporting layer is made up of stromal cells; the cortical cells form the covering of the ovary. Between these two layers the egg cells (follicles) perform the actual business of the ovary.*

ray and looking for teeth within the ovarian mass. Once I had a patient who had a whole palate in a cyst.

Are there tests than can determine without surgery whether or not an ovarian mass is cancerous?

In recent years some fairly effective tests have been developed to differentiate between malignant and benign growths. One is the Doppler flow study, which measures the blood supply to the ovarian mass. If the mass has normal flow characteristics and does not show signs of increased blood flow, it almost always proves to be benign.

The Doppler blood flow test sometimes shows false positives. That is, it will indicate that an ovarian mass has increased blood flow but the mass will turn out to be benign, not cancerous at all. Increased blood flow merely indicates the presence of rapidly dividing cells.

If a physician recommends ovarian surgery, is cancer the likely diagnosis?

While some physicians are beginning to rely more heavily on tests such as the Doppler, often it is difficult to tell with certainty whether a tumor is benign or malignant without resorting to surgery. The only absolutely sure diagnostic method is to remove the tumor or cyst, send it to a pathologist, and let him or her decide what is going on. So if your doctor recommends surgery, there is still a very good chance that what is happening is benign.

When one of my patients has to have ovarian surgery for diagnostic reasons, however, I do prepare her for the possibility of cancer. It is psychologically important to realize that the possibility exists, even though the chances are good that she does not have cancer. In a sense, I am overpreparing her.

What are the stages of ovarian cancer?

The stages of ovarian cancer are similar to those of uterine or cervical cancer. Stage I disease is confined to the ovaries. Stage II disease extends through the pelvis to the uterus. Stage III disease involves spread through the pelvis to more remote pelvic organs such as the omentum, the fat that surrounds the intestines. Stage IV disease has spread beyond the pelvis to distant tissues, for example the lungs.

With endometrial or cervical cancer, the physician can often tell how far the cancer has advanced. Because the gynecologist has already done a D&C or taken a Pap smear, the extent of the disease may be fairly evident before any surgery. Unfortunately, with ovarian cancer this is not the case. Not until the surgery is performed can the physician know the extent of the disease.

If my doctor recommends a "bowel prep" before diagnostic surgery, am I likely to have a colostomy?

Because ovarian tumors can attach themselves to the intestines or other internal organs, I often recommend a bowel prep to clear out the bowel before diagnostic surgery. If someone's tumor has adhered to her intestine, the surgeon may have to peel it off. For that reason it is advisable to have the bowel completely prepared. Very few people end up with a colostomy, even if they have ovarian cancer.

Today, for a bowel prep, most physicians recommend a liquid laxative such as citrate of magnesia or a preparation called Go Lightly. Occasionally a bowel prep will also include oral antibiotics.

What is the usual surgical routine for ovarian cancer?

For the majority of women who are perimenopausal to postmenopausal, most physicians recommend a total abdominal hysterectomy and a bilateral salpingo-oophorectomy—removal of not only the ovaries but also the fallopian tubes and the uterus.

Often women wonder why their uterus and both ovaries are removed because there is a mass on one ovary. There are several reasons. First, most women who are perimenopausal are not interested in reproductive function; if they are postmenopausal, it simply is not an issue.

Suppose the surgeon removes the ovary, sends it down during the operation for what is called a frozen section, and the pathology comes back benign. Later, during full examination of the entire tissue sample, the pathologist finds a spot of cancer somewhere else in the ovary. (In a small percentage of cases that does happen.) Then the patient will be subjected to a second surgery.

It is also possible that cancer is developing in the second ovary, even though that ovary looks normal. In a small percentage of cases the disease is bilateral. And someone who has had an ovarian cancer on one side has a higher chance of developing it on the other side, even if she does not have any active disease at present. So there is reason to remove both ovaries.

Why take out the uterus also? Occasionally there is microscopic spread of cancer to the uterus. But beyond that, many women who have their ovaries removed are candidates for ERT. If their uterus is removed, they will not have to take progesterone to protect them from uterine cancer.

At the beginning of the operation, the surgeon washes the interior of the pelvic cavity with water, which is then recollected and examined for evidence of cancerous cells floating anywhere in the pelvis. Such cells could attach themselves to a different organ and start cancer elsewhere. These floating cells are called washings; their presence suggests higher risk for the spread of disease.

Most surgeons also sample some lymph nodes in the pelvis during the operation. The nodes are sent to the pathologist, and their condition helps to decide the course of subsequent therapy—whether or not to have chemotherapy or radiation. Sometimes the surgeon also removes some of the fat inside the pelvic cavity—but not to make you more beautiful cosmetically. The omentum, a sheet of fatty tissue that lies around the intestines, is a favorite location for ovarian cancer; so the pathologist checks fat cells from the omentum for evidence that the disease is spreading.

If the physician recommends chemotherapy, does it mean that the surgeon could not remove all the cancerous cells?

Many physicians recommend chemotherapy as a preventive step even though they are quite certain that they got all the cancer and even though there is no evidence that the cancer has spread.

In some cases the surgeon is unable to remove all the cancer. Then chemotherapy may well be recommended. It is worth knowing that often chemotherapy makes the remaining tumor dissolve and that there are recently developed chemotherapies to which ovarian cancer is highly responsive.

Still, chemotherapy can be difficult to endure and can have significant side effects. There is no way to prevent hair loss, although lost hair invariably grows back. However, chemotherapeutic agents are changing all the time, and major breakthroughs in nausea medications have occurred. A wonderful new drug called ondansetron almost always prevents nausea in chemotherapy patients. It is extremely expensive, but it works.

What kind of follow-up is done after chemotherapy?

After several rounds of chemotherapy, perhaps six months to a year after the original operation, the physician is likely to want a second look at the interior of the pelvis, to see whether the disease has completely cleared up.

There are two possibilities. Some physicians recommend a laparoscopy, which is basically a "Band-Aid operation," the kind of procedure that is used when someone's tubes are tied with the aid of a laparoscope. The physician makes a small incision, inserts a long tube with a light into the pelvic cavity, and looks around to see what is going on.

The older standard procedure has been a second-look laparotomy. The physician reopens the old incision and looks at the organs in the pelvis, taking biopsies, to see whether any evidence of cancer remains. Even if the second-look operation does not reveal any cancer, the physician occasionally recommends several more rounds of chemotherapy to make sure that there truly is no more cancer.

If the cancer is not gone at the time of the second-look operation, then the physician recommends more cycles of chemotherapy and perhaps a third-look operation. This may seem like heavy-duty therapy, but the reason for the second-look operation is that ovarian cancer is obscure and hard to track. The doctor wants to be certain that the disease is no longer present.

Is recovery from the second-look operation as difficult as recovery from the first?

Generally not, for the surgery is much less intense. With a hysterectomy, I always recommend that women allow at least six weeks for recuperation; after a second-look procedure, women seem to be about their normal activities in three or four weeks.

Can women who have had ovarian cancer ever have children?

Over the past two decades, attitudes toward surgery and ovarian cancer have changed. Twenty years ago, the standard recommendation was that if a woman had ovarian cancer, her ovaries, fallopian tubes, and uterus were removed—no exceptions. Physicians have become more open-minded and try now to adapt their recommendations to the specific circumstances. If a woman still wants to have children, often the surgery can be restricted to removing the diseased ovary and then following her progress very carefully. Many women who have had ovarian cancer can successfully reproduce, even women who have had chemotherapy. Often the physician will recommend that, after she has finished her childbearing, she have her other ovary removed inasmuch as her previous ovarian cancer places her in a higher risk category.

For this reason, younger women should be particularly careful about who operates on a pelvic mass. The surgery is probably best performed by a gynecologist, not by a general surgeon. At some locations in the United States general surgeons routinely do these operations, but they may not be as knowledgeable about the latest thinking on conserving ovarian function as gynecologists, who after all are specialists in this field.

Vulvar Cancer

This form of cancer is very rare, more so than breast, uterine, cervical, and ovarian cancer. The most common symptom of vulvar cancer is itching. Occasionally the cancer will take the form of a lump or tumor, but most frequently it presents with a chronically irritated area that the patient scratches and scratches. It is not the scratching that causes the cancer; it is the cancer that causes the unremitting irritation that causes the scratching.

Who is at risk for vulvar cancer?

Vulvar cancer is one of those diseases to which women become more susceptible as they grow older. Women in their seventies and eighties are more likely to have this kind of cancer than younger women.

Is vulvar cancer curable?

Not only is vulvar cancer rare, it is easily curable if caught early. It is treated by surgery, the extent of which depends on how deep the lesion is. Like other cancers, it has stages. If the disease is superficial, the doctor can just remove a small amount of the vulvar tissue around the lesion. If it goes deeper, the surgeon will do a vulvectomy, cutting into the fat under the vulva. Sometimes the disease spreads into the lymph nodes and a pelvic operation is necessary.

How do I recognize vulvar cancer?

It typically presents with chronic itching that is resistant to the usual medications. Melanoma, a very malignant kind of skin cancer, can appear in the vulvar area. It does not produce itching but rather a dark spot or dark pigmentation on the skin and sometimes also on the mucous membranes.

If you see new dark pigmentation in your vulvar area, you should call your gynecologist to have it evaluated. Not every dark spot that appears on the vulvar tissues is cancerous. I must admit that I have had several patients about whom I was concerned because of dark pigmentation. After doing biopsies and sending off the tissue samples, I was able to come back with the diagnosis of a freckle. It is common knowledge that dark areas called liver spots appear on the hands of older people; they also can appear on the vulva.

What is a vulvar biopsy like?

This procedure is not difficult and can be done in the physician's office. It involves putting a little Novocain in the area and taking a snip of the superficial tissue. Usually there is no scraping, just a little punch of tissue. Your physician may put in a stitch or two, though sometimes the sample is so small that stitches are not needed.

What is colposcopy like?

Colposcopy is a common way of evaluating skin changes in the vulva, so if your doctor wants to use a colposcope to examine you, you should not be alarmed. The colposcope is a kind of giant microscope that the physician uses while you are in stirrups, to check around the vulva. Before examining with the scope, the physician may paint the vulvar area with vinegar. That sounds strange, but the acetic acid of the vinegar highlights certain cells to make changes in them more apparent. Instead of vinegar, the doctor may use a stain (for example, toluidine blue) to make cellular changes more evident.

What kind of doctor should treat gynecological cancers?

If you have stage I disease, your regular gynecologist can probably handle the situation. Most gynecologists feel comfortable and competent performing an ordinary hysterectomy. If you have a satisfactory relationship with your gynecologist, you should be able to ask whether he or she feels comfortable doing the procedure. If the surgery is more complicated, it might be wise to seek out a specialist.

Within the field of gynecology are specialists whose expertise focuses on cancer. They have taken two years of training beyond the regular gynecological residency, training that involves pelvic surgery and radiation therapy, chemotherapy, and other treatments specifically related to cancer.

In my own town we have an active gynecological oncology service. Virtually all our patients who have positive biopsies are discussed by a Gynecological Tumor Board, which then makes recommendations. Recently I biopsied one of my patients and the results showed atypical cells. The board felt it was likely that she had advanced pelvic disease. They recommended that they do the hysterectomy, so I consulted with my oncological colleagues on the board, who performed the actual surgery. In cases where the biopsy suggests that the disease is probably a stage I tumor, the board recommends that I do the surgery but the members remain available in case unusual problems arise.

13 You and Your Doctor

In recent years the health care system in the United States has come under scrutiny and criticism by patients, consumer groups, feminists, the government, the media—in short, by practically everyone. As the old-time family doctor who knew you and your children, and possibly even your parents and your siblings, has evolved into a "primary health care provider," the whole health care system has become more complex and more bureaucratic. This pattern can be expected to continue at a more rapid and more bewildering pace as health maintenance organizations increase in power.

The Doctor-Patient Relationship

At the core of the system remains the doctor-patient relationship. Your own personal dealings with your doctor are certainly among the most important elements of the system. You want competent, intelligent care; you want a physician whose personality you find pleasant and who inspires your trust and confidence. As health care plans limit your choice of personal physician, it may become more difficult to find one who suits your needs and your personality. Nonetheless, the relationship between you and your doctor should remain at the center of your health care plan.

That relationship is really very complicated, both personal and impersonal at the same time. On the one hand, it is a professional relationship, similar to the interaction you might have with a lawyer whom you pay for services and of whom you demand technical knowledge and expertise. On the other hand, the doctor-patient relationship is more than a simple liaison between a buyer and a seller. It contains elements of caretaking, like a relationship between a parent and a child or between a teacher and a student.

In fact, these days it is common to speak of someone's doctor either as a health care provider (a term that emphasizes the marketplace aspect of the relationship), or as a caregiver. The old-fashioned word "doctor" comes from a Latin verb meaning "to teach." The word "patient," another Latinism, comes from a root that means to "suffer" or "endure." So when you spoke of your doctor, the word implied that he or she knew something that you did not and was therefore an authority who taught or told you something you needed to know. You, as a patient, were someone who suffered or endured something; you were basically a passive receptacle for your doctor's wisdom. (The word "client" seems to be coming into use today as a substitute for "patient"—a word that again stresses the impersonal, economic aspect of the relationship.)

Today, however, the relationship between doctor and patient, caregiver and client, is changing, pushed into new shapes by the rise of consumerism and of feminism. Doctors have been toppled from their pedestals and patients have demanded a voice in their own medical care. The previous attitude whereby the physician dogmatically said, "I will tell you what is right and you will listen to me and do what I say," has changed.

Even something as apparently simple as the form of address between doctor and patient has changed. It used to be that the patient called the doctor Dr. So-and-So, while Dr. So-and-So called the patient whatever he (or occasionally she) decided was appropriate. Today our culture has been altered in several significant ways. We are far more informal than we were a decade or so ago: people use first names in relationships where their parents would have used surnames. When rules or customs change, situations can be tricky. Some women, particularly older women who are accustomed to a different tradition, object to being called by their first names; some women prefer the informality. Some physicians do not mind being called by their first names; other do. Many of my patients call me by my first name and I respond in kind. Generally, it is worthwhile to state a preference; if you wish to call your physician something other than Dr. So-and-So, simply ask.

What qualities should I seek in a physician?

As the very bottom line, you want medical competence. How can you find out whether your doctor is competent? First of all, every state has a licensing board and you can call the department of health to determine whether a particular individual is licensed by the state. Most counties in this country also have medical societies, and the county societies too can tell you whether someone is licensed.

Because physicians must do something outstandingly bad to lose their licenses, some less-than-ideal doctors do have state licenses and are in practice. If you do not have the opportunity to get a referral from another doctor whom you trust (if, for example, you have just moved to a new community), you might try calling the county medical society. Talk to the secretaries. Since they are the people registering the complaints, they know who does not have a reputation for competence. Ask them who they would go to if they had your problem.

Another aspect of technical competence is credentials. If you are having a laparoscopically assisted vaginal hysterectomy (LAVH), a relatively new surgical procedure, you want someone who has done that operation successfully many times. As far as new procedures are concerned, reputable hospitals and surgicenters have strict credentialing procedures. Jane Doe or John Doe, gynecologist, cannot just walk in and say, "I am an LAVH surgeon." To be credentialed, doctors must go through a course, usually two to four days long, that teaches them how to perform an LAVH. Most of these courses are sponsored by the various surgical companies. Afterward the physician has to do a preceptorship, performing the procedure in two, four, or six operations overseen by or working with someone who does the operation regularly. The number of cases that the physician in training must perform under the guidance of an experienced doctor depends on the credentialing program. Today, of course, some doctors just coming out of their residencies are routinely trained in such procedures as part of their education. These people are automatically credentialed because they have learned and practiced the technique during their residencies.

It is a truism that any competent and conscientious physician will improve with practice. So when you are contemplating a new or relatively new procedure, ask your doctor whether he or she is credentialed. Ask how many times he or she has done a specific procedure. Most physicians will not take offense.

What qualities are important in a physician besides technical skill?

One of the first things people seek is a physician who will listen to them. Some studies have shown that doctors typically interrupt patients after the first eighteen seconds of an interview; while the physician may be interrupting to get further details or to confirm a hypothesis that he or she is making, you do want your physician to listen as you explain your symptoms or the reason for your visit.

You also want a physician whose personality complements yours, with whom you will feel comfortable discussing what might be significant and even intimate problems. Frequently my own patients come to me with questions about referrals, and I am happy to help. I am also willing to suggest which physicians might appeal to a particular patient in terms of personality. Patients will say, "Well, you know what I'm like; would I do well with Dr. So-and-So?" When it is possible, I will try to match them with someone whose personality will mesh with theirs. This is especially important with regard to an internist, who most often will become someone's "primary health care provider," now that the old-fashioned family doctor no longer exists.

You also will hope to find a physician who respects your own tolerances. For example, people have very different thresholds for surgery. Some have tremendous fear of it, and while no one eagerly seeks major surgery, some would rather have a procedure that causes temporary pain and discomfort in order to gain a long-term benefit. There are women, for example, who absolutely do not want a hysterectomy, so for them I would not encourage surgery except in a life-or-death situation.

Sometimes it is not possible to find the caring practitioner you are looking for in the specialty you need. It is a well-known cliché in the medical profession that few neurosurgeons could be nicknamed "Mr. Personality." For various reasons, this specialty seems to attract people who are brusque (which could be considered the down side of being decisive) and aggressive (the down side of being assertive and self-confident—which seem to be requisite qualities in someone who is going to take a knife to a person's brain).

I will tell a patient looking for a referral to go see Dr. So-and-So; he will not coddle you, and he may not be the friendliest person in the world, but he will give you advice you can trust. If he says you don't need surgery, you can trust that judgment. If he says you do need surgery, you probably do, and he will perform it capably.

The stereotype holds that cardiothoracic surgeons are even more lacking in personal friendliness than neurosurgeons. You will seldom if ever find one who will sit and talk to you about the emotional aspects of your coronary bypass graft. A competent cardiothoracic surgeon will tell you whether you need surgery and give you a good idea of your statistical odds with the procedure proposed; a good CT surgeon will competently perform the operation and may well prolong your life or drastically improve its quality. But you should consider yourself extremely fortunate if your CT surgeon is emotionally supportive as well.

Another vital factor in choosing a physician is your preference for male or female caregivers. Many women today want female physicians. Many men prefer male doctors and feel uncomfortable with a woman physician. These preferences are relevant and should be honored.

Individuals may have preferences about the age of the physician. Some prefer a younger physician, feeling that such a person would be up on current developments and aware of the latest advances. Other people prefer a doctor with more years in practice, someone who has seen more and can rely more on his or her previous experience to make judgments. Doctors vary in their attraction to technology, which might affect your preferences as a patient. Some are drawn to the newest techniques; others are more conservative and traditional in what they recommend. The same doctors who prefer to do LAVHs often control heavy bleeding with endometrial ablation, a technique that uses a laser to burn the lining of the uterus, instead of the old-fashioned D&C.

At a recent medical meeting my female colleagues and I were talking about our practices, asking one another about standard procedures in different parts of the country. From our conversations (and of course these observations are merely anecdotal) it seemed that male gynecologists are more attracted to new high-tech techniques than we women are. Maybe this bias comes from the sex stereotyping in our society: women are encouraged to develop relationships and men are encouraged to take action.

Obviously all physicians should keep up on current developments, but it is not always easy to know whether your own physician does so. If you have an ongoing relationship with your doctor, sometimes conversations can be revealing. He or she may say, "I heard about this at a meeting; let's try it and see whether it works." Or "In England the latest therapy is this, and it sounds promising." When you are looking for a referral, ask whether the doctor in question stays abreast of the new advances; physicians know which of their colleagues do their homework, they know who attends meetings of their professional society and who does not.

The way a doctor runs his or her practice is also important to many patients.

Some physicians are precise and orderly; barring emergencies, they keep everything running smoothly. In other doctors' offices you can count on waiting two hours every time you have an appointment. If you are the kind of person who feels the pressure of time and is annoyed by waiting, find another physician or try making an appointment the first thing in the morning, the first thing after lunch, or the first evening slot if there is one. You can also call the office a while before your appointment to see whether the doctor is on schedule.

Remember, though, that no one can schedule perfectly. Emergencies happen, even in specialties where they are not frequent. If your gynecologist is also an obstetrician and is in solo practice, you should realize that he or she may be performing a delivery when your appointment is scheduled. If you choose a doctor in group practice, you are more likely to be accommodated at the time you have arranged, but your physician still may be away taking care of someone with a ruptured ectopic pregnancy.

I confess that I often run fifteen minutes or half an hour late. But I think that I get behind because I listen to my patients and, statistically, a doctor who listens will run late more frequently than one who does not. My patients come in and tell me things that really need to be listened to; sometimes in the course of an appointment I will hear that someone's husband is beating her or that she is an incest survivor and having flashbacks. These are not trivial problems, and clearly we have to talk about how to get her to appropriate counseling and other issues. Some physicians will say, "Yes, this is obviously bothering you and we need to talk more about it; make another appointment and come back." I can't do that. If somebody is pouring her heart out about having just discovered that she is an incest survivor, I can't tell her to come back next week.

Even if a woman comes in for her regular appointment and tells me that she is feeling seriously depressed because her child flunked math or her dog died or her father-in-law is impossible to deal with, I listen. These may not seem like the world's greatest problems, but people are distressed by different things, and sometimes they need to talk about them.

I always apologize to the next patient, the one I kept waiting. But I expect understanding from that patient too. If I spend a half-hour talking to someone else when I have scheduled fifteen minutes, I will also spend that time with you if you need it. If you are a person who expects her doctor to be absolutely on time, you should not expect that doctor to listen to you if your cat dies or your daughter does not get into Harvard or your mother-in-law is causing you grief.

In general (and I base this generalization only on my own experience), women physicians seem more willing to hear about their patients' emotional problems. If punctuality is important to you, you might think twice about going to a woman health care provider. At the meetings of our local women's medical society, we commiserate about the fact that we all tend to run late.

Once I know what I want, how do I find the right physician?

This is one of the most difficult questions for all of us. If you have a warm relationship with one doctor, for example your gynecologist, you can ask him or her for referrals to other physicians. Suppose you are developing chronically painful knees; call your gynecologist or your children's pediatrician and ask for a lead or two.

Physicians know other physicians. The gynecologists in your area or town know who are the good orthopedic surgeons or the good ophthalmologists practicing nearby. But remember that it is hard for one practitioner to criticize other physicians who practice in their town. So you might want to present an alternative: "Do you think I would prefer Dr. Jones or Dr. Smith?"

If your physician suggests a specialist whom you like, or dislike, you can do your part to keep the network going by providing feedback. When I recommend someone to my patients, I later ask them how they got along with that person. If they did not hit it off, I try to channel them to someone else. My patients' feedback is important to me because people change, doctors included. Someone who might have had an amiable personality five years ago may have burned out, or turned into a money-grubber, or worse.

Choosing a physician becomes truly difficult when you move to a new area where you have not established a relationship with any physician and have no friends or relatives. I have several tricks that I recommend to patients who are moving and will have to find new doctors for themselves. None of these subterfuges, I must admit, originated with me.

If you are going to a location with a medical school nearby, call the school. Find out, if you can, what department in that school is especially good. A number of my patients have moved to Florida, a common relocation area, and although I don't happen to know any physicians in practice on the west coast of Florida, I do know that the University of Southern Florida has a well-respected ob-gyn department. So I tell my patients to call the Department of Obstetrics and Gynecology at the university and ask for recommendations. Frequently the department will know individuals who have been residents in their training program and have settled in the vicinity. Physicians tend to stay in the area where they trained, and it is a statistical likelihood that the school will be able to recommend someone who was an admirable resident. When I first started in practice, I got a number of referrals from the ob-gyn department at Yale, where I had trained. At the time I was one of the few women in practice in the New Haven area, and I had a reasonable reputation; I was flattered that the department thought well of me.

Another trick, helpful for women who are looking for a gynecologist, is one I learned from a colleague who is a nurse-midwife and used to be a labor-floor nurse. Whenever she moved to a new place, which she did frequently as a young woman, she called the labor floor at the local hospital and asked to talk to the charge nurse. She asked, "Whom do the nurses prefer as their ob-gyn?" For the most part, her referrals were quite successful. The nurses in labor and delivery are in the know; they see the doctors delivering babies and they see them operating. Since they are trained caregivers themselves, they know what to look for and fully understand who is a reputable doctor and who is not so great.

What is a normal office schedule?

I schedule patients at fifteen-minute intervals for regular yearly checkups. Some doctors schedule ten minutes. There may be instances when a regular checkup requires more time. When you are attempting to choose a physician, it is worth asking about the routine office schedule. With the changes currently taking place in health care, physicians are under pressure from HMOs and insurance companies to schedule more patients in less time. The standard office visit may be cut to five minutes in the future, which would certainly interfere with the quality of care.

What rights does a patient have?

Patients have a right to the best medical care available. They also have a right to understand their own medical situation and the treatment recommended by their doctor.

My job as a physician is to perform an examination and then explain to my patient, in terms she can clearly understand, what is going on with her body. If I find endometriosis or fibroids or vaginitis, I explain what is happening and tell her whether I think she needs treatment or not. If treatment seems to be indicated, I suggest what that treatment should be and what its risks and benefits will be.

Obviously patients are entitled to have their worries taken seriously. If someone comes to me with concern about a symptom or a physical change that is not harmful or pathological, I need to reassure her and let her know that something either ordinary or nonthreatening is happening. A few years ago the TV show "thirtysomething" had two episodes in which a character developed ovarian cancer. In the area where I practice, the show must have aired on Tuesday evening, because on both of the following Wednesdays virtually all my patients came in suspecting that they had ovarian cancer. While it may have been exasperating to me after the sixth or seventh "case" of this rare Wednesday cancer, the show raised real concerns and fears in the women who watched it. And those anxieties deserved to be taken seriously.

The next step is to decide whether the situation needs intervention. I say to the patient, "Does this symptom drive you crazy? Is it something you can live with, or something you should make a decision about?" If your period is lasting seven days and you are going through six boxes of tampons every cycle, this blood loss may well bother you. If you are happy and keeping up with your blood loss by taking three iron tablets a day, then the situation is under control.

One of my other standard lines goes, "Is the cure worse than the disease?" A lot of people, for example, don't like to take medicine.

Theresa D. has a terrible fear of cancer, actually a phobia about it. She also has a strong family history of cardiovascular disease. Taking estrogen, which would protect her against cardiovascular disease, would make her extraordinarily anxious and might well provoke true disease. At her annual checkup I told her that since she didn't want to take estrogen, she should start exercising—taking a two-mile walk every day instead. I assured her that the walk could give her cardiovascular protection at no risk.

What responsibilities does a patient have?

I in turn expect certain things from my patients. Occasionally people adopt the attitude that they have fulfilled all responsibility for their own health care when they (or their insurers) pay for it. In actuality the process demands work on both sides.

I believe that patients have a responsibility to know what is going on with their own bodies. By this I do not mean that they are expected to examine themselves, diagnose what is wrong, and simply come to me demanding a prescription. I see the procedure as one of give and take.

A decade ago, in a particularly intense period of feminism, some of the women's health cooperatives used to teach women to do vaginal self-examination with a speculum and a mirror. The fact is that women really can't examine themselves very well. Nor can most women be expected to know much about menopausal physiology, although fortunately more information is available to the public nowadays. Examining the patient, I think, is my role.

But I do expect my patients to keep track of what is happening to them. If they remark on heavy periods, they should know how long the periods are continuing and how many tampons they are using. They should write things down. Keeping calendars is helpful both to the patients themselves and to the doctors who take care of them.

I expect patients to follow the advice I give them. If your physician tells you to do something, or stop doing something, because it is important for your health, then you should comply. Of course, I am realistic about the difficulty of some changes. Suppose someone comes to the office who is, say, one hundred pounds overweight. If I say to her, "Please lose a hundred pounds; it would be good for you," it would be unrealistic for me to expect that she will lose that hundred pounds. It has taken her a long time to gain so much weight and she has entrenched lifestyle habits that have brought on her obesity. Still, if she comes in the next year and has lost ten pounds, I congratulate her. She has been trying and is certainly headed in the right direction.

As a physician (and I am sure many other physicians feel this way), I find it distressing when I suggest therapies that a patient rejects yet she still complains about her symptoms. Someone will come in and say, "My breasts are killing me." I advise that she stop drinking coffee and start taking 400 units of vitamin E a day. Neither is difficult to do: there are some flavorful decaffeinated coffees on the market today, and taking vitamin E is certainly painless. (You brush your teeth twice a day; keep the vitamin bottle next to the toothbrush to remind you.) Yet the same woman will call me back the next month with the same complaints. If she hasn't followed my advice, it is distinctly frustrating to me and there is nothing I can do for her.

In contrast, someone else may call and say, "Well, I cut out caffeine. I am down to one cup of coffee a day, which I dilute with decaf and I am taking 400 units of vitamin E. And my breasts still hurt." This is a call I want to receive. We can go on and try the next step. Or someone can say, when I recommend cutting out coffee, "I love my coffee, I love my tea. I've decided that I can live with the tender breasts since they aren't going to cause anything life threatening."

The same is true of PMS. You cannot expect your physician to make something improve if your lifestyle contributes to the problem. If you have PMS and you sit around eating bonbons before your period and don't go out and get a bit of exercise, don't complain. I have one patient who became a marathoner to get rid of her PMS. I grant that this is drastic; most women aren't going to become marathoners, but exercise is a key to controlling PMS. This woman tried running a little and she felt better, so then she tried running farther and felt still better. She has run in the New York marathon five or six times and in the Boston one also. But even someone who regularly walks a couple of miles or joins an exercise class will feel better.

Physicians also are distressed when patients ask the same questions over and over again. I have people who call me on the phone every few weeks with the exact same queries. Now some of these women have Alzheimer's disease, and for them the repetition allows me to keep track of the progress of their disease. I understand their problem and am sympathetic with it. But if you have normal mental capacities and are told something that you do not understand, you should ask questions until you do understand. It is far better to do that than to call repeatedly with what seems to your physician to be the same inquiry.

Doctors also are likely to be upset if patients fail to do the appropriate follow-up. If you are to be responsible for your health care, then you are responsible for getting yourself to the doctor. If your doctor says to call in six weeks, you should call in six weeks. If you are the kind of person who gets mixed up or if you are in the midst of a menopausal period of forgetfulness, write down the need for an appointment on your calendar six weeks or six months ahead. Most physicians send out notices of annual checkups and most physicians have tickler files for appointments at shorter intervals, but patients should realize that the physician's need for such files adds to the cost of health care. Every time I have my nurse or secretary call a patient to remind her of what should have been her own responsibility, it costs money. Too many times I am forced to consider myself a high-class baby-sitter.

You must also realize that your doctor cannot make you feel 100 percent wonderful 100 percent of the time. There are trade-offs, as in everything in life. But you have to know what is important to you, where your tolerances lie. Suppose you love potato chips. If the salt makes you feel bloated, you can try drinking lots of fluids, and maybe this will relieve the discomfort. If not, you are faced with a choice: either give up the chips and live without the bloating, or enjoy your chips and put up with discomfort.

The same can be said for taking medications. Just as you have to be willing to invest in some lifestyle changes that will help you, you have to be willing to take the medications your doctor recommends, or at least to understand that without them your symptoms may not change. I recognize that some women have social or cultural or biological reasons for not wanting to take estrogen. That is their prerogative, and it is my responsibility as a physician to try to help them with their hot flashes and other symptoms in different, nonhormonal ways. It is my responsibility to explain the pros and cons of a medication. But if I suggest a medication that has no social stigma or significant risk, I find it difficult to be sympathetic with a patient who will not at least give it a try.

As a physician, I can make a lot of people feel a lot better, but I cannot make everyone perfectly comfortable all of the time. Nor can I make everything work perfectly for everyone all of the time. This applies both to medical situations, for example where you are taking a medication for some distress, and to surgical situations. If you have an operation and there are complications, it does not necessarily mean that the physician is careless, or wrong, or incompetent. Different procedures have known and accepted complications. In the jargon of lawyers, these events are "maloccurrences," bad things that happen, but they are not malpractice. Patients of the best gynecologists in the world will sometimes get an infection after a hysterectomy, for example; this doesn't necessarily mean that the physician did something wrong.

Are there special considerations to think about if my doctor is a woman?

Many female patients want female caregivers. It is definitely a trend in this country, and understandably so. If you choose a woman caregiver, you should remember that she is a woman as well as a physician: if she is in the appropriate age bracket, she may well get pregnant; if she has young children, she will occasionally be involved in the same situations faced by other mothers of small children.

I have had patients who were very irritated when I took maternity leave, strange though that may seem. I have had patients call and repeatedly tell the office staff that their problem was "special" and needed my personal care. Some went so far that their behavior could be considered harassment. This kind of conduct does not happen frequently; most people are considerate.

If you trust your doctor, you can trust that she will arrange for a competent replacement to handle your problem while she is off having her baby. The substitute will not know your entire sociobiological and ethnic background; still, if you are having a problem with bleeding because of your estrogen prescription or you have had a heavy period that is worrisome, he or she can help you out. If you suddenly discover that you are an incest survivor and are having flashbacks, the interim physician probably cannot deal with it as well as the practitioner who has known you for the last ten years; but in truth your problem might well wait six weeks until your doctor is back from maternity leave. Your physician's partners can probably steer you to appropriate counseling, but if you feel that you really want to talk to your own doctor about it, you will have to wait until she returns from her leave. Just as your physician will understand if you have to cancel your appointment because your six-year-old has chickenpox or your teenager has an emotional crisis, you should extend the same understanding to her.

In recent years I have cut down on my hours. I have not stopped taking care of women who were already my patients, but I have not taken on new patients. Before I was married and before I had my family, I was willing and eager to work sixty hours a week in the office plus many hours on call. Now I want to have some time with my children and my husband; we need one another. Most of my patients understand these feelings, but a few are angry because I will not see their daughter. If I were to take on everyone's daughters and mothers and mothers-in-law, my time would have to be infinitely expandable. Again, if you trust your physician, you can trust her to recommend someone who will be competent to treat your daughter.

So there are problems female physicians have that male physicians do not have, our biology and our society being structured as they are. A few years ago I organized a medical group for women doctors practicing in New Haven. We were all dealing with these issues, with the demands our patients, our children, and our spouses were making on us. We were all feeling that we were alone in coping with these problems, but discovered through the group that the problems are common to us all.

What should I look for in a gynecologist as I approach menopause?

Basically, you should find a doctor or health care provider whom you can trust and who can guide you through the morass of popular knowledge (or rumor) and scientific literature. You need someone who is interested in menopause, who keeps up with the profusion of scientific papers that are published every year, someone who can interpret all these data for you in terms of your own life and help you make good decisions for yourself.

Although I am not yet menopausal, I do feel qualified to talk about menopause. First of all, I have spent almost twenty years listening to women discuss their experiences. So I have considerable secondhand knowledge. I use the analogy of my car to suggest what the doctor-patient relationship is like in many cases. I don't have to know everything about an automobile engine in order to drive a car. I don't have the interest, I don't have the time, I don't even know if I have the ability. But I have a capable mechanic who has never led me astray; who, when something is wrong with my car, will tell me what to do in order to fix it; who gives me the available options and lets me decide: should I scrap the thing, or should I spend money having it repaired? Should I get rust treatment for the underbody, or should I go on as I have been, without it?

The car analogy isn't perfect, because more is at stake with your health than with your car. I have two children. Though I know something about pediatrics, I don't consider myself an expert, and I wouldn't want to be my children's pediatrician. So I take them to a doctor who keeps up in that area and tells me what she would do in certain situations.

Likewise, with menopause I can only tell my patients what I would do in a certain circumstance. Would I take estrogen? If I were menopausal today, yes I would take estrogen. I have big bones, I drink a quart of milk a day, and I run about twenty miles a week, but aside from being a bit fair-skinned, I have absolutely no risks for osteoporosis. Cardiovascularly speaking, my family is very healthy. Still, based on what I know about estrogen, I would take it. If in eight or ten years we find out things that are different, that estrogen does not provide the benefits we think it does, or that it poses risks we have not yet understood, then I will take the new evidence into consideration.

General Health Care

Since menopause is an appropriate time to reevaluate your general well-being it is also an appropriate time to set up a schedule of regular physical exams with your internist, if you have not done so already. The risks of many diseases increase with aging, and the best way to prevent sudden and unexpected problems is to keep up a regular plan of maintenance, just as you do with your car.

As a gynecologist, I serve as the first-line health care provider for many women, because a great many young women in their childbearing years simply do not see other physicians. But there are things that a competent internist can do for you that your gynecologist cannot do as well, and as you get older you perhaps need more attention than you did as a younger person.

When should I establish a relationship with an internist or a family care practitioner?

Although you probably see a gynecologist regularly during your childbearing years, you should establish a relationship with an internist when you are about 35 years old. Many internists feel that certain problems, for example, of sexual dysfunction, come up in her thirties when a woman spends so much time taking care of her children and not enough time taking care of herself and her relationship with her spouse or significant other. Furthermore, it is important to get baseline readings on several factors related to your general health.

How often should I have a physical exam?

A very healthy woman in her thirties should have an exam every three to five years. If you are in your forties, you should be examined every two to three years. After age 50 an annual examination is a good idea. If you are obese at any age (more than twenty to thirty pounds overweight), you should have an annual exam. Some doctors make an exception to the yearly examination rule for women in their thirties and forties who are obese but whose weight is stable and who exercise regularly.

What procedures are recommended for a baseline physical?

First of all, you should have your weight checked. Many women keep the extra weight they gained during pregnancy. Once the pattern of overweight is established and supported by ingrained eating habits, it is much harder to lose the excess poundage. By the time you are 50, losing extra weight that you have been carrying around for fifteen or twenty years is extraordinarily difficult. Therefore many internists feel that early intervention, when you are in your thirties, for example, is helpful.

Interestingly enough, during these baseline exams physicians also identify women who are anorectic. They tend to be borderline anorectics, not in such difficulty that they need hospitalization. Often they are people who have been so involved with their families that they have neglected themselves.

A baseline physical should include a cardiogram. If you don't have any cardiovascular symptoms, it is not necessary to repeat the cardiogram, but obviously if you do, a cardiogram will be part of your routine physical. Internists also recommend a chest x-ray as a screening device for lung disease. If you are not a smoker, you probably won't need another x-ray for five years, but if you do smoke, you probably should have an annual chest x-ray. If you have just quit smoking, for a few years you remain statistically a smoker in terms of your risk for carcinoma of the lung, so an annual chest x-ray for the first three to five years after quitting is in order. After that you can go back to an x-ray every five years.

Also as part of your general screening, a baseline cholesterol check is a good idea. If you are not obese, have no family history of coronary artery disease, and so on, you can probably go three to five years without another screening. But if you are at risk, either because of your family history or because you have high blood pressure, then an annual cholesterol test is quite appropriate.

Nowadays a PPD test for tuberculosis exposure is sensible. It should be repeated annually for people who are at high risk for the disease, for example health care workers, people who ride buses or subways every day, and those who work in soup kitchens and other charitable endeavors. Among my patients are many people who, out of a sense of civic duty, volunteer in hospitals or literacy programs and thereby expose themselves to the possibility of tuberculosis.

Physical examinations can be important for checking up on immunizations. Many women, though conscientious about their children's schedule of shots, are remiss in keeping their own tetanus immunizations, for example, up to date. A tetanus booster every ten years is a valuable precaution. Flu shots, while not recommended for the general population, are worthwhile for many women in their sixties and for younger women, say single mothers, who cannot afford to be laid up for a couple of weeks. Women whose activities or work expose them to large numbers of people (health care workers, teachers, and the same people who are at risk for tuberculosis) should consult their internists about the desirability of flu shots.

Another test that is performed at routine physicals is a CBC (complete blood count). This test turns up a significant amount of anemia. Because people are eating less red meat than formerly, many women are becoming anemic and have to get iron in their diet by other means.

Diabetes screening probably is not necessary as a general measure. If you have a family history of diabetes, a fasting glucose test, which simply tests the amount of sugar in your blood at least eight hours after eating, is probably adequate to determine the presence of diabetes. If your doctor has any misgivings, then a blood glucose measurement two hours after eating or even right after eating (a postprandial glucose) is likely to clear up any doubt. A full formal glucose tolerance test is probably not necessary, even for people with a family history of diabetes.

Are bone density tests a valuable screening device for postmenopausal women?

Many internists recommend bone density studies perimenopausally in women who are not planning to take ERT. If you do plan to take estrogen, you don't have to worry about a bone density study; but if you do not, especially if you are at high risk for osteoporosis, then you should consider having a bone density test.

At what age should people start having tests for bowel cancer?

Most internists feel that checking the stools for blood, the so-called guaiac testing, is an important part of routine screening for everyone in their forties. One major test for bowel cancer is a sigmoidoscopy. A flexible tube is inserted into the sigmoid colon to look for the presence of cancer. Although the test is not particularly uncomfortable if a flexible tube is used, and is not generally risky, it is not a test that people want to have. Internists recommend the test for people between ages 45 and 50 if they have a family history of bowel or colon cancer, especially in more than one relative. Internists start recommending the test universally at the age of 50 and start twisting arms after the age of 60.

What other screening tests are there for cancer?

One of the most crucial tests for women is the mammogram. Blood screening markers for ovarian cancer have been getting a lot of press recently, although these tests are not terribly reliable and many internists do not push them.

Blood screening tests for other kinds of cancer include a CEA (carcinoembryotic antibody) test for cancer of the bowel, which may be useful in checking for recurrences in people who have had bowel cancer. But recent studies are showing that these tests are not sufficiently reliable to be used routinely. So when people say to me that they want blood testing for every possible cancer, I tell them that there are not a lot of tests that are valid for diagnosing different kinds of cancers. One of my internist colleagues believes that if she can get her patients to wear seat belts, she is probably saving more lives than by any blood testing she may recommend.

For men older than 50 (and this is something you should mention to your partner and other significant males in your life), a PSA blood test for prostatic cancer is worth having.

What are the costs of a full physical exam?

The average comprehensive physical exam, including a chest x-ray, an EKG, basic blood work, and the time of the physician, runs somewhere between $300 and $400. Of course, this price varies widely depending on where you live and which doctor you visit. You can expect a routine physical to cost more on Park Avenue in New York than on Main Street in rural Maine. Some insurance plans cover this kind of exam; others do not, even at a time when health care professionals are highlighting the importance of preventive health maintenance.

Remember that for many people a routine physical exam can be considered treatment for a symptom, in which case the care is reimbursable. And almost everybody has some kind of problem. Women with heavy periods often have iron-deficiency anemia, and testing has to be done to evaluate the anemia. Former smokers need to have a follow-up because even though they have quit smoking, they still should evaluate their increased risk of lung cancer from smoking. People with strong family histories of coronary artery disease need to be followed. For some women a baseline bone density test can rule out osteoporosis.

What effects will health care reform have on the practice of gynecology, especially with respect to menopause?

From a gynecologist's point of view, working with menopausal women who have elected to go on ERT is a time-consuming process. Suppose you have decided that ERT is a wise choice for you. You and your doctor should sit down and discuss the pros and cons, what you can and what you shouldn't expect from estrogen. You should know what potential side effects you may experience and what you can do if they occur.

Perhaps you get some bleeding while on ERT. Maybe you are bleeding because you are not taking enough progesterone, or maybe you are bleeding because you are not taking enough estrogen. Maybe you should try a different regimen. Many people bleed while on ERT; in most cases the bleeding does not signify anything serious, but sometimes it is important. The physician, who has to decide whether or not to perform a biopsy, will end up biopsying more women than turn out to have serious disease.

It is a lot easier for your doctor not to give estrogen, because finding just the dosage and just the approach that is right for you is a delicate process. If people are on the wrong dosage, they bleed or they don't feel well; they have questions and want to talk to their physician. If you belong to a health maintenance organization (HMO), you may not be talking to your own doctor all the time, but to someone who has not followed your health year after year.

If under the new health care reform doctors are allowed only five or ten minutes with a patient, they are not going to prescribe ERT. If they are paid per capita, say one hundred dollars a year to take care of Jane Doe, then Jane Doe will probably not get ERT. That would involve much more of her physician's time; she might need a biopsy or two. The per capita fee makes it cost effective for the physician to do as little as possible for Jane Doe in order to have more patients in order to get more per capita fees. The system certainly does not work in Jane Doe's interest. Nor, in truth, does it work in the interest of the physician who really wants to follow patients closely.

Currently, HMOs are run for cost effectiveness; in fact, they are run to make a profit. Is estrogen cost effective? In the short run, perhaps not. Since it is time consuming for a physician to counsel and follow a woman on ERT, that doctor can see fewer patients per hour—a situation that does not benefit the HMO. It is not as efficient as simply saying, "OK, you're menopausal; come back next year for your annual checkup."

But is that approach penny wise and pound foolish? In the long run, estrogen replacement is definitely cost effective. Estrogen prevents coronary artery disease and osteoporosis. If women end up with fewer heart attacks and fewer fractures, they save the health care system a lot of money. Treating a heart attack in a major medical center costs something more than $20,000. Treating a hip fracture is about the same just for the acute event itself, without factoring in that many of these older women must remain hospitalized for a long time. If ERT costs about $1 a day, or $365 a year, then at today's prices you can have ERT for about fifty-five years for the cost of one heart attack or one hip fracture.

There is also the matter of quality of life. When I was a medical student, one of my mentors was John McLain Morris, by then an elderly and well-respected figure in his field. One of Dr. Morris's favorite statistics was that if every American woman took ERT, it would increase the average life span of American women by four months. Four months, of course, is not statistically significant; what *was* important, he said, was the quality, not the duration, of that average American life. If that life, whether four months longer or shorter, is lived in a nursing home, then its quality may be doubtful. But if that life can be lived with the energy and zest that good health provides, there is not much doubt about its quality.

14 Lifestyle

At the turn of the century when the average woman could expect to live only about fifty years, menopause came toward the end of her life. Women who died in their fifties or early sixties survived a few years or perhaps a decade beyond menopause. With increased life expectancy, however, all that has changed. The contemporary American woman can expect to live until about age 80 and will thus spend fully one-third of her life as a postmenopausal woman.

Menopause used to be called the change of life. Although the term was a euphemism, it did express a certain basic truth, for menopause is truly a marker of change. And because it does signal a boundary, as does pregnancy (or even New Year's Day, for that matter), it is a suitable time to take stock, to evaluate your lifestyle and try to prepare yourself for many healthy years to come. It is a time to evaluate your diet, your exercise routine, and your other life habits to maximize the possibility that the ensuing years will be healthy and productive.

Speaking physiologically, the "change" that happens to women at menopause is fairly clear-cut: women who have passed through menopause are no longer producing significant amounts of estrogen on their own. During their reproductive years, estrogen has protected them from certain diseases to which they become vulnerable as they age. Heart attacks and cardiovascular disease are relatively rare in premenopausal women, though they are a threat to men throughout their adult lives. Osteoporosis is not a threat to younger women (or men), but it is a concern for older women and to a lesser extent for older men. So while women do not have to worry much about coronary artery disease or osteoporosis before they are 50, they become more vulnerable to these diseases as they age. Prevention, ideally, should have started years before, with a healthy diet and an exercise regimen, but the years surrounding menopause are critical in paving the way for the future.

In recent years Americans have become more conscious of what they need to do, especially in terms of diet and exercise, to provide the foundation for physical well-being. With the barrage of information in the media, we would have to be willfully ignorant not to know what is good for us. The concepts are simple, at least on paper. Implementing them in your own life may be a lot more difficult.

What can I do to prepare myself for menopause?

Suppose you are a woman in your forties, and you come to my office wondering what you can do to prepare yourself for menopause. My answer is that you should begin the healthy regimens that will stand you in good stead for the rest of your life. My single most important recommendation is that you make sure you are getting adequate calcium, either in your diet or with dietary supplements. The recommended amount for women who are still menstruating is 1,000 mg a day; for postmenopausal women not taking estrogen, the recommendation is 1,500 mg.

To my way of thinking, you should follow two basic principles for a healthy lifestyle, either before or after menopause. First of all, keep yourself in shape by staying close to your ideal body weight and getting enough exercise. The two are related, for numerous studies have shown that you can only maintain desirable body weight by a combination of a moderate caloric intake and exercise. Second, refrain from destructive lifestyle habits: don't smoke, don't abuse alcohol, and don't use illicit drugs.

Diet and Nutrition

What is my ideal body weight?

As far as female body weight is concerned, our society has in recent decades been torn between an unreachable (and ultimately undesirable) ideal and a less-than-healthy reality. In terms of the ideal, society as reflected in the media proposes a slenderness that borders on emaciation. In the fashion magazines the only models we see are barely postpubescent women with prominent cheekbones, protruding collarbones, and thin coltish legs. In reality, however, many Americans are overweight and becoming more so as time goes on. According to the National Center for Health Statistics, which issued a report in 1994 that covered the years 1980–1991, about one-third of the adult population of the United States is obese, with obesity defined as at least 20 percent over desirable body weight. In 1980 only 25 percent of the adult population had reached that unfortunate status, so in the past decade a lot of people have put on a lot of pounds.

The Surgeon General's report of 1988 pointed out that as a statistical pattern the more overweight you are, the greater your risk of premature death. Obese people are at increased risk for diabetes, heart disease, high blood pressure, cancer, back pain, gallbladder disease, and even chronic degenerative arthritis.

In addition to the increased health risks of obesity, enormous social consequences begin in adolescence and continue throughout life. According to a study published in 1993 in the *New England Journal of Medicine*, young women who are overweight are less likely to marry and will have lower household incomes and higher rates of poverty than women of normal weight. These consequences, which hold true regardless of socioeconomic origin and ability as measured by aptitude tests, are only magnified over a lifetime. Since there is a strong cultural bias against overweight people, heavy women are discriminated against in the job market.

That is the bad news. The good news is that our notion of what is defined as overweight has been revised.

How do I know if I'm overweight?

Because overweight increases health risks and lowers life expectancies, some life insurance companies publish charts suggesting appropriate body weights. In the past decade and a half, the Metropolitan Life Insurance Company, whose statistics have become standard throughout the industry, has revised its tables to reflect a wider interpretation of what an appropriate weight might be for a given height. Back in 1968 a woman 5'4" tall with a small frame weighing between 108 and 116 pounds would fall within the guidelines established by the actuarial tables. Today that same woman can weigh between 114 and 127 pounds and still be within the suggested range. If you are 5'8" and have a large frame, nowadays the life insurance companies consider you a good risk, other factors aside, if you weigh between 146 and 167 pounds; in 1968 you would have had to shed 8 or 9 pounds and get down to somewhere between 137 and 154 pounds to meet the requirements.

Table 1. *MetLife Height and Weight Tables [portion for women reproduced here]*
Weights at ages 25–59 based on lowest mortality. Weight in pounds according to frame (in indoor clothing weighing 3 lbs; shoes with 1" heels).

Height Feet	Inches	Small Frame	Medium Frame	Large Frame
4	10	101–111	109–121	118–131
4	11	103–113	111–123	120–134
5	0	104–115	113–126	122–137
5	1	106–118	115–129	125–140
5	2	108–121	118–132	128–143
5	3	111–124	121–135	131–147
5	4	114–127	124–138	134–151
5	5	117–130	127–141	137–155
5	6	120–133	130–144	140–159
5	7	123–136	133–147	143–163
5	8	126–139	136–150	146–167
5	9	129–142	139–153	149–170
5	10	132–145	142–156	152–173
5	11	135–148	145–159	155–176
6	0	138–151	148–162	158–179

Source: *Reprinted courtesy of Metropolitan Life Insurance Company. Source of basic data: 1979 Build Study, Society of Actuaries and Association of Life Insurance Medical Directors of America, 1980.*

Individual differences in bone diameter and in the relative proportions of muscle and fat account for the wide ranges of acceptability on the chart. If you are a strapping, heavy-boned woman of 5'6", you can weigh more than a delicately boned woman the same height and still be close to your desirable body weight. Since muscle weighs more than fat, you will weigh more inch for inch if you are muscular and athletically trained than if you are sedentary.

In addition to the general guidelines established by the chart, there are other tests for overweight. Physicians specializing in weight control sometimes use calipers to measure the thickness of skinfolds on various parts of your body. Another method is to immerse you in a tank of water to find the volume of your body and, relating it to your weight, calculate your percentage of body fat.

The Gerontology Research Center of the National Institute on Aging suggests that as we grow older a certain amount of weight gain is normal. It says that men and women who are just slightly overweight based on the standard height/weight charts have lower mortality rates than those who are precisely on target. Their complex system measures body mass, which involves height, weight, and age, and often gives a higher desirable weight than the actuarial tables of the life insurance companies:

Start with your height in inches and divide by 66. Multiply that number by itself. Then multiply that result by your age plus 100.
Let's say you are 55 years old and 5'4" (64 inches) tall.

Divide your height in inches by the magic number 66: 64 ÷ by 66 = 0.9697.
Now multiply 0.9697 by itself: 0.9697 × 0.9697 = 0.9403.
Now multiply that by your age + 100: 155 × 0.9403 = 145.7 pounds. So your baseline desirable weight is roughly 146 pounds.
You can add or subtract up to 9 pounds depending on whether your bone structure is light or heavy, which gives you a range from 137 to 155 pounds.

If, in fact, you are overweight, you probably already know it and feel guilty about it; a National Institutes of Health study on obesity suggests that of all its effects none is more adverse than the psychological suffering it entails. The most intuitively obvious test is a quick look in your full-length mirror or, even more revealing, in the three-way mirror in your local department store—the one you stand in front of when you try on a bathing suit. If you look fat and flabby to yourself (unless you are anorectic and would look fat to yourself no matter how thin you were), you are probably overweight.

A second test you can perform is the pinch test. Extend one arm and pinch the flesh on its underside halfway between your shoulder and your elbow. If you pinch more than an inch of fat, then you should think seriously about weight reduction.

Is fat distribution important as well as body weight?

Recently scientists have suggested that fat distribution as well as its total amount affects the risk of disease, particularly coronary artery disease.

Researchers have described two general silhouettes in overweight people: the pear and the apple. Pear-shaped people carry their extra weight low, around the hips, buttocks, and thighs; apple-shaped people carry their weight around their waists. Typically, overweight premenopausal women are pear shaped, while overweight men (the sagging belly syndrome) and postmenopausal women (the potbelly syndrome) are apple shaped.

How do you know whether you are an apple or a pear? Measure your waist at the navel. Then measure your hips at their fullest point. If you divide your waist measurement by your hip measurement and the result is less than 1.0, you're a pear. If it is greater than 1.0, you're an apple. For women, if your waist-to-hip ratio is greater than 0.8, you are at increased risk of heart disease.

What is the best way to lose weight?

Although genetic inheritance has a great deal to do with body shape and you can do nothing to change the tendency to heavy thighs that you inherited from Great-Aunt Tilly, with effort you can maintain something close to your ideal body weight.

There are two basic ways to lose weight, and to succeed you have to pursue both: follow a moderate diet with not too many calories, and increase the amount you exercise. While it may be possible to lose weight by doing one without the other, it certainly is very difficult. Restricting calories without exercise usually results in frustration and failure, because the body in its wisdom turns down its metabolic regulator when it senses lowered caloric intake, trying to save you from what appears to be incipient starvation. If you exist on, let's say, a thousand calories a day for a week or so, your body begins to believe that a thousand calories is all it's going to get, so readjusts its metabolic set point to maintain itself on a thousand calories.

Nor does exercise alone seem to do the trick. It is generally believed that just as the body shuts down its metabolic regulator if it becomes accustomed to a low caloric intake, the body will boost its metabolic thermostat if it gets accustomed to a high-energy output, for example needing to supply extra calories for regular exercise. However, there are some data to the contrary. In a 1989 study published in the *International Journal of Sports Medicine*, researchers followed a group of male and female novices who were training for their first marathon. The athletes trained for a period of eighty weeks, with no control over diet. During the training regime, the men lost weight and fat but the women, alas, did not. A study in 1992 reported in the *Journal of Applied Physiology* showed similar results among female runners whose weight was tracked for a year. In a 1984 study in the *Journal of Obesity and Weight Regulation*, both men and women were monitored in a continuous exercise program for twenty weeks, again with no control over diet. The men showed significant decreases in body weight and percentage of fat mass but the women experienced no change. Apparently exercise alone may result in decreased body weight for men, but not for women.

So the only answer has to be the two-pronged attack, controlling caloric intake while increasing exercise. More exercise helps counter the diet doldrums and, we hope, resets the metabolic regulator, helping you to burn more calories for the same amount of physical activity.

You should aim for only a pound or two of loss per week. After all, your objective is a new set of habits that will keep you where you want to be for the rest of your life. If you are losing weight, even though you are doing it slowly and steadily, you will eventually reach your goal and maintain it if you continue your improved habits.

What constitutes a healthy diet?

Just as the notion of ideal body weight has been revised, so has the notion of what we should eat. Most women now approaching menopause were born in the 1940s or early 1950s, when a healthy diet consisted of a lot of meat and potatoes, plenty of milk, cheese, and dairy products, as well as fruit and vegetables. Protein was "in." Starches, as complex carbohydrates were called, were "out" because they were thought to be fattening. Potatoes and pasta were definitely regarded with suspicion. There were seven basic food groups and you were told to eat a certain number of servings of each one.

In 1989 the American Nutrition Society came out with its new guidelines and changed all that. The general structure of the ideal diet is pyramidal, and people are urged to eat more carbohydrates, less fat, and less protein than formerly. In general, the guidelines suggest the following daily intake:

One or two servings of lean meat, skinless poultry, or fish; or, if you prefer a vegetarian diet, nuts, dried beans, peas or lentils, or peanut butter

Two to four servings of fruit

Three to five servings of vegetables, including at least one leafy green vegetable and one orange or yellow vegetable

Two servings of skim or 1 percent low-fat milk, or low-fat dairy products (pregnant and postmenopausal women should have three servings)

Five to eight servings of polyunsaturated or monounsaturated oils, or margarine

Six to eleven servings of bread, cereals, pasta, rice, popcorn, or dried beans or peas

This plan of nutrition is low in cholesterol, low in saturated fats, relatively low in protein, and quite high in complex carbohydrates and calcium. It is a diet healthy for your heart and bones, and one on which it is relatively easy to lose weight if you control portion size and supplement your diet with exercise. It offers a variety of foods and emphasizes fruits, vegetables, and whole grains.

What is an appropriate caloric intake for a 50-year-old woman?

Unfortunately, our caloric needs decline by about 100 calories per day for each ten years of age over 25. So if the average woman at age 25 needs about 2,000 calories to maintain her body weight and keep up her energy, she needs only 1,800 calories for the same activities at age 45. When she is in her midfifties, she needs only about 1,700 calories daily, unless she increases her exercise level.

If you are trying to lose weight, remember that you are working toward slow loss, maybe one or two pounds weekly, which is brought about by a change in your eating habits.

How much calcium should a menopausal woman be getting?

Although the subject of calcium metabolism is complex and the evidence is somewhat ambiguous, it seems estrogen makes it easier for the body to absorb calcium from the diet. Therefore the current recommendation is 1,000 mg daily for premenopausal women and for postmenopausal women who are taking estrogen, and 1,500 mg for postmenopausal women who are not taking estrogen.

What do you have to eat to get 1,500 mg of calcium?

While dairy foods are the main sources of calcium, many other foods are rich in this mineral. Certain green and leafy vegetables, such as broccoli, collard greens, and kale (which may not be a part of your regular menus), are good sources of calcium. Canned fish, such as sardines and salmon (which are canned with the bones), is another source. Any vegetable with high oxalic acid is less desirable as a source of calcium, because the oxalic acid interferes with calcium absorption; among these are spinach, beet greens, rhubarb, parsley, and chard. In case you had hoped to get your calcium from chocolate, you should know that it too is high in oxalic acid. If you don't like milk or dairy products, remember that some orange juice now comes with added calcium.

In order to ensure effective calcium absorption, you must get adequate vitamin D. Good dietary sources include fortified milk, "oily" fish such as sardines and salmon, and cod liver oil, once the bane of millions of American children (a single teaspoon of it contains as much vitamin D as a quart of fortified milk). Another source is sunlight, whose ultraviolet radiation converts a complex fatty component of skin into vitamin D, hence the name sunshine vitamin.

You can see from the accompanying table that you have to be very conscientious if you are to get adequate calcium from your diet: two cups of milk, a cup of yogurt, and a cup of fortified orange juice will give you a baseline 1,320 mg of calcium.

Table 2. Foods High in Calcium

Food	Quantity	Amount of Calcium (mg)
Milk, 1% fat	1 cup	350
Yogurt	1 cup	300
Cottage cheese, low fat	1 cup	120
Collard greens, cooked	1 cup	360
Broccoli, cooked	1 stalk	160
Kale, cooked	1 cup	200
Sardines, canned	8 medium	350
Salmon, canned with bones	3 ounces	170
Tofu (soybean curd)	4 ounces	150
Orange juice, natural	1 cup	30
Orange juice, calcium fortified	1 cup	320

What about calcium supplements?

Since the average calcium intake in the United States is something like 400 to 500 mg daily, only about a third of what a postmenopausal woman needs if she is not taking estrogen, many women who do not like milk and other dairy products find it difficult to get adequate calcium in their diet.

Fortunately calcium supplements are available. A single chewable tablet of calcium carbonate or calcium citrate will supply an additional 200 to 300 mg of calcium beyond what you have in your diet. Some physicians recommend extra-strength Tums, the over-the-counter antacid used by many people to counteract heartburn and indigestion. A single "Tums 500" tablet contains 500 mg of calcium, so if you have one after each meal you will get the 1,500 mg of calcium required by postmenopausal women not taking estrogen.

Since your body best absorbs calcium in an acidic environment, you should take Tums after meals, when your stomach is producing copious amounts of acid to digest your food. Instead of an after-dinner mint patty, try an after-dinner Tums tablet.

Why is cholesterol important?

Cholesterol is a fatty substance that is manufactured by the body. It is present in foods such as red meat and high-fat dairy products and has been linked to coronary artery disease.

Cholesterol in itself is not harmful. It is used by the body to make certain hormones; it helps in digestion; and it is an important building block of bodily tissues. However, cholesterol in the wrong amounts or in the wrong places is dangerous. Coronary heart disease, also called coronary artery disease, happens when cholesterol is deposited inside the walls of the arteries that bring the heart its blood supply. These deposits contribute to buildup of fatty blockage called plaque. Deposits of plaque inside the blood vessels are known as arteriosclerosis, or atherosclerosis, or hardening of the arteries.

Until menopause, women are protected by estrogen and do not have to worry as much about cholesterol and the diseases that result from cholesterol deposits. But postmenopausal women, especially those not taking estrogen, should be aware of the importance of controlling blood cholesterol levels.

In recent years, as research has provided new data, beliefs about cholesterol have changed. Fifteen years ago it was considered all right to have a serum cholesterol of 240 (that is, 240 milligrams of cholesterol per deciliter of blood); ten years ago, 220 mg/dl was acceptable; in recent years, however, physicians and researchers have started looking at a cholesterol level of 200 mg/dl or lower as the desired goal.

What are "good" and "bad" cholesterol?

It is not merely your total serum cholesterol, the amount of cholesterol in your blood, that counts. Because cholesterol is a fatty substance, it does not mix easily with blood and in order to be moved around the body via the bloodstream, cholesterol gets packaged into molecules called lipoproteins. Researchers have identified a number of types of lipoproteins, of which two have received a lot of attention, LDL (low-density lipoprotein, "bad" cholesterol) and HDL (high-density lipoprotein, "good" cholesterol).

Bad cholesterol is bad because it seems to play an important role in depositing cholesterol on the inside of the artery walls. Good cholesterol is good because it seems to help clean out the cholesterol deposits that have already begun to line the artery walls.

Therefore it is the relative quantities of HDL and LDL that are important to the health of your arteries and your heart. These days an LDL level of up to 130 mg/dl is considered fine, 130 to 160 mg/dl is in a gray zone, and anything over 160 mg/dl is anxiety provoking. So if your total cholesterol is 220 but your HDL is 100, then you are in good shape because your LDL is very low.

To complicate this subject still further, levels of HDL and LDL must be taken as relative quantities. It is their ratio that is important. Suppose your HDL is 100 and your LDL is 160, which puts your total cholesterol at something larger than 260 and your LDL at the outer edge of the gray zone. But compare that risk to the risk of someone whose total cholesterol is 190 mg/dl but with an HDL of 20 and an LDL of 170. These people are few and far between, but they are at significant risk for cholesterol problems.

What can you do if your cholesterol levels are high?

Suppose you go to a fair or some public place where cholesterol levels are checked as a public service, and you find that your total serum cholesterol is high. If it is over 300, you should talk soon to your doctor—probably to your internist, since most gynecologists in the country don't feel totally comfortable prescribing drugs to lower blood cholesterol. Various medicines on the market will lower blood cholesterol levels, but all have side effects and all have some toxicity. If your cholesterol is borderline, the two most important things you can do are start exercising and adjust your diet.

How effective is diet in reducing cholesterol?

Fortunately, you can have a significant impact on your cholesterol levels by controlling your diet. If you are overweight, the main factor seems to be not what you eat, but the weight loss that follows a well-designed, controlled diet. The body is able to manufacture cholesterol even though there is no cholesterol at all in your diet. If you live on a diet of all lettuce (which of course you should not) and have an intake of zero cholesterol, your body will still manufacture it for you.

Nevertheless, a diet low in total fat, saturated fat, and cholesterol kills two birds with one stone: it contributes to weight loss (if you need it) and it restricts intake of highly saturated fats, which worsen your blood lipid profile (that is, they increase the relative amounts of bad cholesterol).

Saturated fats, the kind that are solid at room temperature, come chiefly from animal sources. They include milk, cheese, meat, butter, and lard, as well as a few vegetable products, notably cocoa butter and coconut oil. Researchers now believe that saturated fat in your diet is worse for your blood lipid levels than dietary cholesterol. That is why foods such as shrimp (fairly high in cholesterol but lower in saturated fat) have less fearsome reputations than they formerly did.

A sensible low-cholesterol, low-fat diet includes less than 30 percent of total calories from fat and less than 10 percent from saturated fat, which is the kind found in animal products (meat, poultry, fish) and a few vegetable oils (notably palm oil and coconut oil). Adopting this kind of diet will, on the average, reduce total cholesterol 5 to 10 percent. The Appendix shows the fat, cholesterol, and calorie content of some familiar foods.

One important feature of this kind of dietary restriction is that it reduces total calories. Proteins and carbohydrates have 4 calories per gram, whereas fats have 9 calories per gram, more than twice as much. By concentrating on carbohydrates—for example, fruits, vegetables, and grains—you can eat more food while ingesting fewer calories.

Can you control cholesterol by exercising?

The second important factor both in cholesterol control and in weight reduction is exercise. An appropriate aerobic exercise regimen can increase your HDL as much as 20 percent. If a woman comes into the office with a cholesterol level of 260, I don't automatically ship her off to her internist for cholesterol-lowering drugs. Particularly if she is overweight, I try to get her on a suitable diet. I strongly encourage her to get involved in an exercise program. And I strongly encourage her to think about ERT, since we know that ERT can increase HDL by about 20 percent.

Exercise as a Lifestyle Choice

The benefits of physical activity are many and well known both to those who exercise and to those who do not. Exercise improves muscle strength, muscle tone, and flexibility. It promotes a sense of well-being and enhances self-esteem. Weight-bearing exercise helps develop and preserve bone. Aerobic exercise helps stave off cardiovascular disease.

If you are trying to lose weight, exercise depresses appetite, which makes it easier to keep your caloric intake low. Exercise together with calorie restriction encourages the loss of fat rather than muscle, so that you look trimmer, fitter, and healthier as you slim down. Exercise boosts metabolism, enabling you to burn calories faster.

So why don't people exercise? Most women say that the problem is time, but you can make time to exercise if you really are determined.

Basically there are three kinds of exercise, which are important all through life and especially as we get older. The first is aerobic exercise, in which the muscles burn oxygen as fuel. Aerobic exercise, which includes fast walking, jogging, running, aerobic dance, and other forms of rhythmic exertion over fairly long periods of time, is important to cardiovascular health and weight control.

The second type, anaerobic or isometric exercise, involves using particular muscle groups in strenuous bursts for fairly short periods of time. As we age, our muscle mass turns to fat and we get weaker. Very elderly people, both men and women, often have difficulty getting up from chairs or lifting bags of groceries. Anaerobic exercise will help maintain muscular strength so that these activities become easier. Calisthenics, tai chi chuan, yoga, weight lifting, and working out on Nautilus machines are examples of this kind of exercise. The benefits of anaer-

Figure 24. *One way to get adequate aerobic exercise is to raise your heart rate into your target zone and keep it there for thirty minutes at least three times weekly.*

obic exercise include strength, muscle tone, and stamina. If you play golf or tennis, or if you heft grandchildren, improved muscle strength will transfer to these activities. Like aerobic exercise, strength training boosts your metabolic rate, which helps you lose weight, since a trained, muscular body uses more calories than a flabby one, even when sitting still. Furthermore, muscle takes up less space than fat, pound for pound, so if you are more muscular, you will be trimmer.

The third type is exercise for flexibility, which as the years go by becomes increasingly critical to maintaining balance and agility. Muscle stretching before aerobic or anaerobic exercise is important in preventing injury.

Although the ideal exercise program includes all three types, for women in the menopausal age bracket, two points are crucial: getting enough exercise to maintain ideal body weight and keep up cardiovascular fitness, and doing the kind of exercise that promotes healthy bone. One commonly used guideline for

Table 3. Time Needed to Burn Calories from Various Foods

Food	Calories	Type of activity (calories burned)[a]						
		Sleeping (60/hr)	Sedentary (80/hr)	Light (110/hr)	Moderate (170/hr)	Vigorous (250/hr)	Strenuous (350+/hr)
2 8-inch celery stalks	15	15 min	11 min	8 min	5 min	4 min	3 min
2 medium graham crackers	55	55 min	41 min	30 min	19 min	13 min	9 min
2 tbsp fruit-nut snack	70	1 hr 10 min	53 min	38 min	25 min	17 min	12 min
2 tbsp peanuts	105	1 hr 45 min	1 hr 19 min	57 min	37 min	25 min	18 min
1 cup plain low-fat yogurt	145	2 hr 25 min	1 hr 49 min	1 hr 19 min	51 min	35 min	25 min
1 cup split-pea soup	195	3 hr 15 min	2 hr 26 min	1 hr 46 min	1 hr 8 min	47 min	33 min
1 cup fruit-flavored yogurt	225	3 hr 45 min	2 hr 49 min	2 hr 3 min	1 hr 19 min	54 min	39 min
1/3 cup granola with coconut	280	4 hr 40 min	3 hr 30 min	2 hr 33 min	1 hr 39 min	1 hr 7 min	48 min
3-oz hamburger on bun	365	6 hr 5 min	4 hr 34 min	3 hr 19 min	2 hr 9 min	1 hr 28 min	1 hr 3 min
12-oz chocolate milkshake	430	7 hr 10 min	5 hr 23 min	3 hr 55 min	2 hr 32 min	1 hr 43 min	1 hr 13 min

a. All figures are approximate, as energy expenditure varies from individual to individual. The data are calculated on rates for a 123-lb woman; larger, more muscular women will burn calories faster.

Sedentary activity: reading, watching TV, other activities while seated.
Light activity: dusting, ironing, shopping, walking slowly (2¹/₂–3 mph).
Moderate activity: housework, walking more rapidly (3¹/₂–4 mph).

Vigorous activity: gardening, scrubbing floors, golf.
Strenuous activity: bicycling, running, swimming, chopping wood.

Source: Based on data from USDA Home and Garden Bulletin No. 228, Food, pp. 14–15.

cardiovascular fitness suggests raising your heart rate into a target zone, which is somewhere between 60 and 75 percent of its maximum, and keeping it there for thirty minutes at least three times a week. To discover your target zone, subtract your age from 220, then take 60 and 75 percent of that number.

Another way to approach exercise, suggested by the American Heart Association, is to expend at least 2,000 calories weekly in exercise.

The American College of Sports Medicine offers exercise guidelines, which suggest that you alternate aerobic and anaerobic types of exercise, doing strength training (anaerobic exercise) for two or three thirty-minute sessions each week, and on alternate days doing aerobic exercise such as walking, jogging, aerobic dancing, or swimming.

Self-Destructive Habits

One of the hard lessons in life is that to form a good habit, you seem to have to indulge in hundreds and hundreds of correct repetitions. But do something that is bad for you once or twice, and it seems instantly to become a habit of ferocious tenacity.

Smoking
In terms of aging, smoking is a hugely negative factor. It increases the risk of osteoporosis; it increases the risk of cardiovascular disease by causing injury to blood-vessel walls and apparently also by lowering your good cholesterol; it increases the risk of lung cancer and other pulmonary diseases. And, of course, it contributes to early menopause. In short, smoking is bad for everyone and especially poisonous to a menopausal woman.

Do not despair if you are a smoker; there is evidence that if you stop smoking you will regain the advantage that you have lost—almost immediately in terms of your heart, and somewhat more gradually in terms of your lungs.

Alcohol and Middle Age
A second major risk for women is alcohol. Unfortunately, many middle-aged women turn to drinking, possibly because of the stresses associated with this time of life. Women are at double risk, first because pound for pound of body weight they metabolize alcohol less well than men. Blood alcohol concentration after a given number of drinks is related to the body's ratio of muscle to fat; since men in general are leaner, they have relatively more water into which the alcohol

Box 3. Smoking Facts and Figures

Smoking is the most preventable cause of death in our society.

Tobacco use is responsible for nearly one in five deaths in the United States.

The World Health Organization estimates that approximately 3 million people die worldwide each year as a result of smoking.

Smokers lose an average of fifteen years of life.

Female smokers have a risk of dying of lung cancer twelve times higher than women who have never smoked.

Smoking accounts for 30 percent of all cancer deaths; it is a major cause of heart disease and is associated with conditions ranging from colds to gastric ulcers to cerebrovascular disease.

The Office of Technology Assessment of the U.S. Congress estimates that cigarettes cost Americans $68 billion annually in tobacco-related health care costs and lost productivity.

The cost of treating smoking-related disease and lost productivity amounts to $2.59 for every pack of cigarettes sold in this country.

People who stop smoking, regardless of age, live longer than people who continue to smoke.

Quitting smoking substantially decreases the risk of lung, laryngeal, esophageal, oral, pancreatic, bladder, and cervical cancers.

Quitting smoking reduces the risk of coronary heart disease and cardiovascular disease.

Source: Cancer Facts and Figures 1995. Used with permission of the American Cancer Society, Inc.

can be distributed. Second, both men and women tolerate alcohol less well as they age than they did as younger people.

Although alleviating stress with prescription medications has a poor reputation, alcohol is much worse for you. Nutritionally, alcohol is worthless; it is full of those fabled "empty calories" that don't bring the benefits of nutrients along with them. When people drink, they feel full and so they don't eat properly; they have ingested plenty of calories but they have not taken in any vitamins, minerals, or protein.

In addition, alcohol puts you at increased risk for all kinds of diseases. It destroys the liver, so that people who are alcoholic have several different kinds of liver disease, beginning with fatty liver and continuing on to cirrhosis and carcinoma of the liver.

Heavy alcohol consumption boosts your risk for osteoporosis. Whether this additional risk is nutritional because alcoholic women don't eat properly or attributable to some other factor, alcoholic women develop osteoporosis at a faster rate than nonalcoholics.

Some studies in recent years have suggested that very moderate drinking, which for women can be defined as one drink a day, may decrease risk for cardiovascular disease, although the reason is unclear. This research, which has focused only on cardiovascular risk and examined the risks of French wine drinkers and American liquor drinkers, remains controversial. Furthermore, nothing in the scientific literature says that if one or two drinks a day can help you, then three or four can help you more. For many people, particularly those who come from alcoholic backgrounds, drinking one or two often leads to drinking three or four or more. Studies have also suggested that alcohol increases the risk of breast cancer, but this possibility remains ambiguous.

With alcohol, with diet, for that matter with any aspect of your life that you would like to alter, change is certainly possible though usually difficult; replacing destructive habits with healthful ones takes time, discipline, and patience—but it can be done.

The Challenges and the Satisfactions

Biologically, menopause does mark an ending: it signals the close of your reproductive years. Yet it can also be seen as a beginning, a gateway to the second half of your life. Like many women, you may find yourself happier and more content in these middle years than you were as a young woman in your twenties and thirties.

Chances are that you entered adulthood buoyed with energy and youthful optimism. But, lacking in experience, you were probably dependent on parents and mentors, unsure of who you were, of what you wanted to do, of where you belonged in the world around you. By the time you reach the years surrounding menopause, you are a more experienced woman, independent, fortified with knowledge and possibly even wisdom, capable of making the decisions and choices that will shape your future. If you have been a wife and mother, these relationships and the adjustments they require surely have taught you skills of coping and flexibility and have equipped you to distinguish the essential from the peripheral. If you have never married or if you have divorced, you have learned to respect and live by your own values. If you have followed a particular career, you know how to juggle the demands of other people with your own needs and how to channel your energy where it is most required; you undoubtedly have picked up abilities that serve you beyond the boundaries of your job.

Often patients in the menopausal years tell me that while they need reading glasses to check the small print, the big issues in their lives are clear. In their forties and fifties they feel liberated from biological constraints and social expectations. They see this period as a time when they can shape their lives as they want, developing talents and capabilities that were pushed aside earlier in the interest of family or other responsibilities. Other women say that the strands of knowledge they have acquired over the years are suddenly coming together to form a pattern, or that relationships they have cultivated are bearing totally unexpected fruits. No one denies the difficulties of midlife, but for many women the rewards of this stage are extraordinary.

Appendix. A List of Fat, Cholesterol, and Calorie Content of Familiar Foods

Food	Serving size	Calories	Total fat (gm)	Saturated fat (gm)	Cholesterol (mg)
GROUP 1					
Dairy Products					
(2–4 servings)					
Milk, 1% fat	8 fl oz	102	3	2	10
Milk, 1/2% fat	8 fl oz	92	1	1	7
Milk, nonfat	8 fl oz	86	0	0	4
Yogurt, flavored nonfat	1 cup	148	0	0	5
Yogurt, plain nonfat	1 cup	125	0	0	4
Yogurt, flavored low fat	1 cup	229	2	2	9
Cheese, low fat (8% milk fat)	1 oz	54	2	1	13
Cheese, fat free	1 oz	41	0	0	1
Cheese, cottage, 1% fat	1/2 cup	82	1	1	5
Cheese, cottage, low fat	1/2 cup	102	2	1	10
Ice milk, hardened, 5% fat	1/2 cup	92	3	2	9
Ice milk, 1% fat	1/2 cup	81	1	1	2
Sherbet	1/2 cup	135	2	1	7
Frozen yogurt, 1/2% fat	1/2 cup	100	1	1	4

Food	Serving size	Calories	Total fat (gm)	Saturated fat (gm)	Cholesterol (mg)
GROUP 1					
Vegetables (2–3 servings)					
All vegetables are low in fat and saturated fatty acids	1/2 to 1 cup	25	0	0	0
Lean Red Meat, Fish, Poultry (fat trimmed, no more than 6 oz per day)					
Beef, round flank, sirloin	3 oz	176	8	3	64
Pork tenderloin	3 oz	141	4	1	79
Pork, leg	3 oz	188	9	3	82
Pork, ham	3 oz	151	8	3	50
Lamb, leg, loin	3 oz	173	8	3	78
Veal, all cuts except breast	3oz	139	5	2	93
Chicken/turkey, white meat	3 oz	140	3	1	65
Chicken/turkey, dark meat	3 oz	167	7	2	76
Sole, flounder, halibut, perch	3 oz	100	1	0	58
Shark, swordfish	3 oz	128	4	1	62
Salmon, orange roughy	3 oz	157	6	1	42
Tuna fish, canned in oil	3 oz	168	7	1	15
Shrimp	3 oz	84	1	0	166
Frozen dinners, entrees	single serving	140–400	8	3	80
Fruits and Fruit Juices (at least 2 servings)					
All fruits, juices	1/2 to 1 cup or 1 medium	160	0–1	0	0

Food	Serving size	Calories	Total fat (gm)	Saturated fat (gm)	Cholesterol (mg)
GROUP 1					
Breads, Cereals, and Starches, (6+ servings)					
White enriched bread	2 slices	153	2	0	2
Whole wheat bread	2 slices	138	2	0	2
Bagel	1 medium	170	2	0	0
Hamburger bun	1 medium	169	3	1	3
Tortilla, corn, 6" diameter	1	127	2	0	0
Crackers, saltines	1/2 oz	62	2	1	1
Cereal, raisin bran	1 cup	156	1	0	0
Rice, plain, cooked	2/3 cup	181	0	0	0
Spaghetti, plain, cooked	1 cup	197	1	0	0
Dried beans, peas cooked	1/2 cup	117	0	0	0
Potato, white, sweet, yam	1 medium	120	0	0	0
Corn, lima beans, squash	1/2 cup	80	0	0	0
Angel food cake, plain	2" wedge	132	0	0	0
Egg and Egg Substitutes (4 whole eggs per week or less)					
Whole egg, raw	1	75	5	2	213
Egg white, raw	1	16	trace	0	0
Egg yolk, raw	1	63	5	2	213
Fats and Oils (may include 5–8 tsp daily)					
Margarine	1 tsp	34	4	1	0

Food	Serving size	Calories	Total fat (gm)	Saturated fat (gm)	Cholesterol (mg)
GROUP 1					
Fats and Oils (cont.)					
Unsaturated oil (canola, safflower, sunflower, corn, soybean, olive, peanut)	1 tsp	40	5	0	0
Mayonnaise, low calorie	1 tbsp	44	4	1	4
Italian dressing, low calorie	2 tbsp	32	3	0	2
Blue cheese dressing, low calorie	2 tbsp	24	2	1	0

GROUP 2

Higher-Fat Foods

If your caloric needs allow, choose more servings from the basic food groups above. The higher-fat foods listed below may be used once in a while or on special occasions.

3–5 grams total fat

Food	Serving size	Calories	Total fat (gm)	Saturated fat (gm)	Cholesterol (mg)
Milk, 2% fat	8 fl oz	121	5	3	18
Part-skim mozzarella cheese	1 oz	79	5	3	15
Cream cheese, light	1 oz	62	5	3	17
Cottage cheese, creamed	1/2 cup	117	5	3	17
Chicken soup with noodles	1 cup	82	3	1	5
Beef and vegetable soup	1 cup	83	3	1	5
Chocolate chip cookie	1 oz	139	4	4	0

6–10 grams total fat

Food	Serving size	Calories	Total fat (gm)	Saturated fat (gm)	Cholesterol (mg)
Whole milk	8 fl oz	150	8	5	33
Yogurt, plain, whole milk	1 cup	138	7	5	29

Food	Serving size	Calories	Total fat (gm)	Saturated fat (gm)	Cholesterol (mg)
GROUP 2					
Higher-Fat Foods (cont.)					
6–10 grams total fat					
Yogurt, flavored, whole milk	1 cup	268	7	5	22
American cheese	1 oz	106	9	6	27
Cheddar cheese	1oz	114	9	6	30
Ice cream	1/2 cup	135	7	4	30
Ice cream cone	1/2 cup	157	7	4	30
Bacon	2 slices	73	6	2	11
Spaghetti, with meat sauce	1 cup	239	10	2	10
New England clam chowder	1 cup	163	7	3	22
Hamburger, plain	1	274	10	4	30
Frankfurter, chicken	1-1/2 oz	110	8	2	42
Bologna	1 oz	90	8	3	16
Brownie	1 large	172	9	3	34
Sugar cookie	1 oz	137	8	2	0
Biscuit	2 oz	165	7	2	3
Potato chips	1 oz	156	10	2	0
Popcorn, microwave popped	3 cups	118	6	5	0
Oatmeal cookie	1 oz	126	6	1	0
Blueberry or bran muffin	1 large	161	6	2	28
Pancakes, 4"diameter	5	388	7	1	19
GROUP 3					
Even-Higher-Fat Foods					
11–15 grams total fat					
Ice cream bar	3 oz	178	13	10	20
Taco	1	245	15	7	46
Fajita, steak	1	224	11	4	30
Enchilada	1	229	13	7	69
Pork sausage	3 links	144	12	4	32

Food	Serving size	Calories	Total fat (gm)	Saturated fat (gm)	Cholesterol (mg)
GROUP 3					
Even-Higher-Fat Foods (cont.)					
11–15 grams total fat					
Frankfurter, beef and pork	1-1/2 oz	136	12	5	21
Beef stew	1 cup	303	14	5	60
English muffin with egg, cheese, Canadian bacon	1	297	13	6	237
Fried chicken, breast	3 oz	255	15	4	45
Cheese pizza, 6" diameter	1	422	13	8	28
Cheeseburger, single patty	1	326	14	6	44
Chili with beans	1 cup	272	11	4	42
Butter	1 tbsp	102	12	7	31
Italian dressing	2 tbsp	138	14	2	0
Mayonnaise	1 tbsp	99	11	2	8
Croissant	1	172	12	7	30
Waffle, 7-1/2" diameter	1	290	15	5	70
Hot dog with bun	1	264	15	5	23
Peanut butter	2 tbsp	176	15	3	0
Sunflower seeds	1/4 cup	171	15	2	0
French fries	16 medium	210	13	4	0
Doughnut, raised, glazed	1 small	233	14	7	27
16–20 grams total fat					
Macaroni and cheese	1 cup	399	18	5	8
Lasagna, 3" × 3"	1 cup	383	19	9	79
Sandwich, breaded fish	1	424	19	4	37
Peanuts, roasted	1/4 cup	232	20	3	0
Chocolate cake	2" wedge	447	19	8	52
Blue cheese dressing	2 tbsp	154	16	3	5

Food	Serving size	Calories	Total fat (gm)	Saturated fat (gm)	Cholesterol (mg)
GROUP 3					
Even-Higher-Fat Foods (cont.)					
21–26 grams total fat					
Burrito	1	499	23	9	69
Club sandwich	1	483	22	5	65
Pepperoni pizza, 6" diameter	1	653	25	13	72
Tuna salad	1/2 cup	279	24	4	24
Polish sausage	3 oz	277	24	9	60
Spareribs	3 oz	310	26	9	77
Italian sausage	3 oz	275	22	8	66
Bratwurst	3 oz	277	24	8	60
Avocado	1 small	225	21	9	0
31+ grams total fat					
Quarter-pound hamburger	1	572	32	9	77
Quarter-pound cheeseburger	1	629	36	10	90
Chicken salad	1/2 cup	352	32	5	61
Danish w/filling, nuts, icing	1 medium	647	41	15	30
Danish w/filling, nuts	1 medium	565	38	12	48
Submarine sandwich	5-1/2" long	1,242	62	27	148

Note: The American Heart Association's dietary guidelines for adults specify less than 30 percent total fat, less than 10 percent saturated fatty acids, and no more than 300 mg of cholesterol daily.

The foods listed in group 1 form the basis of a nutritious diet, and you should be careful to include the recommended number of servings in each category every day. Foods listed in group 2 are higher in fat; those in group 3 are even higher and should be reserved for infrequent use, perhaps on special occasions.

Source: American Heart Association. Nutrient data from the Minnesota Nutrition Data System, Nutrition Coordinating Center, University of Minnesota, version 2.3; USDA Handbook No. 8. Series: *USDA Provisional Table on the Fatty Acids and Cholesterol Content of Selected Foods*, 1984.

Glossary

acute: Sudden, current, not longstanding.

adenomatous hyperplasia: Excessive growth of the lining of the uterus; potential precursor to cancer of the endometrium.

adenomyosis: A condition in which the glands that line the uterus penetrate its internal muscle walls. Sometimes called internal endometriosis. Often associated with painful and heavy periods.

adhesion: Scar tissue that "sticks" one structure or organ to another to which it should not be attached.

agonist: A chemical that acts in similar fashion to another chemical.

amphetamines: A class of drugs that make people "speed"; often called uppers. Have been used as diet pills; can be addictive and, with overdose, fatal.

anabolic steroids: Drugs of the cortisone family that "build up" tissue. Often used (illegally) by athletes to enhance their performance.

anemia: Low red-blood-cell count. In women, often secondary to heavy periods.

angina: Chest pain associated with lack of oxygen to the heart, usually caused by narrowed coronary arteries.

anovulatory: Associated with lack of ripening and release of an egg from the ovary. Anovulatory menstrual periods are often irregular and heavy.

anterior: Referring to the front or top of the body or an organ.

anticholinergic: Referring to drugs that lower the release of acetylcholine from nerve endings; often used as antispasmodics to calm bowel and bladder activity.

antifungal: Referring to substances that act against yeast and other fungi; often used to fight yeast infections.

anti-inflammatory: Referring to substances that act against inflammation. Frequently applied to drugs used to treat arthritis (for example, Motrin or Anaprox). Anti-inflammatories are sometimes used to combat menstrual cramps.

antioxidants: Chemicals that "eat up" or antagonize free radicals, which are toxic products of cell metabolism. Believed to slow down aging and other toxic cell events.

arrhythmia: Fluctuation of the regular, smooth heartbeat. May originate in the atria (upper chambers) or ventricles (lower chambers) of the heart.

ascites: Fluid in the abdominal cavity. Often seen in people with liver failure or cancer.

atherosclerosis: Thickening of the walls of arteries, primarily composed of fat.

atrophic: Aged, inactive. Relative to tissue of the female genital tract, it means thinned out.

atypia: Condition of having odd-looking cells; sometimes associated with inflammation, sometimes with precancerous changes.

basal metabolic rate: Speed at which the body burns its food. People with a high basal metabolic rate tend to be thin.

basement membrane: A thin layer that divides the superficial cells of an organ from its deeper cells, the "skin" of an organ.

benign: Not malignant. A tumor that is benign does not metastasize (spread to distant organs), but grows only in place.

beta-blockers: A family of drugs that block the activity of adrenaline. Used primarily to slow the heart rate and lower the blood pressure.

biopsy: A sample; or (as a verb) to take a sample of tissue. Often used to determine whether a tissue is cancerous.

birth control pills: Oral contraceptives, also called BCPs. Contain estrogen and progesterone that suppress the release of an egg by the ovary, thus preventing pregnancy.

blood lipids: Fats in the bloodstream; usually refers to cholesterol and triglycerides.

board certified: Most medical specialties require examinations called board exams that test specific bodies of knowledge. Those who pass are board certified or "boarded." Not every physician who hangs a shingle is board certified.

breakthrough bleeding: Bleeding between periods. Usually associated with low-dose usage of birth control pills. Rarely harmful; often a nuisance.

CAD (coronary artery disease): Thickening of the walls of blood vessels to the heart, with obstruction to blood flow. Also known as atherosclerosis. Often leads to angina.

carcinoma in situ: A very localized cancer that has not yet penetrated the basement membrane.

cardiac disease: Heart problems. Usually either CAD or disease of the valves that control the blood in the chambers of the heart.

CBC: Complete blood count, including white and red blood cells.

cerebral cortex: The outer part of the brain. Thinking occurs here; also the processing of complex neurological signals such as vision.

cervix: The neck of or entrance to the uterus. Opens, in labor, to let the fetus out.

chronic: Long-lasting, not sudden.

climacteric: The time frame during which a woman passes from her reproductive to her postmenopausal years; marked by the gradual waning of reproductive function. A more inclusive term than either perimenopause or menopause.

clinical trials: Experiments in which some people are given a drug and some people are given a placebo to check the effectiveness of a new medication.

clotting factors: Proteins in the blood that bring about clotting.

collagen: The substance, which acts like glue, that holds many cells together. Softer than bone; supports the skin and other structures.

colposcope: A giant microscope used to examine and magnify the cervix and vulva. Used to aid in the diagnosis of precancerous and cancerous conditions of the cervix, vagina, and vulva. Can also be used to examine the penis.

cone biopsy: A surgical procedure in which a cone-shaped wedge of tissue is removed from the cervix. Used to diagnose and treat precancerous and cancerous conditions of the cervix.

contraindicated: Term for something that is not a good idea, say a medication or treatment that is absolutely wrong for a certain condition and will make it get worse.

corpus luteum: Literally, yellow body. The cyst that forms after an egg is released by the ovary. Secretes progesterone and readies the lining of the uterus to receive a fertilized egg.

cryosurgery: Freezing. Usually used in gynecology to treat genital warts and precancerous conditions of the cervix. Also known as cryotherapy.

CT scan: Also called CAT scan (computerized axial tomography). An x-ray technique that focuses in at different levels of an organ or body cavity. Allows a three-dimensional visualization of the organ or cavity. Usually fairly expensive.

curettage: Scraping. Usually applied to scraping the uterine cavity.

cystic teratoma: Medical name for a dermoid cyst; a cyst arising from egg cells in the ovary. Can contain hair, teeth, and other formed body parts. Almost always benign.

cystitis: Inflammation of the bladder.

Usually causes frequency of and burning with urination.

cystocele: Bulging of the bladder into the vagina.

cystoscope: A narrow metal tube inserted into the bladder through the urethra to look inside the bladder.

cysts: Fluid-filled growths anywhere in the body. Most often benign.

D&C: Dilatation and curettage. Stretching of the cervix to permit scraping out the inside of the uterus.

dermoid cyst: See cystic teratoma.

detrusor dyssynergia: Irritable or unstable bladder. A condition in which a small amount of urine in the bladder makes the bladder irritable and gives the patient the urge to urinate.

diuretic: A medication that pushes the kidney to excrete water; increases urine output.

drug trials: Comparable to clinical trials, in which patients are randomly given either a new drug or a placebo to assess the clinical effectiveness of the drug.

dysfunction: Abnormal working, as of an organ.

dysmenorrhea: Painful menstrual cramps.

dyspareunia: Painful sexual intercourse.

dysplasia: Abnormal cell growth. Not yet cancer, but different from the usual growth of cells.

electrolyte testing: Usually refers to three elements present in the bloodstream: sodium (Na), potassium (K), and chlorine (Cl). In good health these elements are found at proper levels. Their presence at abnormal levels generally is an effect of medication or disease.

endogenously: Internally; coming from the inside.

endometrial stripe: Usually assessed by ultrasound, the thickness of the lining of the uterus.

endometriosis: Condition in which endometrial-type tissue is found in locations outside the uterus: anywhere in the pelvis, possibly near the bladder or bowel or, rarely, as far away as in the lungs.

endometrium: The lining of the uterus, composed of glandular tissue.

endorphins: Chemicals released in the brain that look like opioids (morphine, for example). Give a sense of well-being and are commonly released with exercise.

epidemiological: Usually referring to data collected from studies of large populations.

epidural: Having to do with the space around the spinal cord. A technique of anesthesia, sometimes used in labor, introducing chemicals into that space.

ERT: Estrogen replacement therapy. Given to women in menopause to replace the hormones they are no longer making. Also called HRT (hormone replacement therapy).

estradiol: A steroid hormone and the major estrogen (female hormone) made by women.

estrogen receptors: Structures on the

surface of tissues to which the hormone estrogen can attach.

euthyroid: Pertaining to normal thyroid function and levels.

exogenously: Coming from outside the body.

exuberant: Very heavy in growth.

fallopian tubes: Narrow tubular structures, attached to the uterus, in which fertilization occurs; conduits for eggs to go from the ovaries into the uterus.

fascia: Sturdy connective tissue that covers muscle.

fibroids: Benign extra growth of the smooth muscle wall of the uterus.

fibroadenoma: Usually refers to a solid but benign breast growth, often seen in women with fibrocystic breast changes.

fistula: A hole, an opening between two structures that are not normally connected.

follicle: The portions of the ovary that surround the eggs and help them mature.

follicular: Referring to follicles; also to the first half of the menstrual cycle before the egg is released from the follicle.

formication: A creeping sensation of the skin, as if it is crawling with ants; sometimes occurs in menopausal women.

free radicals: Toxic chemicals produced during cell metabolism; thought to be associated with aging.

FSH (follicle-stimulating hormone): A peptide chemical made by the pituitary gland; stimulates egg development and estrogen production.

gammalinolenic acid: An essential fatty acid.

GnRH: Gonadotropin-releasing hormone. A chemical produced by the hypothalamus that makes the pituitary gland secrete FSH and LH.

GnRH agonists: Chemicals that act like GnRH, but actually cause the pituitary to make less FSH and eventually decrease estrogen production.

gonad: The ovary or testis.

gonadotropins: Chemicals made by the pituitary gland that stimulate egg or sperm production by the ovary or testis.

granulosa cells: Cells that surround the maturing egg in the ovarian follicles.

hematocrit: The percentage of blood volume that is composed of red blood cells. In women a normal hematocrit is in the range 38-42.

hemoglobin: A measure of the number of red blood cells in the bloodstream. Normal for women is in the range 12-14.

histones: Chemicals found in the seminal fluid with sperm.

HIV: Human immunodeficiency virus; causes AIDS.

HMO: Health maintenance organization.

hot flash (or flush): A sensation of warmth, commonly noted in the upper part of the body, usually associated with dilation of blood capillaries and the rushing of blood through them.

HPV: Human papilloma virus; causes genital warts.

HRT: Hormone replacement therapy; often used synonymously with ERT (estrogen replacement therapy). Women who have not had a hysterectomy are almost always given HRT, both estrogen and progesterone, to protect them from endometrial hyperplasia.

hyperplasia: Benign but excessive growth of tissue, which if left unchecked can occasionally turn malignant.

hypertension: High blood pressure.

hyperthyroidism: Overactivity of the thyroid gland.

hypotensive: Having blood pressure lower than 90/60.

hypothalamus: A portion of the brain that sits on top of the pituitary gland and governs much of the hormonal activity of the body.

hypothyroidism: Condition marked by an underactive thyroid.

hysteroscope: A narrow tube containing a light, which is passed through the cervix and used to look inside the uterus.

incompetent cervix: A weakened neck of the uterus (cervix), which during pregnancy allows the cervix to dilate long before it is supposed to. Often associated with loss of pregnancy in the second trimester.

incontinence: Involuntary loss of urine (or stool).

ischemic: Referring to lack of oxygen. Ischemia (lack of oxygen to tissue) usually gives pain; for example, angina is ischemia of the heart muscles.

IV (intravenous): A small plastic tube inserted into a vein for administering fluids, medications, or anesthetics.

laparoscope: A narrow metal tube, inserted into the abdominal cavity, that allows a look around the inside of the abdomen and pelvis. Can be used to operate without making a large incision.

laser: A highly focused light that delivers so much energy that it can actually cut tissue.

LAVH: Laparoscopically assisted vaginal hysterectomy.

LH (luteinizing hormone): Chemical produced by the pituitary gland that leads to egg maturation and release by the ovary.

lichen sclerosus et atrophicus (LS&A): An inflammation of the vulvar tissue; causes itching.

luteal: Referring to the second half of the menstrual cycle, after ovulation has occurred.

malignant: Cancerous. The character of tumors that can both grow locally and spread widely (metastasize).

mastitis: Inflammation of the breast. Most often seen in women who are breast feeding, but occasionally in others.

melatonin: A hormone manufactured by the pineal gland in the brain. Only some of its functions are known. Levels tend to decrease with age in both men and women.

menarche: The onset of menstrual periods at puberty.

menopause: The cessation of menstrual periods.

menorrhagia: Heavy loss of blood with periods.

metabolic: Referring to the fueling of bodily functions.

metastasis: The spreading of cancerous tissue.

micronizing process: Breaking down a chemical into very tiny pieces, usually to enhance absorption of drugs by the body.

MRI: Magnetic resonance imaging; similar to an x-ray study that allows a detailed look at an organ. Usually expensive.

multifocality: The condition of existing in several places. Dysplasia or cancer can be multifocal.

myoma: Fibroid.

myomectomy: Surgical removal of a fibroid from the uterus.

myometrium: The muscular wall of the uterus.

neoplasia: Literally, new growth. Usually refers to a precancerous or cancerous condition.

neurotoxicity: Harm associated with either pain or loss of function of nerve cells.

neurotransmitter: A chemical messenger released by nerve cells in the brain or in the peripheral nerves, which communicates with other nerve cells or the cells that respond to them.

obesity: Fatness; technically, body weight more than 20 percent above ideal.

omentum: Fatty tissue surrounding the intestines.

opiates: Chemicals such as morphine or heroin, naturally or synthetically produced, that alter moods.

organic depression: Sadness, negative outlook, or melancholy caused not by external events but by chemical imbalances in the brain.

osteoporosis: Loss of bone or softening of bone, associated with increased risk of bone breakage; weakening of bone through loss of its hard inner structure.

ovaries: The female sex organs where eggs are matured, stored, and then released; the primary source of estrogen in the body.

ovulation: The ripening, maturation, and release of an egg by the ovary.

Pap smear: Often used as a test for cervical cancer; involves scraping superficial cells of the cervix. Named for George Papanicolaou.

pathological: Abnormal, associated with disease.

pathologist: A physician who looks at tissue, either through a microscope or with the naked eye, to assess it for health or disease.

PCA: Patient-controlled analgesia; a system, usually with a pump, whereby patients can regulate the frequency with which they receive painkillers.

pedicle: The supporting tissue for an organ or, in surgery, the tissue from which a structure is released. (The stem of a mushroom could be considered its pedicle.)

perimenopausal: Referring to the time "around the menopause." Describes the period when ovarian function and hormone production are declining but have not yet totally stopped.

perineum: One's "bottom." The structure containing the outlets of the urethra, the vagina, and the rectum.

peritonitis: Inflammation of the abdominal cavity; occurs with severe appendicitis or pelvic inflammatory disease.

pessary: A device, usually made of rubber, placed in the vagina and used to support sagging structures (vagina, uterus, or bladder).

phlebitis: Inflammation of the vein wall.

phytoestrogens: Plant estrogens.

pineal gland: A brain structure whose function is still not completely known. Secretes melatonin and is sensitive to light/dark changes.

pituitary gland: A part of the brain, right behind the bridge of the nose. Secretes hormones that regulate the activity of most of the glands in the body.

placebo: A sugar pill. Often used in drug trials to see whether a patient is just thinking herself better or is actually receiving benefits from the specific drug being tested. (Obviously, the patient doesn't know whether she is getting the sugar pill or the real thing.)

placebo effect: See above. In drug trials about 30 percent of those taking placebos feel that they are getting help from them.

PMS: Premenstrual syndrome.

PMZ: Postmenopausal zest; a feeling of liberation and renewed energy experienced by many menopausal women.

polyps: Usually benign outgrowths of normal tissue, they stretch out on a stalk. Polyps in the lining of the uterus may be associated with bleeding.

posterior: Underneath or behind; the back part of the vagina.

posterior repair: The fixing of a rectocele.

potassium: An element in the blood necessary for normal cell functioning. Levels may be depleted by diuretic use.

PPD: Purified protein derivative; a skin test for tuberculosis.

primary care physician: A doctor who takes basic, overall care of a patient. Refers the patient to a specialist if necessary. Women's primary care physicians are usually family practitioners, internists, or gynecologists.

progesterone: A steroid hormone made by the ovary in the second half of the menstrual cycle; stabilizes the lining of the uterus and prepares it for implantation of a fertilized egg.

progestin: One of several synthetic forms of progesterone, made in the laboratory.

prolactin: A hormone made by the pituitary gland, which stimulates secretion of breast milk. When elevated in nonpregnant women, may be associated with infertility.

prostaglandins: A family of hormones, made by the uterus and many other bodily organs, that stimulate the activity of smooth muscle, including the uterine wall. In women their principal role is in labor; also produce menstrual cramps.

pruritus: Itching.

psychotropic: Having an effect on moods and feelings.

receptors: Structures on the surface of cells that bind hormones circulating in the bloodstream.

rectocele: A bulging of rectal tissue into the vagina.

serosa: The tissue on the surface of an organ.

serotonin: A chemical produced in the brain whose levels may influence moods.

sigmoidoscopy: Insertion of a flexible tube to examine the lower bowel.

spina bifida: A congenital separation of the spinal cord, which can be associated with neurological dysfunction of the lower part of the body.

squamous: Referring to superficial cells that line some part of the body. These cells tend to be flat and form the top layer of the skin, vagina, and cervix.

steroids: A family of chemicals whose structure and formation come from cholesterol.

supracervical: Above the cervix. Refers to a hysterectomy where the body of the uterus (fundus) is removed, but the cervix is left in place.

surgicenter: An outpatient surgical facility.

systemic: Throughout the body.

TAH and BSO: Total abdominal hysterectomy and bilateral salpingo-oophorectomy.

testosterone: The "male" steroid hormone. Also made by women, but in much smaller amounts than by men.

thrombosis: The presence of a clot in a blood vessel.

thyrotoxicosis: A very high level of circulating thyroid hormone.

topical: Applied to the surface of the body, as opposed to being taken systemically.

transvaginal: Through the vagina. Ultrasound testing may be done with transvaginal probes; cysts may be drained transvaginally.

tricyclics: A family of antidepressant drugs that raise neurotransmitter levels in the central nervous system.

ultrasound: A diagnostic tool that uses sound waves, not x-rays, to examine the inside of the body. Often used to determine if a mass is solid or fluid filled (cystic). Ultrasound procedures are basically risk free, as they do not involve exposure to radiation.

ureters: The tubes that connect kidneys to bladder.

uterine prolapse: A condition in which the uterus slips downward into the vagina, or in severe conditions actually protrudes outside the body.

urethra: The opening of the bladder to the outside of the body.

vaginal atrophy: The drying and thinning of the vaginal walls because of loss of estrogen.

vaginitis: Inflammation of the vagina.

vasodilation: An opening up or expanding of the blood vessels. Caused by certain drugs, and also associated with the mechanism of the hot flash.

vestibular vulvitis: A painful but benign condition of the outlet of the vagina; associated with nonyeast and nonbacterial inflammation.

vitamin B6: Pyridoxine, a chemical essential for cell metabolism. Has a number of therapeutic uses including diuretic action, decreasing breast discomfort, and treating the nausea of pregnancy and PMS.

vulva: The tissue surrounding the opening of the vagina.

vulvitis: Inflammation of the vulva.

well differentiated: Used to describe a cancer in which the cells look very much like the original tissue. Usually associated with a better outlook than cancers that are poorly differentiated, that is, do not resemble the normal tissue.

Bibliography

These significant books and articles in scholarly journals will give you an idea of current scientific thinking on important topics relating to menopause.

Basic Textbooks and General Studies

Hammond, C. B., Haseltine, F. P., Schiff, I., eds. *Menopause: Evaluation, treatment, and health concerns.* New York: Alan R. Liss, 1989.

Judd, H. L. Hormonal dynamics associated with the menopause. *Clinical Obstetrics and Gynecology* 1976; 19:775–788.

Lobo, R., ed. *Treatment of the post-menopausal woman: Basic and clinical aspects.* New York: Raven Press, 1994.

Metcalf, M. G., Donald, R. A., and Livesey, J. H. Pituitary-ovarian function before, during and after the menopause: A longitudinal study. *Clinical Endocrinology* 1982; 17:489–494.

Mishell, D. R., Jr., ed. *Menopause: Physiology and pharmacology.* Chicago: Yearbook Medical Publishers, 1987.

Siiteri, P. K. Adipose tissue as a source of hormones. *American Journal of Clinical Nutrition* 1987; 45:277–282.

Androgen Therapy

Sherwin, B. B., and Gelfand, M. M. Sex steroids and effect in the surgical menopause: A double-blind, cross-over study. *Psychoneuroendocrinology* 1985; 10:325–335.

———. The role of androgen in the maintenance of sexual functioning in oophorectomized women. *Psychosomatic Medicine* 1987; 49:397–409.

Sherwin, B. B., Gelfand, M. M., and Brender, W. Androgen enhances sexual motivation in females: A prospective, crossover study of sex steroid administration in the surgical menopause. *Psychosomatic Medicine* 1985; 47:339–351.

Breast Cancer

Bergkvist, L., Adami, H.-O., Persson, I., et al. The risk of breast cancer after estrogen and estrogen-progestin replacement. *New England Journal of Medicine* 1989; 321:293–297.

Colditz, G. A., Hankinson, S. E., Hunter, D. J., et al. Use of estrogens and progestins and the risk of breast cancer in postmenopausal women. *New England Journal of Medicine* 1995; 332:1589–93.

Colditz, G. A., Stampfer, M. J., Willett, W. C., et al. Prospective study of estrogen replacement therapy and risk of breast cancer in postmenopausal women. *Journal of the American Medical Association* 1990; 264:2648–53.

Costanza, M. E. Breast cancer screening in older women: Synopsis of a forum. *Cancer* 1992; 69:1925–31.

Dupont, W. D., and Page, D. L. Menopausal estrogen replacement therapy and breast cancer. *Archives of Internal Medicine* 1991; 151:67–72.

Editorial. Oral contraceptives and breast cancer. *Lancet* 1986; 2:665–666.

Key, T. J. A., and Pike, M. C. The role of oestrogens and progestogens in the epidemiology and prevention of breast cancer. *European Journal of Cancer and Clinical Oncology* 1988; 24:29–34.

King, R. J. B. A discussion of the roles of estrogen and progestin in human mammary carcinogenesis. *Journal of Steroid Biochemistry and Molecular Biology* 1991; 39: 811–818.

McPherson, K., and Drife, J. O. The pill and breast cancer: Why the uncertainty? *British Medical Journal* 1986; 293:709–710.

Pike, M. C. Age-related factors in cancers of the breast, ovary and endometrium. *Journal of Chronic Diseases* 1987; 40 (suppl. II):59S–69S.

Stanford, J. L., Weiss, N. L., Voigt, L. F., et al. Combined estrogen and progestin therapy in relation to risk of breast cancer in middle-aged women. *Journal of the American Medical Association* 1995; 274 (2):137–142.

Steinberg, K., Thacker, S. B., Smith, S. J., et al. A meta-analysis of breast cancer. *Journal of the American Medical Association* 1991; 265:1985–90.

Wingo, P. A., Layde, P. M., Lee, N. C., et al. The risk of breast cancer in postmenopausal women who have used estrogen replacement therapy. *Journal of the American Medical Association* 1987; 257:209–215.

Endometrial Cancer

Ettinger, B., Golditch, I. M., and Friedman, G. Gynecologic consequences of long-term unopposed estrogen replacement therapy. *Maturitas* 1988; 10:271–282.

Gambrell, R. D. Prevention of endometrial cancer with progestogens. *Maturitas* 1986; 8:159–168.

Goldstein, S. R., Nachtigall, M., Snyder, J. R., et al. Endometrial assessment by vaginal ultrasonography before endometrial sampling in patients with postmenopausal bleeding. *American Journal of Obstetrics and Gynecology* 1990; 163:119–123.

Granberg, S., Wikland, M., Karlsson, B., et al. Endometrial thickness as measured by endovaginal ultrasonography for identifying endometrial abnormality. *American Journal of Obstetrics and Gynecology* 1991; 164:47–52.

Prough, S. G., Aksel, S., Wiebe, R. H., et al. Continuous estrogen/progestin therapy in menopause. *American Journal of Obstetrics and Gynecology* 1987; 157:1449–53.

Varner, R. E., Sparks, J. M., Cameron, C. D., et al. Transvaginal sonography of the endometrium in postmenopausal women. *Obstetrics and Gynecology* 1991; 78:195.

Estrogen Replacement Therapy

Archer, D. F., Pickar, J. H., and Bottiglioni, F., for the Menopause Study Group. Bleeding patterns in postmenopausal women taking continuous combined or sequential regimens of conjugated estrogens with medroxyprogesterone acetate. *Obstetrics and Gynecology* 1994; 83:686–692.

Bourne, T., Hillard, T. C., Whitehead, M. I., et al. Oestrogens, arterial status, and postmenopausal women. *Lancet* 1990; 325:1470–71.

Brincat, M., Moniz, C. F., Studd, J. W. W., et al. The long-term effects of the menopause and of administration of sex hormones on skin collagen and skin thickness. *British Journal of Obstetrics and Gynaecology* 1985; 92:256–259.

Cardozo, L. D. Oestrogen deficiency and the bladder. In: Drife, J. O., and Studd, J. W.,

eds. *HRT and osteoporosis*. Berlin: Springer-Verlag, 1990.

Lobo, R. A. Estrogen and the risk of coagulopathy. *American Journal of Medicine* 1992; 92:283–285.

Studd, J. W. W. Complications of hormone replacement therapy in postmenopausal women. *Journal of the Royal Society of Medicine* 1992; 85:376–378.

Studd, J., and Magos, A. Oestrogen therapy and endometrial pathology. In: Studd, J. W. W., and Whitehead, M. I., eds. *The menopause*. Oxford: Blackwell Scientific Publications, 1988, pp.197–212.

Versi, E., Cardozo, L. D., Brincat, M., et al. Correlation of urethral physiology and skin collagen in post-menopausal women. *British Journal of Obstetrics and Gynaecology* 1988: 95;147–152.

Wilson, P. D., Paragher, B., Butler, B., et al. Treatment with oral piperazine oestrone sulphate for genuine stress incontinence in post-menopausal women. *British Journal of Obstetrics and Gynaecology* 1987; 94:568–574.

Woodruff, J. D., and Pickar, J. H., for the Menopause Study Group. Incidence of endometrial hyperplasia in post-menopausal women taking conjugated estrogens (Premarin) with medroxyprogesterone acetate or conjugated estrogens alone. *American Journal of Obstetrics and Gynecology* 1994; 170:1213–23.

Fertility and Sexuality

Sarrel, P. M. Sex problems after menopause: A study of fifty married couples treated in a sex counseling programme. *Maturitas* 1982; 4(4):231–237.

Sauer, M. V., Paulson, R. J., and Lobo, R. A.

Reversing the natural decline in human fertility. An extended clinical trial of oocyte donation to women of advanced reproductive age. *Journal of the American Medical Association* 1992; 268:1275.

Semmens, J. P., and Semmens, E. C. Sexual function and the menopause. *Clinical Obstetrics and Gynecology* 1984; 27(3):717–723.

Semmens, J. P., Tsai, C. C., Curtis Semmens, E., et al. Effects of estrogen therapy on vaginal physiology during menopause. *Obstetrics and Gynecology* 1986; 66:15–18.

Sherwin, B., and Gelfand, H. Differential symptom response to parenteral estrogen and/or androgen administration in the surgical menopause. *American Journal of Obstetrics and Gynecology* 1985; 151(2):153–160.

Heart Disease

Barrett-Connor, E., and Laakso, M. Ischemic heart disease risk in postmenopausal women. Effects of estrogen use on glucose and insulin levels. *Arteriosclerosis* 1990; 10:531–534.

Barrett-Connor, E., and Wingard, D. L. Sex differential in ischemic heart disease mortality in diabetics. *American Journal of Epidemiology* 1983; 118:489–496.

Barrett-Connor, E., and Bush, T. L. Estrogen and coronary heart disease in women. *Journal of the American Medical Association* 1991; 265:1861–67.

Brass, L. M., Kisiel, D., and Sarrel, P. M. A correlation between estrogen and middle cerebral artery blood velocity at different times in the menstrual cycle in women with catamenial migraines.

Journal of Cardiovascular Technology 1990; 9:68.

Bush, T. L. The epidemiology of cardiovascular disease in postmenopausal women. *Annals of the New York Academy of Science* 1990; 592:263–271.

Bush, T. L., and Comstock, C. W. Smoking and cardiovascular mortality in women. *American Journal of Epidemiology* 1983; 118:480–488.

Bush, T. L., Barrett-Connor, E., Cowan, L. D., et al. Cardiovascular mortality and noncontraceptive use of estrogen in women: Results from the Lipid Research Clinics Program follow-up study. *Circulation* 1987; 75:1102–9.

Haffner, S. M., Katz, M. S., Stern, M. P., et al. The relationship of sex hormones to hyperinsulinemia and hyperglycemia. *Metabolism* 1988; 37:683–688.

Jacobs, D. R., Mebane, I. L., Bangdiwala, S. I., et al. High density lipoprotein cholesterol as a predictor of cardiovascular disease mortality in men and women: The follow-up study of the Lipid Research Clinics Prevalence Study. *American Journal of Epidemiology* 1990; 131:32–47.

Kannel, W. B., Hjortland, M. C., McNamara, P. M., et al. Menopause and risk of cardiovascular disease. The Framingham Study. *Annals of Internal Medicine* 1976; 85:447–452.

Larsson, B., Bengtsson, C., Bjorntorp, P., et al. Is abdominal body fat distribution a major explanation for the sex difference in the incidence of myocardial infarction? *American Journal of Epidemiology* 1992; 135:266–273.

Manson, J. E., Colditz, G. A., Stampfer, M. J., et al. A prospective study of obesity and risk of coronary heart disease in women. *New England Journal of Medicine* 1990; 332:882−889.

Maynard, C., Litwin, P. E., Martin, J. S., et al. Gender differences in the treatment and outcome of acute myocardial infarction. *Archives of Internal Medicine* 1992;152: 972-976.

Ross, R. K., Pike, M. C., Mack, T. M., et al. Stroke prevention and oestrogen replacement therapy. *Lancet* 1989; 1:505.

Sarrel, P. M. Ovarian hormones and the circulation. *Maturitas* 1990; 12:287−298.

———. Sexuality and menopause. *Obstetrics and Gynecology* 1990; 75:26S–32S.

Sarrel, P. M., Lindsay, D., Rosano, G. M. C., et al. Angina and normal coronary arteries in women: Gynecologic findings. *American Journal of Obstetrics and Gynecology* 1992; 167:467−472.

Stampfer, M. J., Colditz, G. A., and Willett, W. C. Postmenopausal estrogen therapy and cardiovascular disease: Ten-year follow-up from the Nurses' Health Study. *New England Journal of Medicine* 1991; 325:756−762.

Stern, M. P., and Haffner, S. M. Body fat distribution and hyperinsulinemia as risk factors for diabetes and cardiovascular disease. *Arteriosclerosis* 1986; 6:123−130.

Tofler, G., Stone, P., Muller, J., et al. Effect of gender and race on prognosis after myocardial infarction: Adverse prognosis for women, particularly black women. *Journal of the American College of Cardiology* 1987; 9:473−482.

Wren, B. G., and Routledge, A. D. The effect of type and dose of oestrogen on the blood pressure of postmenopausal women. *Maturitas* 1983; 5:135−142.

Zamboni, M., Armellini, F., Milani, M. P., et al. Body fat distribution in pre and post-menopausal women: Metabolic and anthropometric variables and their interrelationship. *International Journal of Obesity* 1992: 16:495−504.

Hot Flashes and Moods

Ballinger, C. B. Psychiatric aspects of the menopause. *British Journal of Psychiatry* 1990; 156:773−787.

Bullock, J. L., Massey, F. M., Gambrell, R. D., Jr. Use of medroxyprogesterone acetate to prevent menopausal symptoms. *Obstetrics and Gynecology* 1975; 46:165−168.

Christy, C. J. Vitamin E in menopause. *American Journal of Obstetrics and Gynecology* 1945; 50:84−87.

Ditkoff, E. C., Crary, W. G., Christo, M., et al. Estrogen improves psychological function in asymptomatic postmenopausal women. *Obstetrics and Gynecology* 1991; 78:991−995

Erlik, Y., Meldrum, D. R., and Judd, H. L. Estrogen levels in postmenopausal women with hot flashes. *Obstetrics and Gynecology* 1982; 59:403−407.

Erlik, Y., Tataryn, I. V., Meldrum, D. R., et al. Association of waking episodes with menopausal hot flushes. *Journal of the American Medical Association* 1981; 245:1741−44.

Fillit, H., Weinreb, H., Cholst, I., et al. Observations in a preliminary open trial of estradiol therapy for senile dementia—Alzheimer's type. *Psychoneuroendocrinology* 1986; 11:337−345.

Greene, J. G., and Cooke, D. J. Life stresses and symptoms at the climacteric. *British Journal of Psychiatry* 1980; 136:486−491.

Kronenberg, F. Hot flashes: Epidemiology and physiology. *Annals of the New York Academy of Science* 1990; 592:52−86.

Kronenberg, F., and Barnard, R. M. Modulation of menopausal hot flashes by ambient temperature. *Journal of Thermal Biology* 1992; 17:43−49.

Kronenberg, F., and Downey, J. A. Thermoregulatory physiology of menopausal hot flashes: A review. *Canadian Journal of Physiology and Pharmacology* 1987; 65:1312−24.

Lock, M., Kaufert, P., and Gilbert, P. Cultural construction of the menopausal syndrome: The Japanese case. *Maturitas* 1988; 10:317−332.

Phillips, S., and Sherwin, B. B. Effects of estrogen on memory function in surgically menopausal women. *Psychoneuroendocrinology* 1992; 17:485−495.

Reid, R. L., and Yen, S. S. C. Premenstrual syndrome. *American Journal of Obstetrics and Gynecology* 1981; 139:85−104.

Sarrel, P. M., and Whitehead, M. I. Sex and menopause: Defining the issues. *Maturitas* 1985; 7:217−224.

Schiff, I., Tulchinsky, D., Cramer, D., et al. Oral medroxyprogesterone in the treatment of postmenopausal symptoms. *Journal of the American Medical Association* 1980; 244:1443−45.

Sherwyn, B. B. Affective changes with estrogen and androgen replacement therapy in surgically menopausal women. *Journal of Affective Disorders* 1988; 14:177−187.

Studd, J. W. W. Complications of hormone replacement therapy in postmenopausal women. *Journal of the Royal Society of Medicine* 1992; 85:376−378.

Tataryn, I. V., Meldrum, D. R., Lu, K. H., et al. LH, FSH and skin temperature during menopausal hot flush. *Journal of Clinical Endocrinology and Metabolism* 1979; 49:152−154.

Tulandi, T., Lal, S., and Kinch, R. A. Effect of intravenous clonidine on menopausal flushing and luteinizing hormone secretion. *British Journal of Obstetrics and Gynaecology* 1983; 90:854−857.

Lifestyle

American College of Sports Medicine. Position stand on the recommended quantity and quality of exercise for developing and maintaining cardiorespiratory and muscular fitness in healthy adults. *Medicine and Science in Sports and Exercise* 1990; 22:265−274.

Baron, J. A. Smoking and estrogen-related disease. *American Journal of Epidemiology* 1984; 119:9−22.

Barrett-Connor, E., and Khaw, K. Family history of heart attack as an independent predictor of death due to cardiovascular disease. *Circulation* 1984; 59:1065−69.

Berta, L., Fortunati, N., et al. Influence of cigarette smoking on pituitary and sex hormone balance in healthy premenopausal women. *Fertility and Sterility* 1991; 56:788.

Cowan, M. M., and Gregory, L. W. Responses of pre- and post-menopausal females to aerobic conditioning. *Medicine and Science in Sports and Exercise* 1985; 17:138−143.

Dawson-Hughes, B., Dallal, G. E., Krall, E. A., et al. A controlled trial of the effect of calcium supplementation on bone density in postmenopausal women. *New*

England Journal of Medicine 1990; 323: 878–883.

Drinkwater, B. L., Nilson, K., Ott, S., et al. Bone mineral density after resumption of menses in amenorrheic athletes. *Journal of the American Medical Association* 1986; 256:380–382.

Dunn, A. L., and Dishman, R. K. Exercise and the neurobiology of depression. *Exercise and Sport Sciences Reviews* 1991; 19:41–98.

Flint, M., Drinkwater, B., and Horvath, S. Effects of training on women's response to submaximal exercise. *Medicine and Science in Sports and Exercise* 1974; 6:80–94.

Friedman, A. J., Ravnikar, V. A., and Barbieri, R. L. Serum steroid hormone profiles in postmenopausal smokers and non-smokers. *Fertility and Sterility* 1987; 47:398–401.

Krølner, B., Toft, B., Nielsen, S. P., et al. Physical exercise as prophylaxis against involutional vertebral bone loss: A controlled trial. *Clinical Science* 1983; 64:541–546.

McKinlay, S. M., Bifano, N. L., and McKinlay, J. B. Smoking and age of menopause in women. *Annals of Internal Medicine* 1985; 103:350.

Shimokata, H., Tobin, J. D., Muller, D. C., et al. Studies in the distribution of body fat. I. Effects of age, sex, and obesity. *Journal of Gerontology* 1989; 44:M66–M73.

Simkin, A., Ayalon, J., and Leichter, I. Increased trabecular bone density due to bone-loading exercises in postmenopausal osteoporotic women. *Calcified Tissue International* 1987; 40:59–63.

Smith, E. L., Gilligan, C., Smith, P. E., et al. Calcium supplementation and bone loss in middle-aged women. *American Journal of Clinical Nutrition* 1989; 50:833–883.

Stillman, R. J., Rosenberg, M. J., and Sachs, B. P. Smoking and reproduction. *Fertility and Sterility* 1986; 45:545–566.

Osteoporosis

Briancon, D., and Meunier, P. J. Treatment of osteoporosis with fluoride, calcium and vitamin D. *Orthopedic Clinics of North America* 1982; 12:629–648.

Cavanaugh, D. J., and Cann, C. E. Brisk walking does not stop bone loss in postmenopausal women. *Bone* 1988; 9:201–204.

Consensus Development Conference. Prophylaxis and treatment of osteoporosis. *American Journal of Medicine* 1991; 90: 107–110.

Cooper, C., Campion, G., and Melton, L. J. III. Hip fractures in the elderly: A world-wide projection. *Osteoporosis International* 1992; 2:285–290.

Cooper, C., Atkinson, E. J., Wahner, H.W., et al. Is caffeine consumption a risk factor for osteoporosis? *Journal of Bone and Mineral Research* 1992; 7:465–471.

Cummings, S. R., Black, D. M., and Rubin, S. M. Lifetime risk of hip, Colles', or vertebral fracture and coronary heart disease among white postmenopausal women. *Archives of Internal Medicine* 1989; 149:2445–48.

Dawson-Hughes, B., Dallal, G. E., Krall, E. A., et al. A controlled trial of the effect of calcium supplementation on bone density in postmenopausal women. *New England Journal of Medicine* 1990; 323: 878–883.

Dempster, D. W. Bone remodeling. In: Coe,

F. L., and Favus, M. J., eds. *Disorders of bone and mineral metabolism*. New York: Raven Press, 1992, pp. 355–382.

Ettinger, B., Genant, H. K., and Cann, C. Long-term estrogen therapy prevents fractures and preserves bone mass. *Annals of Internal Medicine* 1985; 102:319–324.

————. Postmenopausal bone loss is prevented by treatment with low dosage estrogen with calcium. *Annals of Internal Medicine* 1987; 106:40–45.

Genant, H. K., Block, J. E., Steiger, P., et al. Appropriate use of bone densitometry. *Radiology* 1989; 170:817–822.

Heaney, R. P., and Recker, R. R. Effects of nitrogen, phosphorus, and caffeine on calcium balance in women. *Journal of Laboratory and Clinical Medicine* 1982; 99:46–55.

Kiel, D. P., Felson, D. T., Andersen, J. J., et al. Hip fracture and the use of estrogens in postmenopausal women. The Framingham Study. *New England Journal of Medicine* 1987; 317:1169–74.

Lindsay, R. Sex steroids in the pathogenesis and prevention of osteoporosis. In: Riggs, B. L., and Melton, L. J., eds. *Osteoporosis: Etiology, diagnosis and management*. New York: Raven Press, 1988, pp. 333–358.

Lindsay, R., Hart, D. M., and Clark, D. M. The minimum effective dose of estrogen for prevention of postmenopausal bone loss. *Obstetrics and Gynecology* 1983; 63:759–763.

MacIntyre, I., Stevenson, J. C., Whitehead, M. I., et al. Calcitonin for prevention of postmenopausal bone loss. *Lancet* 1988; 1:900–902.

Nelson, B. W., Harris, S. T., Genant, H. K., et al. Intermittent cyclical etidronate treatment of postmenopausal osteoporosis. *New England Journal of Medicine* 1990; 323:73–79.

Reinbold, W. D., Genant, H. K., Reiser, U. J., et al. Bone mineral content in early premenopausal and postmenopausal osteoporotic women: Comparison of measurement methods. *Radiology* 1986; 160:469–478.

Riggs, B. L., Seeman, E., Hodgson, S. F., et al. Effect of the fluoride calcium regimen on vertebral fracture occurrence in postmenopausal osteoporosis: Comparison with conventional therapy. *New England Journal of Medicine* 1982; 306:446–450.

Rigotti, N. A., Nussbaum, S. R., Herzog, D.B., et al. Osteoporosis in women with anorexia nervosa. *New England Journal of Medicine* 1984; 311:1601–6.

Riis, B., Thomsen, K., and Christiansen. C. Does calcium supplementation prevent postmenopausal bone loss? *New England Journal of Medicine* 1987; 316:173–177.

Seeman, E., Hopper, J. L., Bach, L. A., et al. Reduced bone mass in daughters of women with osteoporosis. *New England Journal of Medicine* 1989; 320:554–558.

Slemenda, C. W., Hui, S. L., Longcope, C., et al. Predictors of bone mass in perimenopausal women. *Annals of Internal Medicine* 1990; 112:96–101.

Storm, T. M., Thamsborg, G., Steiniche, T., et al. Effect of intermittent cyclical etidronate therapy on osteoporosis. *New England Journal of Medicine* 1990; 322:1265–71.

Resource List

United States

Alcoholics Anonymous (AA)
General Service Office of Alcoholics
Anonymous
Box 459, Grand Central Station
New York, NY 10163
Tel.: (212) 870-3400
Very successful self-help group, with branches throughout the country; local branches listed in telephone book.

Al-Anon and Alateen
Al-Anon Family Group Headquarters
P.O. Box 862, Midtown Station
New York, NY 10018
Tel.: (212) 302-7240 or (800) 356-9996
Support groups for families, teenaged children, and friends of alcoholics.

Alzheimer's Disease and Related
Disorders Associations (ADRDA)
National Headquarters
919 North Michigan Avenue,
Suite 1000
Chicago, IL 60611
Tel.: (800) 272-3900
National organization; local chapters listed in phone book. Newsletter, pamphlets, and other educational materials. Local chapters sponsor support groups for Alzheimers' caregivers.

American Association of Retired Persons
(AARP)
601 E Street, N.W.
Washington, DC 20049
Tel.: (202) 434-2277 or (800) 424-2277
Provides information and advocacy for people age 50 or older, whether or not retired. Publishes Modern Matu-

rity, a bimonthly magazine, as well as AARP News Bulletin, a monthly newsletter; educational materials on older women and alcohol, insomnia, divorce at 50, retirement planning, etc.

American Cancer Society
1599 Clifton Road, N.E.
Atlanta, GA 30329
Tel.: (404) 320-3333
National organization for research and education; most recent publication, 1995 Cancer Facts and Figures, contains statistics on smoking-related cancers; also publishes guide to quitting smoking.

American Diabetes Association (ADA)
National Service Center
1660 Duke Street
Alexandria, VA 22314
Tel.: (800) 232-3472
National organization with local chapters; offers educational materials, quarterly newsletter, and Diabetes Forecast, bimonthly magazine with articles on diet, peer support groups, research advances.

American Heart Association
7320 Greenville Avenue
Dallas, TX 75231
Tel.: (214) 373-6300 or (800) 242-8721
National organization for education and research on heart disease; local chapters listed in phone book. Information on diet, exercise, smoking, and other facets of heart-healthy living.

Arthritis Foundation
1314 Spring Street, N.W.
Atlanta, GA 30309
Tel.: (404) 872-7100 or (800) 283-7800
National organization with local chapters; publishes educational materials, including newsletter; has developed guidelines for aquatic exercise.

Children of Aging Parents (CAPS)
1609 Woodbourne Road, Suite 302A
Levittown, PA 19057
Tel.: (215) 945-6900
Nonprofit organization that offers guidance and referrals to social service agencies. Publishes newsletter and other educational materials, including guide to starting self-help groups for caregivers of the elderly.

Exceptional Cancer Patients
1302 Chapel Street
New Haven, CT 06511
Tel.: (203) 865-8392
Organization for people with cancer or any devastating illness; support groups and counseling in the New Haven–New York area. Bibliography of books, videotapes, and audiotapes, including those by founder Dr. Bernie Siegel, whose approach integrates self-healing with standard medical treatment.

HERS (Hysterectomy Educational Resources and Services)
422 Bryn Mawr Avenue
Bala Cynwyd, PA 19004
Tel.: (215) 667-7757
Educational organization for women who have had or are contemplating hysterectomy. Physician referral, newsletter.

National Osteoporosis Foundation
1150 17th Street, N.W., Suite 500
Washington, DC 20036
Tel.: (202) 223-2226
Organization for osteoporosis research, education, and support. Publishes quarterly newsletter with information on prevention, exercise, nutrition, rehabilitation.

North American Menopause Society
c/o University Hospitals of Cleveland
Department of Ob/Gyn
11100 Euclid Avenue
Cleveland, OH 44106
Tel.: (216) 844-3334

Professional organization of physicians and researchers who work in the field of menopause. Conducts annual meetings for professionals; publishes bibliography and resource list for nonprofessionals.

PRIME PLUS/Red Hot Mamas
Menopause Management Education
Program
Karen Giblin
23 North Valley Road
Ridgefield, CT 06877
Tel.: (203) 431-3902

Works with physicians and health care professionals to organize programs for menopause education and psychosocial support. Chapters in California, Connecticut, New York, and Pennsylvania.

Resolve, Inc.
1310 Broadway
Somerville, MA 02144
Tel.: (617) 643-2424

National organization that provides support, information, and physician referral for infertility.

Sex Information and Education Council of the United States
130 West 42nd Street, Suite 2500
New York, NY 10036
Tel.: (212) 819-9770

Provides information about sexuality as positive part of healthy life.

Society for Nutrition Education
2001 Kilebrew Drive, Suite 340
Minneapolis, MN 55425
Tel.: (612) 854-0035

Offers educational materials on dietary approaches to good health.

Great Britain

Amarant Trust
11–13 Charter House Buildings
London EC1M 7AN, England
Tel.: 0171 401 3855

Publishes educational materials on menopause and HRT. Has list of menopause clinics.

Breast Cancer Care
15-19 Britten Street
London SW3 3TZ, England
Tel.: 0171 867 8275

Provides counseling, advice, and information on breast cancer and treatment. Telephone helpline: 0171 867 1103.

British Heart Foundation
14 Fitzhardinge Street
London W1H 4DH, England
Tel.: 0171 935 0185

Offers written information about heart health, including exercise and diet.

Faculty of Homeopathy
Hahnemann House
Powis Place
Great Ormond Street
London WC1N 3HT, England
Tel.: 0171 837 9469

Has list of registered homeopaths; educational materials on principles of homeopathic medicine.

Marie Stopes Clinic
108 Whitfield Street
London W1P 6BE, England
Tel.: 0171 388 2585

Offers menopause clinics in London and other cities. Information on sexual and reproductive health.

National Back Pain Association
The Old Office Block
Elmtree Road
Teddington
Middlesex TW11 8ST, England
Tel.: 0181 977 5474

Provides information packet; education on exercise and self-help as well as standard medical treatment.

National Institute of Herbal Medicine
9 Palace Gate
Exeter
Devon EX1 1JA, England
Tel.: 0392 426022

Has national listing of herbalists, send self-addressed envelope for membership list.

National Osteoporosis Society
P.O. Box 10
Radstock
Bath BA3 3YB, England
Tel.: 0761 432 472

Provides information on osteoporosis, including prevention and treatment.

Women's Nutritional Advisory Service
P.O. Box 268
Lewes
East Sussex BN7 2QN, England
Tel.: 0273 487 366

Gives advice on diet, especially in controlling PMS and during menopause.

Index